Philip Burnard is Professor and Vice Dean at The School of Nursing and Midwifery Studies, Cardiff University, Cardiff, UK. He is also Visiting Professor at the Royal Thai Army Nursing College, Bangkok, Thailand, and he has lectured in Finland, Sweden, Malta, Malaysia, the Netherlands, the Czech Republic, China, Africa, Brunei, Australia, the US and the Caribbean. He is the author of 36 books on counselling, communication, ethics, research methods, writing, computing, supervision and mentoring, education and training and has published widely in journals in the UK, USA, Finland, Hong Kong, Romania, the Czech Republic and Italy. Professor Burnard's research interests include stress, culture and communication, AIDS counselling, teaching and learning styles, experiential learning, self-disclosure and cross-cultural views of mental health and mental illness. He is currently engaged in projects in Thailand, Malta, Brunei, the Czech Republic and the UK.

Counselling Skills for Health Professionals

FOURTH EDITION

Philip Burnard, PhD

Professor of Nursing, Cardiff University, Wales, UK and Visiting Professor,
The Royal Thai Army Nursing College, Bangkok, Thailand

Fourth edition published in 2005 by:
Nelson Thornes Ltd
Delta Place
27 Bath Road
CHELTENHAM
GL53 7TH
United Kingdom

05 06 07 08 09 / 10 9 8 7 6 5 4 3 2 1

A catalogue record for this book is available from the British Library

ISBN 0-7487-9384-4

Page make-up by Acorn Bookwork

Printed in Great Britain by Ashford Colour Press

CONTENTS

ACKNOWLEDGEMENTS

I am grateful to the many people who have played a part in the development of this book. Jo Campling was originally responsible for the first edition.

Thanks go to the team at Nelson Thornes who have always been supportive and helpful. I have learned a great deal from the people who have edited and sub-edited my books in this series. Special thanks go to Helen Broadfield and Lisa Fraley for their support for this edition.

Particular thanks goes to my personal assistant, Joy Slack, who has contributed so much to the preparation of this and other texts. I also give thanks to Narakorn Kreokhamla, Wassana Naiyapatana and my other friends in Thailand who have taught me so much about cultural aspects of communication.

The author thanks the British Association for Counselling and Psychotherapy for its permission to reproduce its various codes of ethics and practice for counsellors, trainers and supervisors. It is acknowledged that permission was given on the condition that readers note that the BACP's codes of conduct are updated on a regular basis and that readers should check with the BACP in order to ascertain that the particular code printed is the latest one available.

But you are born
for a limpid day

Hölderlin

INTRODUCTION

This is the fourth edition of a book that I hope continues to be of practical value. For counselling must always be that: practical. No amount of talking, on its own, can really make a difference if people do not end up *doing something* as a result of counselling. The practical thread remains an important one throughout this edition.

In recent years, it has become increasingly important to develop *cultural sensitivity*. All cultures do not share the same ideas, values, beliefs or ways of behaving. Nor do they share the same ideas about counselling or even about talking problems through with another person. To this end, I have included, in this edition, a chapter about culture and communication. It also includes a discussion of the interesting concept of *phatic communication* or 'content-free speech'.

Counselling Skills for Health Professionals is not just a 'how to do it' book: people are probably too complicated for that approach to be of much use. Counselling is never simply a matter of learning a range of skills which you then apply in a range of settings. In the end, counselling is about facing the individuals in front of you, listening to them carefully and then supporting them as they work through their problems. For many problems, there are no easy answers, and counselling doesn't offer any 'quick fixes'. It is essentially a supportive process. There are many things it cannot do. It cannot change certain social and political situations. It cannot cure diseases. On the other hand, what it *can* do is offer people more *hope*. Often, just the fact that there is someone who is prepared to hear your story and to listen to you is all that is needed. I remain convinced that the key issue in all types of counselling is the ability to listen. Some of the best counselling involves the counsellor remaining silent for a lot of the time. In the end, we all need to be listened to.

The basic structure of this book remains unchanged although many new sections, checklists and reports from the theory and research have been added. The first part of the book explores a range of theoretical issues: what counselling is, the issue of self-awareness in counselling, culture and communication, and maps of the counselling process. The second part of the book considers specific counselling skills: listening and attending, counselling interventions, coping with feelings, and support for the counsellor. I sense that there has been a subtle change in counselling theory away from an almost exclusively *client-centred* approach towards one that involves information giving as well as facilitation. I have explored some of these issues in relation to up-and-coming approaches such as the cognitive-behavioural approach.

The last part of the book focuses on practical methods of developing counselling skills and is addressed to three groups of people: those working on their own, those working in pairs and those learning counselling in small groups. Practical suggestions are made about how to set up and run counselling skills groups. The book then offers a range of counselling skills exercises that can be used by any of the aforementioned three groups of people. The emphasis, throughout, has been on keeping things simple without (I hope) glossing over the complexities of the human condition. For this is the paradox: that while simple counselling strategies often make a lot of difference, human beings continue to be as complex and varied as ever.

I hope that the increasing call for health education and for self-direction in health care will mean that the skills explored in this book will be useful to a wide range of people: from the individual who wants to enhance his or her counselling skills to the lecturer or teacher who wants practical ideas about running counselling skills workshops. I know, too, that the book has been useful on some counselling certificate and diploma courses.

We all have problems in our lives, and counselling offers one means of exploring and relieving some of them. While I don't believe that counselling is the answer to all problems, nor do I believe that counselling is something that should and can only be done by trained professionals. After all, we all counsel our friends and families on a daily basis. I do not believe, either, that there is any one right way to go about counselling. We must avoid getting too clever about the degree to which we believe that what we do affects other people. In the end, it is the person referred to as the client who makes a difference to his or her own life. In the end, the client sorts him or herself out. I know, though, that careful and honest listening can make a difference. All health professionals can benefit from training themselves to become better listeners, to avoid rushing in to 'fix' things for other people and from standing back to allow people to sort themselves out. This book is aimed at developing some of those essential skills. I hope it is readable and practical.

Philip Burnard
Caerphilly, Wales, UK

WHAT IS COUNSELLING? 1

If you live in the West, counselling has become a part of everyday life. It is difficult to avoid references to counselling these days. After disasters, after political upheavals, after any group of people has had to face difficult situations, we are informed that the participants in those dramas were 'offered counselling'. We may question the timing. It is debatable whether a person 'needs counselling' directly following a dramatic event, at some time after it, or at all. I suspect that there is a wide range of people from those at one end of the scale who benefit, considerably, from talking things through, to others – at the other end – who prefer to work through their problems and reminiscences in private. At the outset of this book I would like to stress my belief that counselling is not necessarily for everyone and that, clearly, it would be bizarre and presumably unhelpful to foist counselling on those who do not want or need it. If we believe as do many counsellors – that people vary from one another and that, in the end, they are the identifiers of their own solutions to their own problems, then it follows that counselling will suit and help some people and not others. Also, it is not usual in some cultures to adopt counselling as a strategy. In south-east Asia, for example, problems are not normally aired – sometimes not even with family members. The point, there, is often that problems should be accepted as part of life.

In a sense, we are all counsellors. Anyone who works in one of the health professions and comes into regular contact with people who are distressed in any way, whether psychologically, physically, spiritually or practically, offers counselling help. Counselling is something familiar to everyone. There need be no mystique about it. Nor should it be something that is reserved for a particular group of professionals who call themselves counsellors. As we shall see, it is useful to talk about *acting as a counsellor* and *using counselling skills*. Thus the discussion is already focused on familiar territory. Like all such territory, we can always get to know it better. The aim of this book is to explore some of the many facets of counselling and to encourage health professionals to identify ways in which their counselling skills may be improved. All skills are learned. This is true irrespective of any particular psychological point of view we hold. Whether we would call ourselves behaviourally, psychodynamically or humanistically oriented, there is little doubt that we learn and develop skills as we grow, train and live. It is difficult to argue otherwise and to say that we are *born* with counselling skills.

If it is true that we learn skills in this way, then it also follows that we can improve our interpersonal skills. This book focuses on that argument and is a practical guide to enable the already functioning health care counsellor to become a better one. The practical skills described in this book may be used in a variety of situations, from talking through a period of work-related stress with a friend, to coping with a client in emotional crisis. The skills involved in these situations turn out to be remarkably similar. There are basic human skills that can be applied to almost all human situations. In the end, we are always working with another human being who is remarkably like ourselves underneath the skin.

There are also pitfalls to be avoided. These are also discussed. Human problems are rarely profession specific. Whilst the doctor deals with aspects of the human situation differently from the physiotherapist, and the nurse and speech therapist are responsible for different aspects of care, in the end, the difficulties that arise through the process of living turn out to be the domain of all health professionals. We all suffer from the same sorts of problems, or as Carl Rogers, the founder of client-centred counselling, noted, 'What is most personal is most universal' (Rogers, 1967). The fact that we live at all, gives us a clue to the sorts of problems that anyone can suffer. The fact that we live at all also gives us the clue to how others overcome their problems. This is not to say that everyone perceives their problems in the same sorts of ways, but to note that suffering is universal. Anyone concerned for another person's health and well-being needs, necessarily, to be concerned for what may be called that person's *problems in living*. It is towards these problems in living that counselling is directed. On the other hand, we live our lives differently to each other too, and cultural differences are important. These are also discussed in a new chapter on culture and communication. We would do well to remember that we are *not* 'all the same under the skin'.

The *process* of counselling can be defined as the means by which one person helps another to clarify his or her life situation and to decide further lines of action. Lack of clarity often brings anxiety. We are frightened by what we do not know or understand. Such fear and lack of clarity often lead, in turn, to inaction. This is often true in health care settings. The patient or client who is suffering from chronic illness often finds it difficult to plan ahead, often through fear born out of lack of information about his condition. The aim of counselling must be to free the person being counselled to live more fully, and such fuller living comes through *action*. In the end, counselling must have a practical aim. It can never be 'only talk'. It must seek to empower the client to become confident enough to choose a particular course of action and see it through. In this sense, counselling is also a form of *befriending*, of supporting the other person. Again, such befriending is familiar to us all and is a vital part of any person's job in the health professions. The nurse befriends the psychiatric patient when in the role of community psychiatric nurse. The social worker very clearly befriends the families with whom she works, and the GP becomes a friend to many of his patients. It is clear that an immediate requirement of anyone who seeks to work as a counsellor is that he or she must *like* people. This concept of befriending is discussed further in Chapter 5, under the heading of the qualities of an effective counsellor.

The British Association for Counselling and Psychotherapy (BACP) defines counselling as follows:

Counselling takes place when a counsellor sees a client in a private and confidential setting to explore a difficulty the client is having, distress they may be experiencing or perhaps their dissatisfaction with life, or loss of a sense of direction and purpose. It is always at the request of the client as no one can properly be 'sent' for counselling.

By listening attentively and patiently the counsellor can begin to perceive the difficulties from the client's point of view and can help them to see things more clearly, possibly from a different perspective. Counselling is a way of enabling choice or change or of reducing confusion. It does not involve giving advice or directing a client to take a particular course of action. Counsellors do not judge or exploit their clients in any way.

In the counselling sessions the client can explore various aspects of their life and feelings, talking about them freely and openly in a way that is rarely possible with friends or family. Bottled up feelings such as anger, anxiety, grief and embarrassment can become very intense and counselling offers an opportunity to explore them, with the possibility of making them easier to understand. The counsellor will encourage the expression of feelings and as a result of their training will be able to accept and reflect the client's problems without becoming burdened by them.

(BACP, 2004)

Although there is a wide range of books available that contains various approaches to defining counselling, perhaps one of the most all-encompassing and exhaustive of definitions is that offered by Feltham and Dryden. They suggest that counselling is:

A principled relationship characterised by the application of one or more psychological theories and a recognised set of communication skills, modified by experience, intuition and other interpersonal factors, to clients' intimate concerns, problems or aspirations. Its predominant ethos is one of facilitation rather than of advice-giving or coercion. It may be of very brief or long duration, take place in an organisational or private practice setting and may or may not overlap with practical, medical and other matters of personal welfare. It is both a distinctive activity undertaken by people agreeing to occupy the roles of counsellor and client ... and it is an emerging profession ... It is a service sought by people in distress or in some degree of confusion who wish to discuss and resolve these in a relationship which is more disciplined and confidential than friendship, and perhaps less stigmatising than helping relationships offered in traditional medical or psychiatric settings.

(Feltham and Dryden, 1993)

In this book, we will discuss each of the various issues that arise out of Feltham and Dryden's definition.

Definitions of *counselling* on the Web

Something that provides direction or advice as to a decision or course of action.

www.cogsci.princeton.edu/cgi-bin/webwn

The opportunity to talk things over with a trained counsellor. This can help you make sense of your feelings and offer you encouragement. It does not tell you what to do, but it can offer new ideas for coping.

www.macmillan.org.uk/glossary/

Intervention involving the provision of advice or support on a personal basis, by someone who has been trained to provide that support.

www.standards.dfes.gov.uk/research/glossary

Generally refers to one-on-one assistance with personal issues.

students.ubc.ca/current/glossary.cfm

An interaction with a mental health professional who offers guidance and advice on matters of education, marriage, work, relationships.

www.mindful-things.com/Glossary/glossary_c.html

Counselling is a process where clients are helped in dealing with their personal and interpersonal conflicts by a third-party therapist.

www.mediate.ca/shortglossary.htm

Within these procedures, counselling means a confidential discussion in a one-to-one situation.

www.churchschools.co.uk/subscribers/churchschools/level3/staff/staffmatrix/
gdcprocs/gdcdefns.htm

Advising or giving counsel to.

www.emerys.com.au/glossary.htm

COUNSELLING OR COUNSELLING SKILLS?

This book is about counselling skills. It is not, necessarily, about the process of becoming a counsellor. What's the difference? Some people work as full- or part-time counsellors. Their job is to counsel other people, and if they were asked what they did, they would say that they were a counsellor. Many other people use a range of skills associated with counselling in their everyday work as health professionals. Thus, a distinction can be made between *working as a counsellor* and *using counselling skills*. Not all health professionals who use counselling skills will work as counsellors although *all* counsellors will obviously use counselling skills. The prime aim of this book is to encourage those working as health care professionals to think about ways in which they can use counselling skills in their everyday practice. It is not assumed that everyone reading it will want to function, primarily, as a counsellor – although, clearly, the book will have relevance to professional counsellors as well. The appendix offers the BACP framework for counselling and pyschtherapy.

AN ACT OF FAITH

Counselling is also much more than just skills, processes and procedures. It is more, even, than words, plans and actions. It is also about *faith*. Whilst the efficacy of counselling, from the point of view of research, has not been established, those who practise it do so, I suspect, because they *believe* in other people and in the power of helping people to tell their stories. We counsel, I suspect, because we have faith in it:

> *And how shall we be able to administer help to others without the Faith of the Counsellors?*
>
> (Halmos, 1965)

Nor are we born equal. This is as much true of our personality structures as it is of any other social, physical or cultural variables. William James, one of the founding fathers of modern psychology, made this observation, which seems to sum up the vagaries of human nature:

> *Some persons are born with an inner constitution which is harmonious and well balanced from the outset. Their impulses are consistent with one another, their will follows without trouble the guidance of their intellect, their passions are not excessive and their lives are little haunted by regrets. But there are others whose existence is little more than a series of zigzags, as now one tendency and now another gets the upper hand. Their spirit wars with their flesh, they wish for incompatibles, wayward impulses interrupt their most deliberate plans, and their lives are one long drama of repentance and effort to repair misdemeanours and mistakes.*
>
> (James, 1890)

In particular, we are born into certain cultures, and that fact alone makes us view the world and our own problems differently.

Fortunately or unfortunately, it is these differences which make us human. However, it also remains the case that, at some point, we need to undertake thorough 'outcome' studies to identify whether or not counselling really makes a difference to people in the long term. Whilst counselling has become a popular activity, there has been relatively little research undertaken to prove or disprove the ultimate value of it. One of the problems of such research is allowing for what are sometimes called 'confounding variables'. In the end, there are so *many* things that impinge on any particular person's life that it is probably impossible to say, one way or the other, that it was *counselling* that made the most important difference to a difficult life situation. However, we live in a time when health care has to be shown to be cost-effective. It cannot be long before those who encourage counsellors to use their skills or who buy the skills of counsellors for their health

why limited research.

care programmes begin to demand a means of proof of those counsellors' effectiveness.

If counselling is sometimes an act of faith, it also, sometimes, brings fear to the counsellor as well as it might to the client. Reporting on a study of counsellors' experience of fear, Smith cites one of his respondents' experiences as follows:

> *My fear is of some clients' states of mind and the ideas that they are formulating. Sometimes people with paranoid thoughts and ideas have been describing events outside of the session, which they then bring into the session. One client has this idea that people outside were either in the blues or the blacks. People fell into two separate camps. He put himself in the black camp and attributed all kinds of negative attributes to those in the blues. The question then came around as to whether or not I was in the blues or the blacks. You're trying to put across you're neither, but, according to his reckoning, everyone's either in the blues or the blacks and the whole thing is spiralling downwards and your explanation can never be satisfactory. Suddenly it's in the room, it's come alive and you're having this debate about what camp you're in.*

(reported in Smith, 2003)

Perhaps an overall 'faith' in what we do must also be tempered with caution. We must not become too zealous in our work at the expense of some long, hard, rational thinking about what we do and at the expense of appropriate support and supervision. It is when we are scared or nervous that our 'faith' in counselling is tested.

THE WILL TO CHANGE

Perhaps one of the most important concepts in counselling, from the client's point of view, is the *will to change*. Sigmund Freud is often accredited with saying that the last thing a neurotic person wants to lose is his or her symptoms. So it can be with those who seek counselling. If counselling is to be effective, then the client has, to a greater or lesser extent, to *change*. Sometimes, people come to counselling expecting that either (a) the counsellor will somehow change them or (b) the process of counselling itself will change them. What has to happen, of course, is that the client has to change: nothing will come of counselling if the only change is the counselling itself. We might put it, oversimply, as follows: the client, during the process of counselling, needs to be able to identify:

- those things that he or she has to *do*;
- those things that he or she has to *stop doing*;
- those things that he or she needs to *continue to do*;
- those things that he or she needs to *accept*.

These points can become concrete aims in any counselling relationship. The counsellor can help the client to identify those things that he or she has to do, stop doing, continue to do or accept. It seems likely that almost all counselling involves a mix of these things. There is, perhaps, much truth in those old US saws, 'If it ain't broken, don't fix it' and 'If it works, do more of it'.

Also important, is the *rate of change* or the slope at which change is introduced. Too much change, too quickly, is likely to overwhelm the client and force him or her to see his or her 'new life' as too painful or dramatic. On the other hand, too slow a rate of change and the client may feel that nothing is happening. Most of us resist change. It needs, perhaps, to be introduced slowly, reinforced often and, most of all, *practised*. This process is not dissimilar to learning to play an instrument. The more we practise working at change, the better we are likely to be at it. Nor is the change that emerges out of a counselling relationship a once-and-for-all thing. It is likely that most of us very frequently have to review our lives and make adjustments and alterations or, perhaps, learn to acknowledge that certain things about us and our lives *cannot* be changed. In this case, we need to be able to learn acceptance.

On the other hand, all of this depends on our own idiosyncratic view of the degree to which we can change. If we *believe* that we can only change slowly, then probably that is the case. However, it is equally possible to believe that we can 'change overnight' and do it. For some, it certainly seems possible to step out of one behaviour or one mindset or one emotional state and adopt another. Much depends, perhaps, on the degree to which we believe we are 'plastic' and changeable.

WHO SHOULD COUNSEL?

As we have noted, in a sense, everyone is involved in counselling at some level. On the other hand, as we have also seen, not everyone would formally call themselves 'counsellors'. In an effort to offer an answer to the question, 'Who should be trained as counsellors?', Pearce offers this useful list for consideration:

- Counselling skills training should be a normal and necessary part of the training of all professionals. The depth of training in those skills is likely to be greater for those engaged in the helping professions such as nursing, teaching, and social work than those who are lawyers, dentists, estate agents and so on.
- At a lower level the foundation for counselling skills training should be laid in schools with an increasing emphasis on providing training for students in active listening and on helping them to understand and practise the concepts of respect, empathy, and genuineness which contribute towards building effective relationships.
- Managers in industry and elsewhere need counselling skills training in order to understand how counselling integrates with their other functions in working with people (Pearce, 1989).

Elsewhere, counselling has been advocated in at least the following settings:

- helping those with serious disabilities (Herbert, 1996; Mullins *et al.*, 1997; Swain, *et al*, 2003);
- sex education for young people (O'Driscoll, 1997);
- empowering oncology rehabilitation patients (Smith *et al.*, 1998);
- enabling student midwives (Crowley, 1997);
- preparing people for retirement (Langer, 1997);
- enabling older people to cope with change (Sennott-Miller, 1992);
- helping people through writing (Wright, 2002);
- informing people about contraception (Moskowitz and Jennings, 1996);
- breaking bad news (Winbolt, 1997);
- teaching spiritual care to health care students (Bradshaw, 1997; Gallia, 1996; Ross, 1996);
- health promotion amongst those who are HIV in the community (DiScenza *et al.*, 1996);
- helping people to cope with bereavement (Youll and Wilson, 1996);
- helping those who are incontinent (Langley, 1995);
- helping in mentoring (Stokes, 2003);
- advising in dietetics (Licavoli and Hahn, 1995);
- coping with sudden infant death syndrome (McClain and Mandell, 1994);
- helping with giving up smoking (Hurt *et al.*, 1994; Leininger and Earp, 1993);
- helping to educate those working in the cancer and palliative care fields (Faulkner *et al.*, 1991);
- pastoral counselling (Woodruff, 2002);
- help in armed conflict (West, 2003).

THE ETHICAL DIMENSION

All health professionals work in situations in which others have to trust them. Those who counsel or who use counselling skills are also in positions of considerable trust. Often they will be listening to people who are very vulnerable or are listening to stories which are very personal. It is essential that anyone who undertakes counselling or who uses counselling skills does so *ethically* and does not abuse his or her situation in any way. The British Association for Counselling and Psychotherapy lays down ethical guidelines for counsellors and for those using counselling skills, and these are reproduced as an appendix to this book. It is notable, too, that almost all health professions have their own codes of conduct which will apply just as much to the use of counselling skills as to any other aspects of care or work with clients.

One aspect of maintaining an ethical relationship involves the ability of those using counselling skills to monitor themselves. Counselling relationships often become close ones. It always remains the responsibility of the health professional using counselling skills to ensure that a reasonable and therapeutic *distance* is maintained. Without that distance, boundaries – both professional and personal – can become blurred. It is often, when this blurring of boundaries occurs, that ethical dilemmas arise. None of this is to assume that health professionals and clients should not become close but simply to acknowledge that there is an important difference between a personal relationship and a professional one. In a personal relationship, usually, two people meet as equals in status and they choose, jointly, whether or not to enter into a deeper relationship with each other. This is not the case in a professional relationship, where one person is already designated 'a professional' and, by definition, is expected by the other person to be professional, reliable and trustworthy.

It is possible to read, in the literature on counselling and therapy, of counsellors and clients who fall in love with one another. It is possible to argue, though, that such relationships are never ones of equality but are based rather more on a power dynamic, with the counsellor always being in a 'one-up' position in relation to the client. It is also possible to argue that the client falls in love with the counsellor AS counsellor and not as just another human being. Later in such a relationship, both would have to face that the original designations of 'client' and 'counsellor' are no longer there, and that each is, arguably, not in love with the person they perceived each other to be when they occupied those roles. From being in a 'one-up', 'one-down' power relationship, they suddenly have to face each other as equals and, arguably, the 'healing' aspect of the relationship is potentially lost, as the counsellor becomes just another person with many of his or her own personal and life problems. Nor is it simply a case of dismissing the power relationship and declaring that 'I treat my clients as equals, anyway'. This may or may not be the case but it does not allow for how each *client* may perceive the *counsellor* or health professional. Simply by being a helper or carer, the health professional is already cast in a certain light by his or her clients. This is not to suggest, in any way, that counsellors and health professionals have 'special powers' in any sense, but to acknowledge that they are always acting out a role that is constantly being defined for them by their clients and by themselves. In another sense, however, the issue is very much about power. For a counsellor to encourage an emotional and romantic relationship is for him or her to abuse his power. For, at some level, the client is likely to see the counsellor (temporarily at least) as a more able and more powerful person. In this sense, the client is likely to 'look up' to the counsellor and to admire his or her skills. The counsellor always abuses that set of relationships once he or she develops or encourages a romantic or even sexual attachment. The counsellor who does develop such relationships should question, very seriously, his or her motivation for being a counsellor at all. In a sense, then, the counsellor, like any health care professional, must be beyond reproach and always acting in the primary interests of the client. All other things come secondary to this.

Finally, West raises the ethical issue of the degree to which those engaging in counselling, for the first time, do so from a position of true 'informed consent'. He notes the following:

> *How can clients consent to counselling, especially if they have had no previous experience of counselling? How can this possibly be informed consent? Even if the client has had some previous experiences, say of the CBT (cognitive behavioural therapy} therapist down the road or a colleague of mine who describes her practice in the same way as I do, how can I accurately convey to this would-be client what counselling from me would be like? If my would-be client is seeking counselling because of some life crisis, does this not affect his or her ability to give consent?*
>
> (West, 2002)

West has no answer to his own dilemma. Given that we cannot leap ahead and see what happens in future counselling sessions, perhaps the best we can do is to make sure that the prospective client is aware of our *intentions* as a counsellor, and that he or she can reserve the right, at any time, to withdraw from the counselling relationship.

COUNSELLING AND THE HEALTH PROFESSIONAL

Counselling involves listening, helping, empowering and befriending. In these respects, it is the central feature of the work of all health professionals. Examples of the application of counselling skills are numerous, and some examples are identified as follows. These examples of health professions and applications are not claimed to be exhaustive:

1. *Medicine*
- helping patients and clients to describe their symptoms;
- helping clients experiencing emotional, social and relationship problems;
- facing family crises and difficulties;
- helping and empowering the 'worried well';
- advising people who are worried about HIV/AIDS.

2. *Nursing*
- helping to plan nursing care;
- identifying the patients' needs and wants;
- coping with dying and bereaved people;
- reassuring relatives and colleagues;
- handling other people's anger and fear;
- helping students to work through their courses.

3. *Occupational therapy*
- talking through personal issues with clients, individually and in groups;
- discussing coping strategies;
- enabling clients to regain their ability to live independently;
- helping clients to talk about their reactions to their disabilities.

4. Physiotherapy
- helping clients to adapt to long-term disability;
- helping people to cope with their treatment;
- helping people to regain their motivation in the rehabilitation process.

5. Teaching
- talking through course work and academic problems;
- helping students to write essays and dissertations;
- vocational guidance;
- pastoral work;
- helping students to reflect.

6. Voluntary work
- listening to clients' problems in living;
- supporting other health professionals;
- coping with other people's emotional release;
- learning more about yourself.

7. Social work
- enabling the client and family group to clarify problems and identify goals;
- helping parents and their children;
- enabling client advocacy.

8. Speech therapy
- discussing problems with clients;
- talking to parents and other relatives;
- working with other health professionals.

Many of these aspects of health professionals' role overlap with each other and interrelate between professional roles. It is also clear, though, that counselling skills form an integral part of the daily work of all health professionals. The skills described and discussed in this book will enable all professionals to enhance their daily practice, whatever their particular focus. Thus the skills may be used by nurses working with the elderly and the mentally ill as well as by those working in rehabilitation and general medicine. Physiotherapists will find the sections on listening, client-centred counselling and on coping with emotion useful when helping both the acutely and chronically ill. Occupational therapists may well find that what are described as counselling skills in this book are skills that can be used daily when working with both the individual and the group in psychiatric and general practice.

Davis and Fallowfield identified the following list of 'deficiencies in professional communication' which they use to preface their work on developing counselling skills in the health professions. They offer a useful set of points to consider in the context of *any* health care professional's work:

1 failure to greet the patient appropriately, to introduce themselves, and to explain their own actions;

2 failure to elicit easily available information, especially major worries and expectations;

3 acceptance of imprecise information and the failure to seek clarification;

4 failure to check the doctor's understanding of the situation against the patient's;

5 failure to encourage questions or to answer them appropriately;

6 neglect of covert and overt cues provided verbally or otherwise by the patient;

7 avoidance of information about the personal, family and social situation, including problems in these areas;

8 failure to elicit information about the patient's feelings and perceptions of the illness;

9 directive style with closed questions predominating, frequent interruptions and failure to let the patient talk spontaneously;

10 focusing too quickly without hypothesis testing;

11 failure to provide information adequately about diagnosis, treatment, side-effects or prognosis, or to check subsequent understanding;

12 failure to understand from the patient's point of view and hence to be supportive;

13 poor reassurance (Davis and Fallowfield, 1991).

Although their list refers to 'doctors' and 'patients', Davis and Fallowfield's points could be applied to *any* health care situation and any set of relationships between health care professionals and the people with whom they work.

VARIETIES OF COUNSELLING

In order to identify the variety of aspects of the counselling process, it will be useful to identify different sorts of counselling. Counselling is not one set of skills to be used in a narrow range of situations but a differing and often idiosyncratic mixture of personal qualities, practical skills and interpersonal verbal and non-verbal behaviours that combine to make up a particularly caring aspect of the health professional's job. Later, it will be necessary to consider how the counsellor needs to take care of herself: human caring of the sort being described here takes its toll. We cannot be involved with others without that contact touching our own lives, our belief and value systems and our emotional make-up. Counselling is a remarkably personal activity which not only changes the client but also changes the counsellor. As carers, we need to take care of ourselves.

Supportive counselling

One of the most common forms of counselling is when we are asked to support people. This may take the form of acting as a sounding board for their ideas, plans or suggestions. The primary skill required in acting in this way is the skill of listening. To really listen to another person is the most caring action of all. Listening is more fully discussed in Chapter 7 of this book. In that chapter, various aspects of the listening process are explored, and readers are offered practical suggestions about how to improve their listening skills. Whilst we all have experience in listening, so do we all have experience of only half listening – of being so caught up with our own concerns and of rehearsing our answers. All of these things distract us from the process of offering true support to another person. If we are to offer supportive counselling, we must learn to give ourselves almost completely to the other person for the period we are with them. Not really an easy task.

Supportive counselling also calls for more than just the ability to listen. It calls for the capacity to imagine how the world seems to the other person. It is to offer what Rogers called 'empathic understanding' (Rogers, 1983). This is similar to the old Indian idea that you shouldn't criticise a person without having first walked a mile in his moccasins. To support is also to understand what the other person is feeling. The degree to which it is possible to offer this sort of empathy is open to question, and this, too, is taken up in a later chapter.

Another important aspect of any discussion about offering support on a professional basis is the question of *commitment* to the process. Alistair Campbell discusses this issue eloquently in his book *Paid to Care?* (Campbell, 1984a). There seems to be something curious about the fact that each of us is involved in caring for others in a way that involves deep understanding, whilst also doing a job of work. We need, as users of counselling skills, to consider our motives. Whilst altruism and true caring for the needs of others must be at work in the counselling process, it is also reasonable to assume that in supporting others, we are also getting something out of the process for ourselves. Social exchange theory offers the slightly cynical view that there is *always* a 'payoff' in human relationships. Homans goes as far as to suggest that:

> *The open secret of human exchange is to give to the other man behaviour that is more valuable to him than it is costly to you and to get from him behaviour that is more valuable to you than it is costly to him.*

> (Homans, 1961)

Nothing, perhaps, is free. We need to be clear about our motives when offering support, and clear about why we are offering support to the other person. If it *is* part of a professional commitment and part of our job, then we need to work through the implications of that, too. We need to make sure that we can be both sincere in our work and fully aware of the cost as well as the benefits, to ourselves.

Supportive counselling occurs in a variety of settings. The physiotherapist who sees a client through the lengthy rehabilitation process is also offering a type of supportive counselling. It is she who often has to listen to the client's darker thoughts and feelings during the inevitable troughs in the process of rehabilitation. The voluntary worker in a general hospital often undertakes supportive counselling as a very specific part of her role. Very often, she has the time that other health care professionals do not have (or do not claim to have). Also, perhaps, because she is doing the job 'for love', her motives for supporting may be clearer. She is taking on the role of counsellor simply because she wants to. General practitioners, in allowing their patients to verbalise their personal and family problems are also offering supportive counselling. Student nurses working in a wide range of settings, from working with the mentally handicapped to caring for the terminally ill, regularly face situations in which they are asked to be supportive.

All health professionals have to help patients and clients adapt to various situations, from learning to live with paralysis to coping with a colostomy. In many of these situations, patients and clients have to adjust to a different body image, a changed perception of self. Fortunately, such adaptation *can* be made but the health professional who is able to offer adequate and appropriate support can do much to smooth the process.

The skills outlined in this book can enable health professionals to survive the pressures of such situations. Health care, particularly in the UK, has changed dramatically in the past 10 years. The provision of care, the means of financing it, the numbers of people involved as carers – all of these factors have put pressure on health care professionals as well as on the clients who are recipients of care. Such factors can be emotionally exhausting and undermining. In the past, it was usual to encourage health professionals to 'grin and bear it', to hide their feelings wherever possible. Today, the situation is somewhat paradoxical. On the one hand, there is intense pressure on health professionals to economise and make sure that they offer 'value for money'. On the other, they are more readily encouraged to express their feelings about caring. Thus the 'hard-nosed' and the 'softer' approaches seem to have come together. We all have to be sound business people and, at the same time, remember our humanity and frailty.

Informative counselling

Health professionals develop a considerable amount of knowledge about the domain in which they work. Some of this is 'formal' knowledge: knowledge learned from books, lectures and through the educational processes of colleges and universities. Lots of it, though, is 'experiential' or personal knowledge that is gained through the process of living and working with other people. Much of this knowledge relates directly to how people function and feel. Different sorts of health practitioners have different sorts of very specific knowledge about physiology, disease and health. Many have a wealth of 'ingrained' knowledge that involves intuition as well as rationality. Clients often ask for very specific information about the nature of their health or lack of it, and such information is clearly what makes up informative counselling. Clearly, clients require accurate and understandable information, and information on which they can *act*. A current example of how people may require informative counselling is in the field of HIV and AIDS. People require an understanding of how they should conduct their sexual relationships or manage the administration of intravenous drugs. All of this requires a considerable knowledge base. It is not a simple matter of knowing about using condoms or of needle-exchange schemes. It is also just as much about relationships, both gay and straight, and about people's feelings and fears.

People, then, need information. Someone else has that information. All that is left is for the information to be handed over. In reality, of course, it is rarely as simple as that. Any information concerning me and my body or my life concerns me. Not in a detached, academic way but in a very personal sense. Anyone who has been a patient in hospital or who has been given advice in a GP's surgery will know the difference between what information 'means' to the medical profession and what it means to the person who is hearing it. Thus, the giving of information in the health professions is unlike the giving of information in, say, estate agency. In the latter, we are dealing, at least to some degree, with impersonal, objective facts. In the former situation, the case is overloaded with an emotional aspect that calls at once for sympathy, empathy, tact and considerable skill. To give another person information about themselves or their relatives is an emotional process. Whilst the information must be accurate, the delivery of that information must be appropriate to the needs of the receiver.

Another problem arises here. Giving information about illness, health or physiology seems to be reasonably straightforward if we develop the skill of giving it sensitively. With *problems in living*, alluded to previously, the situation is different. When it comes to giving another person information about how to live his or her life, we are on much less certain ground. Some would argue that the only person who is truly able to furnish information about another person's problems in living is that person himself. It would seem prudent to avoid offering information about other people's life situations unless it is directly asked for by the client, and then only tentatively. The temptation is often great to suggest to clients what *we* think they should do. Or perhaps we offer them suggestions as to what we would do given their situation. Such advice is not usually very helpful but, fortunately, rarely dangerous. It would seem that people are relatively self-protecting in this respect and they do not accept advice that they cannot use. On the other hand, this may be a reflection on the way in which clients choose the people they seek out to be counselled by. Jean-Paul Sartre (1973) suggested that one person goes to another for advice already knowing the sort of advice that he will receive. He may not do this consciously, but it would seem that this process of selection does take place on some deeper level. As a demonstration of this, in your own life, reflect for a moment on whom you would choose to talk to about the following: problems about money; sexual problems; problems of self-confidence. Now ask yourself what *sort* of advice you would be likely to receive from the people you have chosen. It seems likely that you select out the people who will tell you what (at some level or another) you already know.

Informative counselling, then, is best restricted to relatively concrete situations, where expert information can make a direct contribution to the person's well-being. We have noted that this is rarely the case: better and more effective methods of counselling exist, and the skills involved in these methods are easily learned. However, there are exceptions to all this, and these are also explored in a later chapter.

It should be noted, too, that just because someone is given up-to-date and expert advice does not automatically mean that the person will *take* and *act on* that advice. Being given information does not, necessarily, lead to behaviour change. A good example of this is in the field of smoking. Although most people today are offered detailed accounts of why smoking is bad for you, those accounts do not themselves automatically lead to the giving up of smoking. There are plenty of examples of people in the health care professions who know all the reasons not to smoke and yet continue to choose to do so. There is even a possibility that people are put into 'information overload' in the health care services. Most drugs dispensed carry lengthy descriptions of what those drugs contain, how they should be used and how they should not be used. Pharmacists, who dispense those drugs, currently give out further information when the drugs are purchased. It seems possible that people may find themselves overloaded and even confused by being given so much information and in such a short space of time. Similarly, many doctors have now been trained to 'explain' everything that is to happen to a patient. There remains little evidence, to date, that all such information giving, either relieves anxiety or leads to behavioural change – even though the motives behind such information giving are benign.

Informative counselling in practice

Sally is a physiotherapist who is visiting an elderly patient, Jean Andrews, in the ward prior to her having an operation for a hip replacement. During the process of being taught breathing exercises, Jean asks Sally about her operation. Sally uses client-centred counselling interventions to establish what Jean has and has not been told about her coming operation. She is then able to offer clear and precise information about what may be expected, being careful not to use jargon or to 'talk down' to Jean. In this way, Jean's anxieties are relieved and she is better prepared for her operation because of her increased knowledge. There is evidence to suggest that patients who are given sufficient information about surgery and its possible outcomes, suffer subjectively less pain than do those who are not prepared in this way (Hayward, 1975). In this example, too, the information given is of a concrete and practical nature that will enhance the patient's comfort and relieve her anxiety.

On the other hand, in a cultural context, information giving – even in the case of personal problems – may be seen as appropriate. In Muslim countries, typically, a person would not see a counsellor but go to a religious advisor who would offer a view from the Quran on matters of personal issues.

Educational counselling

Health professionals are often to be found in educational settings. Most of the professions employ people trained in those professions as educators to the next generation. A number of the caring professions operate an apprenticeship type of training in which work in the field is combined with blocks of academic study. This format, however, is changing rapidly. The nursing profession, for example, used to use an apprenticeship approach to training but has replaced it with a scheme in which all trainee nurses are full-time students in colleges and universities and spend short periods in clinical practice with supernumerary status.

People who work in an educational capacity frequently find themselves in the role of personal tutor to one or more students. Such tutoring combines both the educational aspect of the student's life and also the personal. It is this dual function that can combine both types of counselling discussed previously – the supportive and the informative. It is usually useful, however, to establish some parameters to the student–tutor relationship, and the use of a *contract* is helpful here.

In contract setting, the tutor negotiates the following with the student:

- the amount of time that they will spend together (e.g. 1 hour per week);
- the type of counselling relationship that is required (e.g. academic and course related and/or personal);
- whether or not some of the academic counselling will take place in small groups to include other personal tutees. Whilst this may not suit all students it is certainly more economical in terms of the tutor's time;
- what both student and tutor expect of the relationship.

There are occasions on which the personal aspects of a student's life will shade into his or her academic life. On the other hand, to keep a counselling conversation focused on one or other of these topics can enable both tutor and student to clarify what it is they want from the relationship at that particular time. Hopefully, too, the distinction can enable some objectivity about a student's academic work to be maintained by the tutor, although this can be a problem. When personal issues are discussed alongside academic issues, the problem of how to assess written and project work can become difficult, as the tutor may be too distracted by the personal issues that are involved. In some cases, this may constitute an argument for personal tutors *only* being concerned with academic and work-related issues. Some might argue that if such tutors begin to help on personal issues then they are likely to lose the ability to stay objective about students' academic work. To this end, many colleges and universities employ student counsellors who will see students to talk about personal issues. Unfortunately, it remains the case that such counsellors are sometimes stigmatised: some students still see it as something of a personal weakness if they have to consult the college counsellor. The ideal picture, perhaps, is of a personal tutor who can move freely between academic work and personal issues, whilst retaining a certain objectivity about course work. This is, in practice, harder than it sounds.

The skills of educational counselling and coaching turn out to be very similar to those of other sorts of counselling. This is illustrated, quite dramatically, by the late psychologist, George Kelly, in his description of the various facets of his work as a teacher and as a therapist:

> *One of my tasks in the 1930s was to direct graduate studies leading to the Master's Degree. A typical afternoon might find me talking to a graduate student at one o'clock, doing all those familiar things that thesis directors have to do – encouraging the student to pin-point the issues, to observe, to become intimate with the problem, to form hypotheses either inductively or deductively, to control his experiments so that he will know what led to what, to generalise cautiously and to revise his thinking in the light of experience.*
>
> *At two o'clock I might have an appointment with a client. During this interview I would not be taking the role of the scientist but rather helping the distressed person work out some solutions to his life's problems. So what would I do? Why, I would try to get him to pin-point the issues, to observe, to become intimate with the problem, to form hypotheses, to make test runs, to relate outcomes to anticipations, to control his ventures so that he will know what led to what, to generalise cautiously and to revise his dogma in the light of experience.*
>
> (Kelly, 1963)

So was born Kelly's personal construct theory, in which Kelly maintained that 'people are scientists' who are continuously developing hypotheses about how they and the world around them will be, and then testing those hypotheses against how the world actually turns out.

Counselling in crisis

Another aspect of counselling is helping the person who suddenly finds himself in crisis. Murgatroyd and Woolfe (1982) have characterised a crisis in the following ways:

- Symptoms of stress – the person experiences stress both physically and psychologically.
- Attitude of panic or defeat – the person feels overcome by the situation and experiences both helplessness and hopelessness.
- Focus on relief – the person wants, more than anything else, relief from the feeling of being in crisis.

- Lowered efficiency – in other areas of their life, apart from the crisis, the person's functioning may be impaired.
- Limited duration – because the experience is psychologically painful, it does not last long and can be viewed as an acute experience of limited duration.

There are many different sorts of crises that occur in people's lives, ranging from sudden death to the realisation of child abuse in a family. Differences occur, too, with regard to the point at which individuals perceive themselves to be in crisis. Thus, the point at which counselling interventions are offered will vary from person to person. Sometimes that intervention is offered through access to a crisis intervention team of one sort or another. Usually such teams are multidisciplinary and offer the services of a range of practitioners. At other times, crisis counselling is offered through telephone counselling and through a range of helplines. Clearly, telephone counselling calls for a very different range of skills than does face-to-face counselling, in that the immediate presence of the person in distress is missing. In such a situation, all non-verbal means of communication between the two people are lost and verbal intervention is almost the only means of interchange available. The word 'almost' is used deliberately here, for even on the telephone, an intuitive sense of a situation may be grasped by the effective counsellor. General guidelines in counselling on the telephone include the following:

- Allow the caller to talk freely. Try not to interrupt them but keep them talking.
- Take the lead from the caller. Explore the issues *he* wants to talk about.
- Once you have established rapport, try to make sure that the caller (or other people in his company) are out of direct danger.
- Use occasional 'minimal prompts' to indicate that you are listening ('mm' or 'yes') but use them sparingly.
- If appropriate, make sure that you have the caller's name and a contact phone number. Make sure that the caller knows your name.

Crisis counselling calls for swift action in helping the person to function effectively. Schwartz (cited by Murgatroyd, 1986) offers some suggestions as to how such action may be initiated. Amongst other things, Schwartz suggests the following steps that the counsellor may take:

- Help the person face up to the crisis – discourage denial and attempt to help him to be objective.
- Break up the crisis into manageable doses – most people can deal with serious problems more easily if they are not overwhelmed by the sheer magnitude of the situation.
- Avoid false reassurance – the counsellor should resist the temptation to prematurely assure the person in crisis that 'Everything will work out OK'.

- Help and encourage the person to help himself – if the person in crisis can actively use the help of friends or family this will cut down the dependence on the counsellor and increase decision-making.
- Teach the person in crisis coping skills – once the immediate danger has past, the individual needs to develop a repertoire of coping strategies to help ward off future and similar situations.

Crisis counselling is demanding work and the urgency of the situation often calls for quick decisions to be made. In such situations it is easy to take over too quickly and for the counsellor to try to take control of the situation. Whilst this may help in the first instance, such an approach does not help the person in crisis in the longer term. Sometimes, crisis counselling calls for considerable constraint on the part of the counsellor, and it is often emotionally draining. For this reason, it is often helpful, wherever possible, for crisis counselling to be conducted in pairs or by a small group of people. In this way, mutual support is offered by the counsellors to each other: the responsibility for the situation is shared and more objective help can be offered. However crisis counselling is organised, the counsellor should have available a list of names and telephone numbers of other agencies who are likely to be able to help. Knowing that you have a referral number to the local social services, police, rape crisis centre or other agency means that you are more readily able to offer concrete and practical help to defuse the situation.

There are numerous examples of crises that health care professionals may have to help their clients or patients through, and a short list of examples of such crises would include, at least, the following:

- rape or sexual assault;
- sudden death of a partner or spouse;
- child abuse;
- sudden death of a child;
- trauma caused by accident or injury;
- sudden onset of acute psychological or emotional distress;
- suicide or attempted suicide;
- fear of death or the process of dying;
- concern about HIV/AIDS;
- fear of surgical intervention;
- sudden and acute physical pain;
- acute anxiety about the future;
- panic attacks.

Post-trauma counselling

In the past few years, as in other decades and centuries, we have witnessed large-scale wars, disasters and personal tragedies. The sort of counselling that is undertaken to help someone after a major trauma is similar, in a way, to that used to help the bereaved (Parkinson, 1993). He suggests that there are four main tasks in post-trauma counselling:

1 To help people to accept the reality of their experiences and to counteract the defence of denial.

2 To encourage them to feel the pain and to provide reassurance of the normality of their reactions. This also deals with the problem of denial.

3 To help them adjust and adapt to the changes which have taken place in their lives.

4 To help them redirect their emotions and their lives so that they can move to acceptance and healing (Parkinson, 1993).

In the end, as in all forms of counselling, the person has to find his or her way through. Brian Keenan, for nearly five years a hostage in the Middle East, wrote the following in an article in *The Guardian* on Friday, 9 August 1991, soon after the release of his friend and fellow hostage, John McCarthy:

> *Each man must find within himself the various methods to contain and control the pain and confusion within. There are no ready-made answers. It is a slow process of rediscovery, where denial or flight from the inward turmoil is the antithesis of self-healing. We go that road alone. We may be helped but we cannot be pushed or misdirected. We each have the power within us to re-humanise ourselves. We are our own self-healers.*

Keenan was writing about the after-effects of trauma but he might have been writing about anyone who experiences profound personal and emotional problems, and his words summarise well the central issue in counselling: self-healing.

There is a question here, too, about *time*. It is possible to believe, from the media, that the time that people require counselling, after a tragedy, is *immediately*. It is arguable, however, that people, in some situations, may need *time* in order to reflect on what has happened to them and to allow the healing processes of rationalisation to take their course. Perhaps, people do not always need immediate counselling after a life-shattering event.

Counselling in spiritual distress

Spiritual distress is the result of total inability to invest life with meaning. It can be demotivating, painful and can cause anguish to the sufferer. Counselling people who experience such distress presents a considerable challenge to health professionals who care for them.

It would seem that the need to find meaning in what we do is a very basic human need (Bugental and Bugental, 1984). Such meaning may be framed in the context of a set of religious beliefs that can take very varied forms (Wallis, 1984). Alternatively, meaning may be found through adherence to a particular ideological viewpoint: philosophical, psychological, sociological or political. Others take the view expressed by Kopp (1974) that there is no meaning to life except what we as individuals invest in it. Those with a positivistic scientific view of the world may dismiss the metaphysical altogether, and thus the notion of a spiritual problem does not arise for them. We should, of course, be open to this too. Not *everyone* needs spiritual care or finds the world of the spiritual of importance to them.

The first qualification for engaging in spiritual counselling may be the development of an understanding of a wide range of religious doctrines, philosophical and political systems of thought and an appreciation of how various thinkers throughout history have approached the ultimate questions of life. Such an enterprise can be humbling. It can enable us to understand that not everyone views the world as we do and may guard against any temptation on the part of the counsellor to proselytise. As Jung pointed out (Fordham, 1966), the counsellor needs to be a 'wise' person, not only trained in counselling methods but also widely read, experienced and open-minded.

Counsellors also need, perhaps, a highly developed intuitive sense: the ability to see and understand beyond the words that people use to attempt to express themselves. Carl Rogers noted that he felt himself to be functioning best as a counsellor when he paid full attention to this intuitive sense (Rogers, 1967). Counselling in the spiritual domain, then, is far more than the development of a range of counselling skills. It involves the whole person and can, at times, tax the counsellor's own belief and value system. Indeed, the counsellor must be prepared to 'live on the edge' when counselling in spiritual distress and acknowledge that there are times when there are no answers to the taxing problems of meaning.

Who, then, are the people likely to require spiritual counselling? The range of those who experience spiritual problems is wide and includes adolescents suffering from identity crises (Erikson, 1959), those in middle age who may suddenly be faced with the difficulty of individuation (Storr, 1983), and the older person who may fear death. Along this age dimension are those of any age who suddenly find themselves confronting the issue of personal meaning. This may happen as part of a depressive illness but it may also happen when depression is not present. Dispiritedness, or the failure to find meaning, has been described as a state of mind separate to depression and identified as the questioning of the point of life in someone who is otherwise functioning 'normally' (Bugental, 1980; Tillich, 1952). It may occur, for instance, in the person who up to that point has held well-defined religious beliefs but who now has doubts about them. It can happen in those who are faced by some sort of extreme challenge in life and are left questioning the reasons for such an occurrence. It can occur, also, as a result of the crisis described in the previous section and should be looked for as a possibility after the immediate crisis has abated. Clearly, it can occur in a great number of situations that are found in hospitals: during sudden, severe and life-threatening illness; following surgical intervention that causes changes in body image (mastectomy, for example), following the death of a child or a close relative and numerous other situations in which the person may call into question the issue of meaning.

In later life, the problem of individuation described by Jung (Storr, 1983) as the quest for finding and understanding the self, may be preceded by a feeling of vacuum, pointlessness and lack of ability to be self-motivated. The psychoanalyst, Victor Frankl, has described this feeling as an 'existential vacuum' (Frankl, 1959, 1969, 1975). He argues that this is characterised by despair, distress and a feeling of emptiness. Frankl is clear, however, that this is not a neurotic condition but a very common human experience. Indeed, such a feeling is well described in works of literature that are concerned with the human condition. It occurs in the hero of Sartre's *Nausea* (1965) and Hesse's *Steppenwolf* (1927) and is addressed extensively in Colin Wilson's survey of such literature, *The Outsider* (Wilson, 1955). It is the darker side of the human situation.

The whole issue of dispiritedness, existential vacuum or spiritual collapse presents a great challenge to the health professional who meets people suffering from such life crises. How, then, may we help the person who, almost by definition, seems beyond counselling? Perhaps the first thing that we can do is to *listen* to the person. It is tempting when we are threatened by the content of another person's conversation to refuse to let him talk. Somehow, the despairing content of his conversation seems to call into question our own beliefs about life. This may indeed be the case and it suggests that before we engage in counselling of any sort, we therefore clarify our own belief and value systems (Simon *et al.*, 1978). If we are clearer about our own view of life, we may find that we are less threatened by the views of others. There is, however, no guarantee. We enter into every spiritual-counselling situation in something of an act of faith: there can be no absolute certainty that we will not be changed by the encounter. It may be important that this is the case. If we are so secure in our own belief system, we may also become closed minded and less questioning: such a position is probably not the best one from which to work as a counsellor.

Apart from listening to the person who is experiencing spiritual distress, we need also to *accept* what he says: if someone expresses particularly negative thoughts, the temptation is to try to persuade him to think otherwise. In counselling, however, the aim is to listen and to accept and not to argue. Often this means that the person being counselled needs to talk quietly through something, sit in silence for some time and generally to acknowledge and face the blankness that he feels. It is often the case that the very facing of the blankness can lead to an apparent paradoxical change. It is as though through allowing and accepting the feeling, the feeling itself changes. Sometimes those who face complete meaninglessness, find meaning. This accent on accepting rather than fighting feelings is described in detail by Reibel (1984) who calls it the homeopathic approach to counselling. She adopts the metaphor of homeopathy to describe this process of 'allowing' a condition or state of mind rather than fighting it. In homeopathic medicine, small doses of toxins that cause an illness may be given as a remedy for the illness. So, in homeopathic counselling, the thoughts and feelings that are troubling the spiritually distressed person are encouraged rather than argued against. Sometimes by such encouragement the dispirited feelings are transformed or transmuted and replaced by more positive, life-asserting feelings.

Closely allied to this homeopathic approach is that which involves the use of paradoxical strategies. These are variously described as paradoxical intention (Frankl, 1960, 1969, 1975), paradoxical interventions (Tennen *et al.*, 1981) and paradoxical therapy (Fay, 1976, 1986). These constitute a cluster of techniques whose essential element is an unexpected reversal of the anticipated procedure. Thus, instead of joining forces with the client to tackle his dispiritedness, the practitioner suggests a continuance or even an intensification of the negative feelings. This curious about-turn in counselling can, again, sometimes encourage a contrary alleviation of the negative feelings. It is as though by being implored to get worse, the client gets better! On the other hand, such an approach will not work with everyone, nor will it suit every practitioner. It is, however, an approach that may be considered as one or more means of helping the distressed person.

This is, perhaps, the crux of spiritual counselling and, for that matter, of any sort of counselling – that no one approach works for everyone. Health professionals engaged in spiritual counselling need to remain sensitive to personal needs and differences. Indeed, if they can develop the deeper listening approach alluded to previously and described in more detail in Chapter 7, they may enter the client's world view and discover, through the client, the right approach. The client, in other words, is telling the counsellor what help he needs. The difficulty lies in being receptive to that description. There are times when clients have great difficulty in articulating what their needs are, but such articulation is nearly always possible given time and sensitivity and also a considerable amount of humility on the part of the counsellor.

Health professionals acting as counsellors always need to know their limitations. They need to know when to call in other help agents, whether those agents are doctors, clergy, other members of the family or other health professionals. There are times, too, when counsellors have too close a relationship with the client and find their own judgement clouded by this closeness. If they are supported by other colleagues, such a period can be worked through to the benefit of both client and counsellor.

The skills involved in counselling the person who is spiritually distressed may serve as a template for the sorts of skills required in all counselling situations. Perhaps because of the extreme nature of the person's feelings, counselling in this situation calls upon certain aspects that we shall encounter again and again in later chapters – the ability to listen, to accept and to have some self-understanding.

It should be noted, too, that the word 'spiritual' used in this context, is not necessarily synonymous with the word 'religious'. Spiritual concerns, as they are described here, are concerns about *meaning*. The quest for meaning is probably a universal one and is just as much the domain of agnostics and atheists as it is of believers. On the other hand, McLeod notes counselling's historical links with religion, as follows:

> *Another field of study which has a strong influence on counselling theory and practice is religion. Several counselling agencies have begun their life as branches of the Church, or have been helped into existence by founders with a religious calling. Many of the key figures in the history of counselling and psychotherapy have had strong religious backgrounds, and have attempted to integrate the work of the counsellor with the search for spiritual meaning. Jung made the most significant contribution in this area. Although the field of counselling is permeated with Judaeo-Christian thought and belief, there is increasing interest among some counselling in the relevance of ideas and practices from other religions, such as Zen Buddhism.*
>
> (McLeod, 1998)

Counselling in spiritual distress in practice

Sian is a senior nurse in a large psychiatric hospital. Whilst talking to Ann, a ward sister, during her staff-appraisal meeting, she discovers that Ann finds it difficult to sustain interest in her work as person in charge of an acute-admissions ward. At first, this lack of motivation appears to be a result of having worked on the ward for two years. After further discussion, however, Ann talks of her difficulty in seeing the 'point' of her work and talks of a general disenchantment with life itself. Sian and Ann meet regularly and Ann is allowed to talk through her feelings. Gradually, she discovers a sense of purpose again, although there are times when both Sian and Ann are uncertain about the possible outcome of their discussions. Sian notes, too, that earlier in her career as a psychiatric nurse, she would have tended to dismiss Ann's problem as symptoms of depression.

Counselling in emotional distress

Frequently, there are times when the counselling relationship can evoke emotion in the client. Sometimes this occurs out of the discussion that the client is having – the very nature of the material under discussion is painful and brings to the surface a great deal of bottled-up feelings. At other times, the client comes to the practitioner in distress.

In the first instance, when the client is stirred up by the nature of the discussion, the most helpful thing that the counsellor can do appears to be to *allow* the full expression of those feelings (Heron, 1977a). However, this allowing goes against the cultural grain. We are more readily moved to cheer the person up or to help him to stop expressing strong feeling, even more so when that person's expression of emotion stirs up feelings in us as counsellors. It is arguable, however, that it is exactly because the person has been encouraged to bottle things up that he perceived himself as having problems. It is as though the bottled-up emotion changes the person's perception and tends to make for more negative perceptions. On the other hand, if those emotions are fully released, the person's impression of the situation will often change to the more positive. Clearly, this is not always the case. People in all walks of life experience real and distressing situations that cannot easily be resolved: death in the family, unemployment, illness, financial problems and so forth. None of these situations can be changed easily by the process of counselling. Even though this is true, the individual's perception of his situation can still change through counselling and, in this case, through expression of pent-up emotion. In a sense, there are no good or bad life situations: what is good and bad is the way that we view those situations – the sense we make of them. Whilst counselling may not be able to halt the fact of much of life being intractable, it can help in encouraging a more positive and life-assertive world view.

In the situation where the client comes to the practitioner in a distressed and emotional state, a decision has to be made as to whether to distract that person and move him away from his emotional release or whether to accept the release as outlined previously. Much will depend here on what the client is asking of the counsellor. Is he asking for help to control his emotional state? Is he asking that the counsellor hear him and allow him his expression? As we noted in the section on counselling in spiritual distress (pp.21–5), the counsellor must learn to read the signs and to hear what is being requested. If there is still ambiguity and the client's needs and wants are not clear, the counsellor has the option of asking the client what he wants. At first, this may seem like an uncomfortable option. In practice, it is quite possible to say to the other person, 'Do you want to continue crying or would you like me to help you stop?' Again, such an intervention is counter-cultural. Normally we do not ask such questions! The question can do much to help the client to determine exactly what is needed at this particular time. It is easy to imagine that because a person is crying, he is out of control in every other respect. The person who is crying is still able to be self-determining and still able to make decisions about what it is he does or does not want of another person.

There is a cultural aspect to all of this. It should be noted that, while in the 'West' the expression of emotion is seen as therapeutic and even to be recommended, this is not the case in many parts of south-east Asia. In much of Asia, there is a social taboo on the expression of strong feelings. To lose one's temper or even to cry, in company, is to risk losing considerable 'face'. Thus, the task of a helper in those countries is *not* to help the client to express feelings but to encourage him or her to restrain themselves and thus to maintain face. The job of the helper, in these contexts, is often simply to 'jolly along' the other person, to distract them away from the emotional turmoil they experience.

Those born into a northern European or US context are likely to find this apparent 'suppression' of emotion all wrong – or at least, unhelpful. However, it is vital that we do not impose our values on others or come to believe that our values are somehow 'right', over and against other people's. The wise counsellor will know something of these cultural variations and act accordingly. It is no use, for example, encouraging a Thai person to 'let go' and to cry. This is just the thing that the Thai person does not want to do and is trying hard *not* to do. Further aspects of culture, as they related to counselling and care, are described in a later chapter of this book.

The stranger-on-the-train phenomenon

Perhaps a reason counselling in emotional distress 'works' is that it can feel comfortable disclosing problems to a complete stranger. While it may be difficult to talk to someone you know really well, paradoxically, it can be easy to self-disclose, in some depth, to a complete stranger. Sometimes, the counselling can fulfil the role of the complete stranger. This tendency to disclose in this way has been called the 'stranger-on-the-train' phenomenon and, ironically, it is perhaps best described by the travel writer and novelist, Paul Theroux:

> *The conversation, like many others I had with people on trains derived an easy candour from the shared journey, the comfort of the dining care, and the certain knowledge that neither of us would see each other again.*

> (Theroux, 1977)

The specific skills involved in helping the person who is experiencing emotional release are described in Chapter 9. This section has merely opened up the question of what to do when someone is in emotional distress. Again, it would seem, the accepting method has much to commend it as a style of counselling

Confessional counselling

There are times when people need to talk, in confidence, about things that they feel unable to talk to almost anyone about. This might be called *confessional counselling* and it can take a number of forms. Sometimes, it is the case that a person has a particular habit or way of thinking that he feels to be somehow 'odd' and that he seeks reassurance that it is quite OK to be odd. Sometimes, relief comes simply from someone else having 'heard' him – that he has been able to disclose. At other times, the 'confession' may take the form of disclosure of something that proves to be contrary to the law – child abuse, certain sexual acts and so on. This type of disclosure may change the dynamics of the counselling relationship, for what is said cannot be unsaid. The counsellor, in a very clear way, is to some degree party to the act that has been described. The issue of confidentiality in counselling is discussed later in the book but anyone working in the counselling field should be aware of the possibility of sitting and listening to someone who tells things that causes the listener, as counsellor, to receive a certain responsibility from the client. For if I tell you that I have committed an obviously illegal act, then you also shoulder some of the responsibility. The act of telling becomes one of sharing responsibility.

The experienced counsellor may well have a strong sense of when such disclosures are being edged towards. He or she will need to make a decision about the implications of hearing such a decision and may even decide to discuss, with the client, the implications of that client making such a disclosure. It seems reasonable, to me, to be prepared to say something to the effect that 'I think you want to tell me something very serious about your life and I want us to talk about the implications of what your telling me might be'.

It must be borne in mind that the counsellor does not somehow stand outside of the law and cannot claim particular immunity for knowing certain things about another person if those things are of an illegal nature. Nor is this a debate about morality in the broader sense. The issue at stake, here, is whether or not by knowing something 'illegal' about another person, we are forced to act on that information. An extreme example may help here. If a person were to tell you that he or she had murdered someone and intended to kill again, one would, presumably, be in no doubt that action was required on your part to try to prevent this happening. Another example, although perhaps a little less black and white, is the person who discloses that he sometimes has suicidal feelings. In this case, the counsellor is required to make some sort of judgement about whether or not it is *always* appropriate to pass this information on to another person. The author was once faced, on a Friday afternoon, with a student who discussed the possibility of suicide. As I was likely to be the last person in the college to see her that afternoon, I had to weigh up what my responsibilities were towards her and towards her family and friends. In the end, I talked her into letting me go with her to her GP.

The point of this debate is to be prepared. People who counsel or use counselling skills must have thought through, *beforehand*, the implications of other people telling them things which they may not want to hear or may not want to have shared with them.

Again, this version of counselling may be very culture-specific. Not all people, in all cultural contexts, want to confide in another person or 'confess'. Again, the wise counsellor will note cultural differences and act accordingly.

COUNSELLING CONTEXTS IN THE HEALTH CARE PROFESSIONS

The range of situations in which health care professionals may be called to counsel is vast and no one list is likely to cover every possibility. It is interesting, however, to note the contexts described in Davis and Fallowfield's (1991) book and to attempt to add to it:

- counselling and renal failure;
- counselling and disfigurement;
- counselling in head injury;

- counselling with spinal cord injured people;
- counselling people with multiple sclerosis and their families;
- infertility counselling;
- counselling in gynaecology;
- genetic counselling;
- neonatal intensive care counselling;
- counselling families of children with disabilities;
- counselling in paediatrics;
- counselling patients with cancer;
- counselling in heart disease.

Other contexts in the health care professions that might be added to this list would include, at least, the following:

- HIV and AIDS counselling;
- counselling gay and bisexual people;
- counselling in sexual disfunction;
- career counselling;
- racial counselling;
- counselling in mental health settings;
- rehabilitation counselling;
- cultural counselling.

COUNSELLING AND PSYCHOTHERAPY

The differences between counselling and psychotherapy are often blurred. Nelson-Jones offers this distinction:

> The term 'counselling' is used in a number of ways. For instance, counselling may be viewed: as a special kind of helping relationship; as a repertoire of interventions; as a psychological process; or in terms of its goals, or the people who counsel, or its relationship to psychotherapy.
>
> (Nelson-Jones, 1995)

However, Davies is less sure about the relative differences between the two and she suggests that:

> The only difference between definitions of counselling and psychotherapy according to the perspectives of writers such as Nelson-Jones is essentially one of emphasis rather than there being any definitive or absolute differences in the definitions. Differences in emphasis may be seen in the nature of the relations, in the theoretical orientation of the activity, in the setting in which the activity takes place and in the different client populations.
>
> However, even this distinction appears relative rather than absolute. Consider the point about the settings in which counselling and psychotherapy take place: definitions of counselling tend to point out that counselling is more likely to take place in non-medical settings rather than medical settings. In terms of client populations, definitions of counselling tend to indicate that

counselling focuses on moderately to severely disturbed clients. However, it should be emphasized that any such distinctions are relative rather than forming mutually exclusive categories. Carl Rogers, himself, worked with clients who had been diagnosed as schizophrenic, while many of the therapies which come under the term psychological therapy, such as the cognitive and behavior therapies, are viewed frequently as the therapy of choice for less distressed clients. Further, counsellors are increasingly being employed to work in such medical settings as general practice or in health centres, as well as in clinical psychology departments and in psychotherapy departments within the NHS. Generally, it may still be the case that counsellors in these settings tend to be referred less chronically disturbed clients.

(Davies, 1987)

THE RANGE OF COUNSELLING INTERVENTIONS

Whatever sort of counselling is undertaken, certain skills and processes are involved. Counselling skills can be divided into two groups:

1 listening and attending;
2 verbal-counselling interventions.

In other words, the counsellor listens to the client and responds verbally. The skills involved in listening are described more fully in Chapter 7. It may be useful, however, to identify the range of counselling interventions that may be used in any counselling situation. John Heron, a UK philosopher and humanistic therapist has devised a valuable division of all possible therapeutic interventions called 'Six category intervention analysis' (Heron, 1986). The analysis transcends any particular theoretical stance adopted by the counsellor and has many applications. The six categories described in Heron's analysis are as follows:

1 prescriptive interventions;
2 informative interventions;
3 confronting interventions;
4 cathartic interventions;
5 catalytic interventions;
6 supportive interventions.

These six categories will be described in further detail but it is important to note that Heron further subdivides the categories into those he calls authoritative (the first three) and those he calls facilitative (the second three). Authoritative counselling interventions are those in which the counsellor plays a directive role in the counselling relationship and guides it in a fairly structured way. Facilitative counselling interventions are those in which the counsellor plays a less directive role and enables the client to take more control over the relationship. Another way of describing the difference is that authoritative interventions are 'I tell you' interventions and facilitative ones are 'you tell me' interventions. Heron argues that the skilled counsellor is one who can use a balance of the two types of interventions appropriately and skilfully in a wide range of counselling situations. It is not, then, a question of using all of the different types of interventions in all counselling situations but of consciously choosing the right intervention for the right occasion. What, then, are examples of the six categories of therapeutic intervention?

Prescriptive interventions

Prescriptive interventions are those in which the counsellor's intention is to suggest or recommend a particular line of action. Thus, if the counsellor says, 'I recommend you talk this over with your family', she is making a prescriptive intervention. Heron suggests that when prescriptive interventions are clumsily used, they can degenerate into heavy-handed, moralistic patronage. Certainly they can be overused in counselling, very easily.

Examples of how prescriptive interventions may be effective in the health care setting are when a physiotherapist offers a recently paralysed person practical suggestions as to how he may increase his mobility with the use of a wheelchair, or offers the elderly person advice about how to correctly use a walking frame.

The ethical issue is an important one here. We must ask ourselves the degree to which we have the right and the authority to recommend action to others. Do we seek to offer ethical guidance? Do we imagine we are able to suggest the 'right' thing for people to do? Clearly, any amount of prescription must be done with both humility and tact.

Informative interventions

Informative interventions are those in which the counsellor informs or instructs the client in some way. If, for example, the health professional says, 'You will probably find that you will have some discomfort in your leg for about three weeks', she is using an informative intervention. Heron notes here that unskilful use of informative interventions leads to dependence on the counsellor, and the relationship can degenerate into the counselling situation becoming one of overteaching on the part of the counsellor. As we have seen from the previous discussion on informative counselling, information is best limited to concrete situations and should not extend to 'putting your life right' information.

The nurse who instructs a patient to complete a course of antibiotics is offering informative help. It is notable that such information is limited to concrete, practical issues. As we have noted, it is easy to take over a patient's life and create dependence through offering too much information. It is also vital that the information that is given is accurate and up to date. Here, the counsellor should ensure that she supports her counselling practice from an *evidence base*. The counsellor working in the health care field is duty-bound to keep herself up to date with current literature and research. One useful means of doing this is via the Internet. While the Net gains a considerable amount of criticism, there is no doubt that it also contains a huge amount of useful information on just about any topic. Access to bibliographical search engines such as MEDLINE is also invaluable to the health care counsellor who is looking to maintain her own evidence base, from which to advise clients.

Confronting interventions

Interventions of this sort are those that challenge clients in some way or draw their attention to a particular type of repetitive behaviour. An example of a confronting intervention may be, 'I notice that you frequently complain about the way your wife talks to you ...'. If confrontation is used too frequently in the counselling situation, it may be perceived by the client as an aggressive approach. Clearly, confrontation needs to be used appropriately and sensitively. This issue is addressed more specifically in Chapter 11.

Once again, confrontation is a cultural issue. Whilst it is deemed reasonable to become an assertive person and to learn how to confront in the 'West', this is not the case in many other cultures – particularly those in south-east Asia. Confrontation, of any sort, is rarely acceptable in these cultures and is a major cause of loss of face to the person being confronted. The wise and skilled counsellor knows this and avoids using confrontational techniques with a client group from this cultural context.

Cathartic interventions

These are interventions that enable the client to release tension through the expression of pent-up emotion. Thus an intervention that allows a person to cry may be termed a cathartic intervention. The counsellor may give the client permission to cry by saying, 'You seem to be near to tears ... it's all right with me if you cry ...'. Cathartic interventions may be misused when they force the client to release feelings when that person is clearly not ready or willing to express them. It is sometimes tempting but rarely appropriate to anticipate that it will 'do the client good' to express bottled-up feeling. More appropriately, perhaps, it should be the client who decides when and if such release of emotion occurs. The issue of emotional release and cathartic skills is discussed in greater detail in Chapter 9.

There are very many situations in health care when effective use of cathartic skills is valuable. A short list would include, at least, the following:

- supporting the recently bereaved person;
- helping the person who is adjusting to new, yet profound, disability;
- assisting people to cope with shock after trauma;
- helping the person to express his or her feelings after assault, rape or accident;
- enabling the depressed person to release pent-up feelings of anger or self-doubt.

All carers need cathartic skills and yet, perhaps, they are the most difficult to develop. They require considerable self-awareness on the part of the professional and a willingness to explore our own emotional make-up. Once again, as we shall see, expressing emotion is not, universally, seen as being a 'good thing'. We will note in a later chapter the need for all counsellors to choose interventions to suit the client. In the case of clients from south-east Asia, cathartic interventions are only *very rarely*, if at all, going to be appropriate. For to express strong emotion in south-east Asia, is to lose face.

Catalytic interventions

Catalytic interventions are those that draw the client out and encourage him to discuss issues further. Thus, any sorts of questions are examples of catalytic interventions. Again, used inappropriately, questions can appear interrogative and intrusive. They need to be well timed and sensitively phrased. Certain other forms of catalytic intervention may be more appropriate than questions and these are discussed further in Chapter 8.

Catalytic interventions are perhaps the most useful of all interventions to the health professional. Often it is essential to explore how much a patient or client knows about his condition, prior to offering further information. The person skilled in catalytic counselling can discreetly and tactfully help the person to express his own wants and needs. Thus, catalytic counselling can become an integral part of health care *assessment*.

Supportive interventions

These are interventions that support, validate or encourage the client in some way. Thus, when the counsellor tells the client, 'I appreciate what you are doing', she is offering a supportive intervention. Used badly, supportive interventions can degenerate into patronage. Often, too, they are symptomatic of the counsellor's need to quickly reassure the client – perhaps evidence of the counsellor being a 'compulsive helper'.

These, then, are short descriptions of the six categories. Heron (1986) suggests that they are exhaustive, as a set of categories, of all possible therapeutic interventions. Thus, anything a counsellor can say to a client will fit under one of those six headings.

The category analysis has a number of applications. First, it can help us to appreciate a wide range of possible interventions to use in the counselling relationship. In everyday conversation, we tend to limit ourselves to a particular and often rather limited range of expressions, questions and verbal responses. The category analysis offers the chance to identify other interventions that we could use. Further, we can learn to make use of what Heron (1977b) calls 'conscious use of self'. In other words, we learn to take responsibility for what we say and choose to make a particular intervention at a particular time. At first, this obviously feels unnatural and clumsy. It is, however, the key to becoming an effective and appropriate counsellor. If we do not reflect on what we say and how we say it, we limit our competence. If we consciously choose what we say, then we stand to broaden our repertoire.

Second, the analysis can make us aware of alternative interventions. There are occasions in counselling, as in every other situation in life, where it is possible to think, 'What do I say now?'. Reference to the category analysis offers further possibilities of response: this must be the case if Heron's claim that it is exhaustive of all possible therapeutic interventions is valid.

Further, the analysis can be used as a research tool for identifying how groups of people view their own counselling skills. In a study of 93 trained nurses in the UK who were asked to rate themselves on their own perception of their levels of counselling skills using the analysis, most said that they were most effective at being prescriptive, informative and supportive, not as skilled at being catalytic and least skilled at using confronting and cathartic interventions effectively (Burnard and Morrison, 1987). Such research is easily carried out and can be used, at a local level, to determine training needs in the interpersonal domain, in much the same way as has been previously recommended.

Becoming aware of the range of counselling skills available is the first step towards becoming an effective counsellor. The next stage is to consider when and how to use those skills effectively.

COUNSELLING OR EVERYDAY COMMUNICATION SKILLS?

There comes a point in any debate about counselling as to when counselling skills can be differentiated from the skills used by a person who is a very effective communicator. Clearly, there is an overlap between the skills of a counsellor and a person with everyday interpersonal skills (see Figure 1.1). The person with 'everyday' skills will probably be a good listener. He or she is likely to be able to see the other person's point of view and will be little inclined to force his or her views on the other person. Perhaps the thing that marks out the person with counselling skills is his or her ability to focus, almost exclusively, *on the other person*. For this is what counselling involves. It means leaving behind your own interests, opinions, needs and wants, and giving your time completely to the other person.

To look at the other side of the argument, it does not follow that the person with counselling skills *also* has effective interpersonal skills in a range of other settings. It is quite possible to imagine – and to meet – people who are useful and helpful to others in the structured, one-to-one atmosphere of the counselling situation but less comfortable dealing with others on a more informal basis or with people in groups. There may be something of a contradiction here. If we were to argue that what is important in counselling is an inherent 'humanness' in the counsellor, then we might expect that humanness to spill over into other, everyday, situations. Ironically, though, this does not always seem to be the case.

Trying to stand outside of the debate for a moment, it seems likely

Acting as an ambassador for the organisation
Admitting you were wrong
Answering the phone
Apologising
Arguing
Attending a tribunal
Avoiding certain topics
Being a go-between
Being an advocate
Breaking bad news
Breaking up arguments
Chairing a conference
Chairing a discussion
Chairing a formal meeting
Chatting
Controlling feelings
Correcting another person
Countering someone else's argument
Criticising
Defending a colleague
Defending an idea
Defending an opinion
Describing
Disagreeing
Disciplining
Dissuading
Distracting
Encouraging
Expressing feelings
Giving a conference paper
Giving a presentation to colleagues
Giving a report
Giving advice
Giving an opinion
Giving information
Giving instructions
Helping
Instructing
Interrupting
Introducing self
Inviting ideas
Listening
Mediating
Negotiating
Offering a verbal assessment

Participating in a group
Passing judgement
Passing on information
Passing the time of day
Persuading
Reasoning
Receiving bad news
Receiving good news
Rectifying a mistake
Remaining silent
Returning goods
Saying 'no'
Saying 'sorry'
Saying good-bye
Saying good-bye to a group of people
Seeking opinions
Selling an idea
Sharing a joke
Sharing feelings
Sharing good news
Sharing ideas
Sharing self
Sharing thoughts
Showing appropriate anger
Speaking over an intercom system
Sticking to a point of view
Supporting
Supporting relatives
Supporting someone else's argument
Switching your viewpoint
Taking instructions
Talking on radio/television
Talking to colleagues
Talking to patients
Talking to people from other disciplines
Talking to the press
Talking whilst carrying out a procedure
Teaching patients/clients
Teaching peers
Teaching students
Thanking an individual
Thanking people in a group
Using the telephone
Welcoming guests

Figure 1.1

A comprehensive list of interpersonal/communication skills in the health care professions (Burnard, 1996).

that almost *all* health care professionals require effective communication and interpersonal skills in order to do their jobs. On the other hand, only relatively few will be required to be skilled as *counsellors*. In the middle of all this is the value of having both general communication skills and some counselling skills. Presumably, people in the health care professions who have both of these sets of skills are likely to function best of all. I have discussed elsewhere, in more detail, the acquisition of general interpersonal and communication skills (Burnard, 1996; 1997).

THE OUTCOME OF EFFECTIVE COUNSELLING

Clearly, different people respond differently to being counselled but it is worth considering what Carl Rogers noted was the general outcome of effective counselling. His list of the changes that may take place is based on observation and evaluation of numerous people 'getting better' in counselling and may serve as a useful indicator of the personal changes that can be achieved:

> *The person comes to see himself differently. He accepts himself and his feelings more fully. He becomes more self-confident and self-directing. He becomes more flexible, less rigid in his perceptions. He adopts more realistic goals for himself. He behaves in a more mature fashion ... He becomes more acceptant of others. He becomes more open to the evidence, both to what is going on outside of himself and to what is going on inside of himself. He changes in his basic personality characteristics in constructive ways.*
>
> (Rogers, 1967)

We must, however, remember that these *were* Rogers' observations and not ones based particularly on research. It is possible to view these 'outcomes' as, perhaps, rather too optimistic. In the latter part of the 20th century, it may be reasonable to settle for less. Sometimes, the fact that *one part* of a person's life has been helped by counselling is enough and sometimes it is all that we can expect. Perhaps, regrettably, too, there are going to be times when counselling *cannot* help and we would do well do bear this in mind too: counselling can never be a panacea.

PSYCHOLOGICAL APPROACHES TO COUNSELLING

2

In recent times, a huge range of different types of counselling and therapy has developed. The general consensus – although it is a culture-specific one – is that 'It is good to talk'. If we look at advertisements for counsellors, we find that they range from the 'traditional' to the 'new age'. The former will tend to be aligned to particular psychological schools of psychology while the latter will often adopt what they call an 'eclectic' approach, drawing from a range of different perspectives. How 'pure' a psychological approach to counselling should be is a matter of debate, as is the degree to which it is possible to use the word 'eclectic' to mean the equivalent of, 'I act as a counsellor in the way that I feel like acting at the time'. Eclecticism could be an excuse for having no particular 'school' to follow or it could be a demonstration of open-mindedness and a willingness to try to offer the client exactly what he or she needs. It is worth taking a little time to reflect on these two possible situations, yourself. Which position do *you* favour: adherence to one particular approach or the use of a wide number of approaches?

It is also worth noting that the approaches identified here are only *some* of the possible approaches to counselling. Feltham notes:

> *Estimates vary as to the number of different theoretical approaches to counselling and psychotherapy but the figure of 300 is often agreed as representative. Textbooks aiming to represent the field usually find it necessary to include between 10 and 20 mainstream approaches.*

(Feltham, 1995)

In this book, considerably fewer than '10–20 mainstream approaches' are considered.

Anyone who acts as a counsellor does so from a position of having certain assumptions about the nature of the person. We all carry with us a certain set of beliefs about the psychological make-up of ourselves and other people. Often this belief system is only hazily articulated. Sometimes it is not articulated at all. However vague that system is, it motivates us and helps us in our decision-making about how to help other people. In this chapter, some formalised belief systems about the person are briefly explored, drawn from a variety of schools of psychology. It is suggested that in exploring this variety of approaches to the person, we may be able to clarify our own set of beliefs. Harrow offers a useful checklist for considering our own beliefs, values and theories about counselling:

1 Explore your personal values and convictions about human beings and life in general. Do not be afraid to test your personal values and beliefs. Any value or belief worth having is one that can withstand close scrutiny.

2 Explore the major theories of counselling and psychotherapy. Choose the one that most closely resembles your own personal values and beliefs. That's your first approximation, your base.

3 Study your chosen theory in depth. Read all you can by its founder and by those who have developed it further. Take any available workshops to get supervised practice with associated techniques. Identify what draws you to this theory, and why. Identify also your areas of disagreement, and the reasons for them. If you find that disagreement outweighs agreement, begin the process again from the beginning.

4 Apply what you've learned in your work with clients. Observe how well this approach works for you. If you feel uncomfortable or ineffective working this way, it might mean you need to study the theory and its applications more thoroughly. Or you might simply be discovering your limits, identifying those situations where this theory doesn't seem to work well for you. If, on balance, this way of working doesn't suit you after all, begin the process again from the beginning.

5 When you are feeling well grounded and comfortable working with your theory of choice, re-examine some of the other theories that you considered. Do they seem to offer any technique that fits well with your chosen theoretical base? If you can explain these techniques in terms of the theory you are working from, try them and see how they work in practice.

Do any of these other theories offer any explanatory concepts that are philosophically consistent with your base theory, and perhaps cover situations in which your base theory seems weak to you? Be mindful of philosophical and theoretical consistency, and of consistency of theory and practice.

6 Keep learning about ways of understanding and working with people. Keep checking theory against your own lived experience. Keep cycling through these steps. Gradually, through them, you will discover your own personal working style (Harrow, 2004).

It is only through clarifying what we believe that we can hope to change or modify our practice. What follows, then, is a brief exploration of some psychological approaches to counselling. Some will seem to be congruent with what we believe ourselves. Others will seem quite alien. The skill may be to try to adopt the psychological approach least like our own and to suspend judgement on it for a while. In trying out a new set of ideas in this way, we are already developing a skill that is vital in the process of counselling – that of adopting a frame of reference different from our own. This is a process that is fundamental to counselling. As we listen to the other person, we must try to enter a theoretical approach that is different from our own in order to try to understand it.

There is also a practical reason for adopting this approach. As we sit with clients, reflecting upon what they say in terms of the belief system we have about the nature of persons, so they, too, sit with their own belief system about the nature of the person. Clearly, there is no reason to suppose that the belief system that the client has, however hazy or well articulated, will correspond to our own. We cannot guarantee that the client has the same set of views about human nature that we do. It is important, then, to consider a range of ways of making sense of human beings and a range of ways of allowing theory to inform our practice. What follows does not claim to be an exhaustive classification of all possible views of the person, but will allow the individual reader to draw his or her own conclusions about why people may do the things they do and how best to help them in the counselling situation. The discussion here of the various approaches is necessarily brief and the reader is referred to the considerable literature on the topic for a more detailed exposition.

THE PSYCHODYNAMIC APPROACH

Sigmund Freud is usually viewed as the father of the psychodynamic school of psychology (Hall, 1954). Essential to the approach is the notion that people are, to a greater or lesser extent, affected by unconscious motives and drives. That is to say, we cannot clearly give an account of why we are behaving, thinking or feeling as we are, at any given time, because there are forces at work beneath the level of conscious awareness that cause us to act in a particular way. This unconscious level of the mind is developed out of experiences that happened to us in earlier parts of our lives that we were unable to deal with at the time. When we encounter an experience in the present that is in any way similar to that past event, we experience anxiety – we are unconsciously reminded of the situation.

For psychodynamic psychologists, then, the key to understanding a person's present behaviour is through a thorough exploration of his past. Thus, the psychodynamically oriented counsellor will usually choose to explore the client's past history and help him to identify and, if necessary, to relive various painful, past events in order to make him less anxious and more able to make rational decisions about the present. In essence, then, the psychodynamic approach is a deterministic one. *Determinism* is the notion that every event has a cause and, in this case, every aspect of a person's behaviour has a cause and that cause is buried in the person's personal history. If you want to understand the person in the present, you must first understand his past. Essentially, too, a person's behaviour is basically understandable once these links to the past have been made. The process of counselling from the psychodynamic point of view may be likened to a jigsaw. Once all the pieces are put together, the whole thing makes sense. It is notable that many health professionals, particularly those in social work and certain types of nursing may have been 'brought up' on the psychodynamic way of understanding people. It may be useful for them to explore other ways.

The psychodynamic approach has come under considerable criticism in recent years (Masson, 1990; 1992). In particular, Masson – in his study of Freud's archives came to question Freud's 'seduction theory'. In early writings, Freud took the view that many women *imagined* that they had been sexually assaulted as children. Masson believes that Freud realised, later in his career, that many women *were* assaulted in this way but that his idea of these remembrances being 'fantasies' was never corrected in classical psychoanalytical theory. In questioning classical theory in this way, Masson found himself out of favour with the psychoanalytical movement and subsequently gave up undertaking any types of psychotherapy and counselling. An important lesson for counsellors in all this, would seem to be that clients should, first of all, be *believed*. Given the levels of child abuse that have been 'discovered' in recent years, this would seem to be particularly important.

Psychological mindedness is described by Coltart (1993) as crucial if clients are to make use of psychoanalytic psychotherapy. If it is necessary for clients using this model, it must also be required of their therapists. Coltart lists nine qualities that she suggests add up to psychological mindedness, which she looks for when assessing patients for psychotherapy. They are:

- an acknowledgment, tacit or explicit, by the patient that he has an unconscious mental life, and that it affects his thoughts and behaviour;
- the capacity to give a self-aware history, not necessarily in chronological order;
- the capacity to give his history without prompting from the assessor, and with some sense of the patient's emotional relatedness to the events of his own life and their meaning for him;
- the capacity to recall memories, with the appropriate effects;
- some capacity to take the occasional step back from his own story and to reflect upon it, often with the help of a brief discussion with the assessor;
- signs of willingness to take responsibility for himself and his own personal evolution;
- imagination, as expressed in imagery, metaphors, dreams, identifications with other people, empathy and so on;
- some signs of hope and realistic self-esteem. This may be faint, especially if the patient is depressed, but it is nevertheless important;
- the overall impression of the development of the relationship with the assessor.

In a study of women with postnatal depression, 193 women were enrolled to receive one of four interventions, routine GP care, non-directive counselling, cognitive-behaviour therapy, and psychodynamic therapy (Cooper *et al.*, 2003). The women were assessed immediately after the end of treatment, and at 4.5 months, 9 months, 18 months and 60 months. All three psychological treatments were equally effective and had similar effects on maternal mood. The only variation was that psychodynamic therapy relieved symptoms of depression more.

The psychodynamic approach in practice

The health professional who adopts the psychodynamic approach to counselling will tend to:

1 highlight the relationship between past and present life events;
2 acknowledge that unconscious forces are at work that affect the client's behaviour;
3 encourage the expression of pent-up emotion.

Examples of practical applications of this approach in the health care field include:

1 helping with long-term emotional problems;
2 coping with anxiety;
3 helping the client who talks of having had an unhappy childhood.

THE COGNITIVE-BEHAVIOURAL APPROACH

While Freud was developing his theories in Europe around the turn of the century, John Watson in the US was developing a different and opposing view of the person (Murphy and Kovach, 1972). He was adamant that the study of the person should be a scientific enterprise. To that end, he felt it should abandon the introspective methods suggested by Freud and concentrate on the arguably more objective study of human behaviour. Developing this theme, Watson argued that all human behaviour was learned and therefore could, if necessary, be unlearned. Such learning took place through the process he called *positive reinforcement*. Essentially, we learn those behaviours that we get encouraged to learn, and forget those behaviours for which no such encouragement is forthcoming. For the behavioural counsellor, then, the important issue is not the recollection of painful, past events but the identification of what the client sees as undesirable behaviour. Once those undesirable (or uncomfortable) behaviours have been identified, the next step is to organise a scheme whereby more positive behaviours will be encouraged (or, in behavioural terms, a 'schedule of reinforcement' is drawn up). The client is then encouraged to go away and work at developing the desired behaviours through the scheme organised with the counsellor. No attempt is made, in the behavioural approach, to understand the cause of behaviours in terms of the past as no such theory of causation is mooted.

The behavioural approach may be described as a *mechanistic* approach in that it tends to view the person as a highly complex machine – perhaps rather like a computer. And just as a computer responds only to its programming, so the person responds only to the learning he has achieved through reinforcement. The key issues in the behavioural approach, then, are learning, unlearning and relearning. The behavioural approach is frequently used as the basis for the training of psychiatric nurse therapists.

Mehrabian highlights some of the advantages to this approach thus:

> *If we can find a way to expand the statement of a problem to a concrete list of specific behaviours which constitute it, one major obstacle to the solution of the problem will have been overcome. In other words, the initial ambiguity with which most people analyse their interpersonal problems tends to contribute to their feeling of helplessness in coping with them. Knowing which specific behaviours are involved, and thereby what changes in those behaviours will solve the problem, provides a definite goal for action – and having that goal can lead to a great sense of relief.*
>
> (Mehrabian, 1971)

Further, two other writers in the field indicate how important changes in *behaviour* are in helping people to change their perceptions of their situation:

> *Much of what we view clinically as 'abnormal behaviour' or 'emotional disturbance' may be viewed as ineffective behaviour and its consequences, in which the individual is unable to resolve certain situational problems in his life and his inadequate attempts to do so are having undesirable effects, such as anxiety, depression, and the creation of additional problems.*
>
> (D'Zurilla and Goldfried, 1971)

In recent years, the strict form of behaviourism with its insistence on the primacy of *behaviour* as a matter for scientific investigation has given way to the *cognitive-behavioural* approach, with its accent on the fact that the way we *think* also affects our behaviour.

The cognitive-behavioural approach to counselling takes the view that what we think about ourselves affects the way we feel about ourselves. Thus, if we change our way of thinking, we can modify our feelings. Further, the argument is that many people hold exaggerated or incorrect beliefs about themselves that nevertheless affect their self-image. Examples of such false beliefs include, 'No-one likes me', 'Everyone thinks I'm stupid' and 'I can't cope with anything'. These 'globalisms' or very general statements can have a negative effect on the person's functioning. The aim of the cognitive counsellor is to challenge these inaccurate and negative statements in order to modify the way the person thinks about himself and thus how he feels about himself.

Albert Ellis (1962), who developed 'rational emotive therapy', a particular sort of cognitive therapy, argued that there were twelve typical irrational beliefs that people could hold about themselves. They were not intended to be an exhaustive list of all the possible irrational beliefs that people can hold but represent commonly held erroneous beliefs that may have a profound effect on how a person thinks, feels and acts. The twelve beliefs that Ellis identified are:

1 It is a dire necessity that I be loved or approved of by everyone for everything I do.
2 Certain acts are wrong and evil and those who perform these acts should be severely punished.
3 It is terrible, horrible and catastrophic when things are not the way I would like them to be.
4 Unhappiness is caused by external events – it is forced upon one by external events, other people and circumstances.
5 If something is or may be dangerous or fearsome, I should be terribly concerned about it.
6 It is easier to avoid or replace life's difficulties than to face up to them.
7 I need someone or something stronger or greater than myself upon which I can rely.
8 I should be thoroughly competent, adequate and achieving in all the things I do and should be recognised as such.
9 Because something in my past strongly affected my life, it should indefinitely affect it.
10 What people do is vitally important to my existence and I should therefore make great efforts to change them to be more like the people I would like them to be.
11 Human happiness can be achieved by inertia and inaction.
12 I have virtually no control over my emotions and I just cannot help feeling certain things.

Ellis claimed that anyone who holds any one or more of these beliefs is likely to experience distress inasmuch as they affect the way that person acts on those beliefs. Clearly this is a contentious list, but it is interesting and perhaps salutary to reflect on it and to reflect on the degree to which we ourselves hold any of these beliefs!

In the cognitive-behavioural approach, the style of counselling is one of challenging and confronting the client's belief system. In this respect, it is almost diametrically opposed to the style of counselling advocated by Carl Rogers – the client-centred approach. In the latter, the aim is to fully accept whatever the client says as a valid point of view about how that person views the world at that time. In the former approach, the aim is to call into question any number of beliefs that may be stopping the client from living fully and effectively. The approach has been used effectively with people who suffer from depression and other debilitating problems in living, and practical examples of how the approach is used in practice are well described by Beck *et al.* (1979) and also in Grant *et al.* (2004).

King *et al.* (2000) found that in a primary care setting 'non-directive counselling' and cognitive-behaviour therapy (CBT) were *both* significantly more effective clinically than usual GP care in the short term. At four months the mean scores on the Beck depression inventory were 4–5 points lower than the mean scores of the patients in the GP care group. There were no differences in outcome in the two therapies when they were compared directly using all the 260 patients randomised to a psychological therapy by either the patient preference method or the routinely randomised method. At 12 months the patients who had received the 'non-directive counselling' were more satisfied with the treatment they had received compared to those patients who had received CBT. The costs of providing therapy were recouped 'due to savings in visits to primary care, medication and other specialist mental health treatments'. All the three groups had the same outcomes at 12 months.

Technique and methods of cognitive-behavioural counselling

John McLeod offers a useful list of the approaches used by some cognitive-behavioural counsellors:

1 Establishing rapport and creating a working alliance between counsellor and client. Explaining the rationale for treatment.
2 Assessing the problem. Identifying and quantifying the frequency, intensity and appropriateness of problem behaviours and cognitions.
3 Setting goals or targets for change. These should be selected by the client, and be clear, specific and attainable.
4 Application of cognitive and behavioural techniques.
5 Monitoring progress, using ongoing assessment of target behaviours.
6 Termination and planned follow-up to reinforce generalisation of gains (McLeod, 1998).

He also suggests that the following techniques are commonly used:

- Challenging irrational beliefs.
- Reframing the issues: for example, perceiving internal emotional states as excitement rather than fear.
- Rehearsing the use for different self-statements in role plays with the counsellor.
- Experimenting with the use of different self-statements in real situations.
- Scaling feelings: for example, placing present feelings of anxiety or panic on a scale of 0–100.
- Thought stopping: rather than allowing anxious or obsessional thoughts to 'take over', the client learns to do something to interrupt them, such as snapping a rubber band on his or her wrist.
- Systematic desensitisation: the replacement of anxiety or fear responses by a learned relaxation response. The counsellor takes the client through a graded hierarchy of fear-eliciting situations.
- Assertiveness or social skills training.
- Homework assignments: practising new behaviours and cognitive strategies between therapy sessions.
- *In vivo* exposure: being accompanied by the counsellor into highly

fearful situations: for example, visiting shops with an agoraphobic client (McLeod, 1998).

The cognitive-behavioural approach in practice

The health professional who adopts the cognitive-behavioural approach to counselling will tend to:

1 rely less on personal warmth and more on confrontation in the counselling relationship;
2 use a logical and rational approach to problem-solving;
3 encourage the client to develop a realistic and pragmatic outlook on life.

Examples of practical applications of this approach in the health care field include:

1 helping the person who is depressed;
2 helping the person who has multiple problems;
3 encouraging rational thinking in someone who is highly emotional;
4 working with the person who has extreme anxiety by helping him or her to 'reframe' the emotion and to experience it as something else, such as excitement.

THE HUMANISTIC APPROACH

In the late 1940s and 1950s and perhaps reaching a peak in the 1960s, a movement began in psychology in the US that challenged the determinism of psychodynamic psychology and the mechanism of behavioural psychology (Shaffer, 1978). This was what came to be known as the 'third force' in psychology – humanistic psychology. Drawing heavily on the field of existential philosophy, humanistic psychology argued that people were essentially free and responsible for their own condition. They were neither 'driven' by an unconscious mind nor were they only a product of what they had learned. Essentially they were *agents*. The fact of consciousness gave them the ability to determine their own course of action through life, and they were the best arbiters of what was and what was not good for them. In humanistic psychology there could be no 'grand plan' of how people's minds work or how their behaviour could be manipulated. Humanistic psychology stressed individuality and individual differences in the human condition.

It was out of the humanistic school that the client-centred approach to counselling developed (Rogers, 1951). Rogers consistently argued that what made for effective counselling was trusting the individual's ability to find his own way through his problems. Rogers believed to this end that people were essentially life-asserting and 'good', by nature. In this respect, he drew from the philosopher Rousseau and, perhaps more directly from the US pragmatist and philosopher of science, John Dewey (1966, 1971). The aim of counselling for Rogers, then, was not necessarily to explore the person's past nor to necessarily try to modify his behaviour but to accept the person and to help him to progress through his difficulties by his own route. Counsellors, then, were not experts in other people's problems but individuals who accompanied other people on their search for personal meaning. The client-centred approach has been pervasive in the counselling world and has been adopted as a starting point for many training courses for counsellors, and used in a variety of contexts in the health professions in the UK, from psychiatric nurse training (ENB, 1982) to the training of marriage guidance counsellors (Marriage Guidance Council, 1983).

Arguably, it is out of the humanistic school of psychology that many of the 'alternative' counselling and therapy styles have arisen. A number of reasons for this development may be advanced. First, the humanistic school is an intensely *optimistic* one: it offers the individual the chance to take control of his or her life and does not posit the need to spend years of soul searching in order to do that. Secondly, historically, the humanistic school has developed alongside other changes in attitudes towards schooling and health care both in the US and the UK. It seems almost inevitable that the humanistic approach would gradually find more popular acceptance amongst the 'new age' forms of therapy. Thirdly (and this is by no means an exhaustive list), the methods used in the humanistic approach are relatively easy to learn and to put into practice. There is not a huge body of knowledge to absorb – as is the case with the psychodynamic approach, nor are there very particular skills to be learned – as is the case with the cognitive-behavioural approach. This latter point may also be one of criticism. Sometimes, the methods forwarded under the heading of humanistic psychology are so vague or so abstract that it would be very difficult to assess the degree to which they are or are not effective.

The humanistic approach to counselling is, essentially, an optimistic one. Humanistic psychology (as opposed to, for instance, psychodynamic psychology – and many religions) concentrates on the positive aspects of the human being. Whilst this is sometimes refreshing, it also has its own problems – especially when attempting to account for very disturbed behaviour and very serious mental illness – or even the 'problem of evil'. In noting the limitations of 'positive psychology', Lazarus has this to say:

> *However, it might be worthwhile to note that the danger posed by accentuating the positive is that if a conditional and properly nuanced position is not adopted, positive psychology could remain at a Pollyanna level. Positive psychology could come to be characterized by simplistic, inspirational and quasi-religious thinking and the message reduced to 'positive affect is good and*

negative affect is bad'. I hope that this ambitious and tantalizing effort truly advances what is known about human adaptation, as it should and that it will not be just another fad that quickly comes and goes.

(Lazarus, 2000)

The humanistic approach in practice

The health professional who adopts the humanistic approach to counselling will tend to:

1 avoid 'interpreting' the client's behaviour;
2 seek to encourage the client to identify his or her own solutions to his or her problems;
3 acknowledge that every individual is to some degree responsible for his or her own behaviour.

Examples of practical applications of this approach in the health care field include:

1 dealing with spiritual distress and problems of meaning;
2 helping with problems of self-image;
3 helping to free the client who believes that he or she is somehow controlled by circumstances.

THE TRANSACTIONAL-ANALYSIS APPROACH

Transaction analysis may be described as a neo-Freudian approach to therapy. Transactional analysis offers an economical way of describing and discussing people's relationships with one another. Formulated by the American psychotherapist Eric Berne (1964, 1972), the analysis suggests that we all relate to other people (and the world) from three distinct 'ego states'. These ego states are described as the Parent, the Adult and the Child. When we operate from the Parent (which is developed through the early absorption of parental and judgemental attitudes), we tend to talk down to others, feel superior to them or patronise them. On the other hand, when we operate from the Child (which is mainly developed through our experiences of being a child), we tend to adopt a subservient relationship *vis-à-vis* other people. Thus, we become dependent upon them or submit too readily to their demands and feel uncomfortable as a result. Berne argues that the most appropriate method of relating to others is through the Adult, which is to say that we meet others as mature, equal beings.

Beyond this first formulation, it is possible to map the ways in which people relate to one another from ego state to ego state. Thus a husband, for example, may relate to his wife from his Adult to her

Child. Now if she is satisfied with this relationship, all well and good. Problems start, however, when the wife tries to relate to her husband on an Adult–Adult basis! This represents what Berne calls a 'crossed transaction' and will tend to lead to problems in the relationship (see Figures 2.1 and 2.2). The aim of transactional analysis is to enable clients to identify the sorts of relationship 'games' that they play with one another via these ego states and to learn more readily on an Adult–Adult basis.

The transactional-analysis approach in practice

The health professional who adopts the transactional-analysis approach to counselling will tend to:

1   notice the interpersonal 'games' that people play;
2   encourage the client to remain Adult in his or her relationships;
3   encourage the client to try new strategies in his or her relationships.

Examples of practical applications of this approach in the health care field include:

1   marital and relationship difficulties;
2   encouraging the client to become more assertive;
3   identifying more adult ways of dealing with problems.

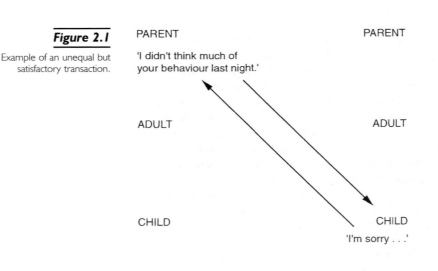

Figure 2.1

Example of an unequal but satisfactory transaction.

PARENT   PARENT

'I didn't think much of
your behaviour last night.'

ADULT   ADULT

CHILD   CHILD
                                          'I'm sorry . . .'

Husband   Wife

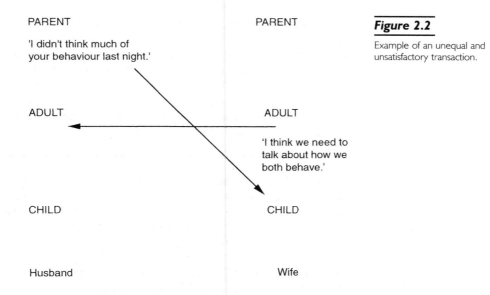

PARENT   PARENT

'I didn't think much of
your behaviour last night.'

ADULT   ADULT

'I think we need to
talk about how we
both behave.'

CHILD   CHILD

Husband   Wife

Figure 2.2

Example of an unequal and
unsatisfactory transaction.

THE PERSONAL-CONSTRUCT APPROACH

The personal-construct approach was developed by George Kelly
(1955). Kelly used the metaphor of the scientist to describe how the
person progresses through life. Thus, what we do is to predict how
things will be in the near future (we develop a hypothesis). Then we test
out that hypothesis in terms of what actually happens. As a result of
what happens, we either consider our hypothesis confirmed or we
discard it in favour of a revised hypothesis. Thus, according to Kelly,
life is a series of personal predictions and confirmations or reconstruc-
tions. Our view of the world and of ourselves changes according to
what happens to us and what sense we make of what happens to us.

Secondly, argues Kelly, we tend to view the world through a series of
'constructs' or 'ways of viewing' that colour our vision of how the
world is. These constructs may be likened to a series of pairs of goggles
that we put on at various times in order to make sense of what we
perceive. An important point, here, is that the 'goggles' that people wear
are not inaccurate or accurate or right or wrong: they merely represent
different aspects of the world that stand out or are important for us.

Kelly devised an interesting way of exploring people's personal
constructs, and the following activity demonstrates how such constructs
or ways of seeing can be elicited. Try the exercise now.

Activity————————————————————

An exercise to explore personal constructs

Think of three people that you know. Choose people from different aspects
of your life. You may, for example, choose (a) someone you live with,

(b) someone you know at work and (c) a close friend, though any three people will be fine. Now consider a way in which two of those people are similar and different from the third. This quality, behaviour or characteristic is what Kelly would call a *construct*. Now consider what you take to be the opposite of that quality, behaviour or characteristic. There are no right or wrong answers, but Kelly considers that this opposite characteristic represents another aspect of a person's construct system. Now consider to what degree you tend to view other people in terms of those two qualities, behaviours or characteristics.

You may like to try the activity again with a different trio of people and see what constructs you elicit in this case. If the process is repeated a number of times, you will tend to see a pattern of responses emerging. For Kelly, these represent something of your particular and idiosyncratic way of viewing the world.

It is important to say that no one can interpret anything from your responses but they may give you some clarification as to what stands out about other people in your life experience.

For Kelly, then, the process of counselling can concern itself with exploring the ways in which the client construes the world around him. Gradually through such exploration, the person can come to modify or change his construct system in order to make his life more liveable.

Personal-construct psychology views the person as an evolving, dynamic subject who is continuously modifying his view of the world in the light of what happens to him. Thus, as we have seen, that person may be likened to a scientist and the person's constructs as the set of criteria, rules or methods of interpretation through which that person modifies or changes his picture of the world. Epting (1984) and Stewart and Stewart (1981) offer practical methods of using the personal-construct approach in counselling.

The personal-construct approach in practice

The health professional who adopts the personal-construct approach to counselling will tend to:

1 acknowledge that people differ from one another in fundamental ways;
2 look for the client's belief and value system as a clue to problem-solving;
3 avoid interpreting the client's problem.

Examples of practical applications of this approach in the health care field include:

1 helping the client to enhance self-awareness;
2 coping with marital and relationship difficulties;
3 'unpacking' complex and multifaceted problems.

THE GESTALT-THERAPY APPROACH

The gestalt approach (it is usually spelt with a lower-case 'g', perhaps to distinguish it from Gestalt Psychology – a different thing altogether!) was devised by Fritz Perls (1969) who drew from a number of influences, including psychoanalysis, phenomenology, existentialism and Eastern philosophy (Smith, 1976). The German word *gestalt* is not easily translatable but roughly corresponds to the notion of wholeness or completeness. The gestalt approach emphasises the interplay between psychological or mental state and the state of the body, thus pointing up the totality of personal experience. It also concentrates on the changing and fluctuating nature of mental and physical states and concentrates most particularly on what is happening to the person now. It argues, reasonably, that the past is past and the future unknowable, therefore the focus of counselling attention should be the present moment. Thus, the gestalt approach encourages clients to become aware of what they are thinking, feeling and sensing, physically, in the here and now, and how they restrict or limit themselves by making continuous reference to the past or how things may be in the future. Further, it uses a particular set of sometimes startling interventions to enable clients to explore various aspects of what is happening to them. As with the personal-construct and humanistic approaches, the emphasis is on the client interpreting or making sense of what is happening to him or her: it is not the counsellor's place to do that. The following dialogue may give something of the unique flavour of the gestalt approach:

Counsellor: What are you feeling at the moment?

Client: Nervous, odd.

Counsellor: Where in terms of your body do you feel that nervousness, oddness?

Client: (rubs his stomach)

Counsellor: Can you increase those feelings?

Client: Yes, but what a strange thing to ask! Yes, they're spreading up into my chest.

Counsellor: And what are you feeling now?

Client: It's changing ... I'm feeling angry now!

Counsellor: Who are you angry with?

Client: Me! I realise that I've been bottling up my feelings for months!

Counsellor: OK ... Just imagine that your bottled-up feelings are sitting in that chair over there ... what do you want to say to them?

Client: Go away! You stop me getting on with what I want to do!

Counsellor: And what do the feelings say back to you?

Client: I keep you in check! I stop you from getting too involved with people!

Counsellor: And what do you make of all that?

Client: How odd! I realise how much I restrict myself by holding on to everything – it's becoming convenient! I feel different again, now ... something else is happening.

And so the dialogue continues. The counsellor's aim is to stay with the client's moment-to-moment phenomenology or perception of himself and to help him to explore it. As we have noted, the counsellor does not interpret what the client says nor offers suggestions as to how he may 'put his life right'. These are important principles in this person-centred and present-centred approach. Perls *et al.* (1951) offer a manual that, besides outlining the principles and theory of the gestalt approach, suggests a wide range of do-it-yourself gestalt exercises to increase self-awareness and clarify perception. A number of colleges and extra-mural departments of universities both in the UK and the US offer short and extended courses in the gestalt approach.

The gestalt-therapy approach in practice

The health professional who adopts the gestalt-therapy approach to counselling will tend to:

1 treat each counselling situation as unique;
2 deal with issues as they arise and in the here and now;
3 notice small, non-verbal behaviours exhibited by the client.

Examples of practical applications of this approach in the health care field include:

1 helping the client who bottles up emotion;
2 helping the person who has difficulty in verbalising his or her problems;
3 coping with problems of self-image and self-confidence.

WHICH IS THE *MAIN* APPROACH USED TODAY?

The answer to this does, of course, depend on where you are standing and on your particular point of view. In general terms, though, there is a tendency towards counsellors being able to *demonstrate* that what they do is effective. In the 'purchaser–provider' climate of the new health care service in the UK, this demand for evidence-based practice is likely to become more acute. To this end, there is evidence that, currently, the cognitive-behavioural approach to counselling is becoming more popular – perhaps at the expense of the psychodynamic approach. The humanistic approach remains popular given the fact that its methods are relatively easy to teach and learn and, perhaps, because, historically, they have been used for so long. It seems, to this writer – writing in the early part of the 21st century – that the emphasis will continue to be on establishing forms of counselling that are economical, able to be practised over a relatively short space of time and which can be *demonstrated* to be effective. At the time of writing, the counselling approach that seems most likely to meet these criteria is the cognitive-behavioural approach or a variant of it.

THE ECLECTIC APPROACH

In the end, what we do in counselling depends upon a number of issues: our skill levels, what we feel comfortable with doing in the counselling relationship, our belief and value systems as they relate to how we view what people are 'about', our level of self-awareness, our mood at the time, our present life situation, our perception of what (if anything) is wrong with the client, current work load and time available and many other factors. Thus, it is reasonable to argue that no one set of counselling tools or no one particular approach can be appropriate in every counselling situation. What is perhaps more useful is that the health professional considers a wide range of possibilities, tries out some of the approaches (first, perhaps, with a willing colleague and in return, having that colleague try them out on the health professional!) and slowly incorporates the approaches that most suit that person, into a personal repertoire. This personal repertoire or personal style offers the most flexible approach to counselling – the eclectic approach. Further, it is in line with Heron's argument in Chapter 1 (p.31) that the counsellor becomes skilled in a wide range of possible counselling interventions in order to help a wide range of people. After all, health professionals meet a wide range of clients varying considerably in their cultural backgrounds, their personal experience, belief systems, needs, wants and wishes, political persuasions and personal psychologies. It is important that we offer clients what they want and not necessarily what we perceive that they want. The counselling relationship belongs to the client and not to the counsellor: we should not be dazzling them with a range of counselling interventions but finding out what they really want. In a sense, this is almost overwhelmingly simple for, as Epting notes, echoing the social psychologists, Allport, Kelly and others, 'If you want to know something about someone why not ask them: they might just tell you!' (Epting, 1984).

In keeping with this idea of an eclectic approach, Egan (2002) offers the following suggestions for content in a training programme for helpers. He suggests that in addition to a working model of helping, a fuller curriculum for training professional helpers might include the following:

- A working knowledge of applied developmental psychology – how people develop or create their lives across the life span and the impact of environmental factors such as culture and socioeconomic status on development.
- An understanding of the principles of cognitive psychology as applied to helping, because the ways people think and construct their worlds has a great deal to do with both getting into and out of trouble.

- An understanding of the dynamics of the helping professions themselves as they are currently practised in our society together with the challenges they face.
- An understanding of clients as psychosomatic beings and the interaction between physical and psychological states.
- The ability to apply the principles of human behaviour – what we know about incentives, rewards and punishment – to the helping process, because wrestling with problem situations and undeveloped opportunities always involves incentives and rewards.
- Abnormal psychology – a systematic understanding of the ways in which individuals get into psychological trouble.
- An understanding of the diversity of age, race, ethnicity, religion, sexual orientation, culture, social standing, economic standing and the like among clients.
- An understanding of the ways in which people act when they are in social settings.
- An understanding of the needs and problems of special populations with which one works, such as the physically challenged, substance abusers, the homeless.
- Applied personality theory because this area of psychology helps us understand in very practical ways what makes people 'tick' and many of the ways in which individuals differ from each other (Egan, 2002).

The eclectic approach in practice

The health professional who adopts the eclectic approach to counselling will tend to:

1 believe that no one approach to counselling suits each situation;
2 read widely and learn a variety of different sorts of counselling skills;
3 run the risk of being 'jack of all counselling skills and master of none'!

Examples of practical applications of this approach in the health care field include:

1 everyday counselling practice;
2 working with the client who does not respond to a particular counselling approach;
3 helping the person who has very varied problems in living.

IS IT POSSIBLE TO DO WITHOUT A THEORY OF THE PERSON?

In this chapter, we have reviewed various ways of thinking about how people 'work'. Is it possible, then, to do counselling *without* any particular theory of the person? In the strict sense, probably not. The very fact that we choose to say, 'I do not have any particular theories about human beings' is a theoretical stance in itself. However, I believe that it is possible to manage with *minimal* theory. If we think about it for a moment, we will, perhaps, appreciate that all of the aforementioned theories are, to a greater or lesser extent, empirically untested. It would be difficult, in the end, to decide, once and for all, that one theory approaches 'the truth' more nearly than another – although, arguably, some theories are more open to testing than others.

We can, however, take the view that, as people vary widely and as it is impossible to understand, completely, other people's minds, then we can use theory *parsimoniously* and use as little theory as possible in order to work as counsellors. To this end, I would like to suggest the following principles as ones for reflection and discussion:

- It may be best not to make any particular assumptions about *why* the person in front of us does the things that he or she does.
- It may be best to *believe* what other people say to us – at least until they contradict themselves or indicate otherwise.
- The person in front of us may be similar to us or very different from us and we should, perhaps, not make any assumptions about those similarities or differences.
- It is possible that people do things *for no particular reason at all*. This, too, is important in counselling.
- It seems probable that some people find talking about their problems useful and that some people do not.
- It may or may not be true that past experiences influence the way we are today. It is also possible that some people are more affected by their past than others. It is not proven as to the *importance* of recalling the past and linking it to present-day events and actions.
- Given that memories are often faulty, it may be better to be *future focused* rather than focused on trying to work out *why* any given person is the way that he or she is. After all, we live our lives *forward*.

Herein lies the paradox: these statements could be construed as the beginning of a theory! My point, though, is that we need, perhaps, to theorise about other people as *little* as possible, to listen to them, to focus on the future and to worry less about the 'why' than the 'what comes next'. It is, if you like, a pragmatic approach to counselling.

PSYCHOLOGICAL APPROACHES TO COUNSELLING AND THE HEALTH PROFESSIONAL

As we have noted, no one school of psychology or theoretical approach to counselling offers *the* way of viewing the person. The approaches offer different ways of looking at the person and those ways of looking are not necessarily mutually exclusive. Which of the approaches the health professional chooses to use as a guide to understanding the process of counselling will depend on a number of factors, including, at least, her original psychological training that accompanied her basic professional training, the influences of any workshops, study days or further training, exposure to colleagues and friends who offer different points of view, further reading around the topic and so forth.

Another deciding factor may be the type of relationship that the health professional has with her client and the amount of time they spend together. The social worker, the speech therapist and the psychiatric nurse may all spend considerable time building up a relationship that, itself, may last for months or even years. On the other hand, the physiotherapist and the occupational therapist may have a shorter if quite intense relationship. It may be that the shorter relationships require a pragmatic psychology that allows for goals to be set and to be achieved: in this sense, the behavioural approach offers usable concepts that can help to structure the relationship. Or, if a longer-term relationship is being developed, a 'process' model may be more applicable and the health-professional-as-counsellor may wish to consider those models that emphasise the quality of the relationship and an analysis of what is going on in that relationship. Here, the psychodynamic and humanistic approaches may help. In the end, too, what will determine what any health professional adopts as a psychological model for understanding the counselling relationship will depend on her own beliefs about the nature of people. In order to clarify what our beliefs are, we need to develop a degree of self-awareness – the topic of the following chapter.

We have noted, also, in this chapter, that the health care climate is changing – at least in the UK – towards the need for *evidence-based practice* and for the need for counsellors and those who use counselling skills to *demonstrate* that what they do is effective.

COUNSELLING AND SELF-AWARENESS

3

The idea of having a 'self' – some sort of stable, inner core, appeals to those who live in Western countries. As we shall see elsewhere in this book, the notion is culture-bound. Although everyone, supposedly, is aware that he or she functions autonomously, other cultures do not pay such attention to the idea of 'self' as do people in the West.

Generally, it would seem reasonable to say that if we are to help others, we should know something, first, of ourselves. Self-awareness is an essential component in the counselling process. It is necessary for a number of reasons. These will be discussed first before the questions of self-awareness itself are addressed.

Firstly, self-awareness allows us to discriminate between our own problems and those of the client. If we do not have at least a minimal self-awareness, it is easy for us to identify with the other person's problems and to imagine that they are similar to, or even the same as, our own. The reverse of this situation is also possible. Without self-awareness it is possible to imagine that everyone else (and particularly this client) has the same problems as we do. In this way, our own problems are projected onto the client. We need to be able to identify clear 'ego boundaries': to make a clear distinction between ourselves and our client. As a matter of fact, what the client is describing at any particular time is never the same as a situation we have found ourselves in. It may be similar to it, but it can never be the same. Self-awareness can enable us to mark out our ego boundaries and successfully discriminate between what belongs to us and what belongs to the client. Haydn describes the problem well when he writes:

> *Day by day, hour by hour, we misunderstand each other because we cross well-marked boundaries; we blur the sense of you out there and me here; we merge, frequently very sloppily, the subjective with the objective, in various ways. We make of the other person simply an extension of self, either through the attribution of our own thoughts and attitudes to the other person, or by too facile a decision about his nature, after which we go on responding to him as though he were the character we invented.*

(Haydn, 1965)

Such demarcation is also an essential part of the counsellor's taking care of herself. When ego boundaries become blurred, considerable emotion is invested in the relationship by the counsellor and the net result can be *burnout* – emotional and physical exhaustion as a result of work-related stress. Burnout manifests itself in the following sorts of ways:

- disillusionment with the job;
- a feeling of hopelessness and inability to cope;

- a need to get away from people;
- a loss of ability to empathise with others.

Burnout can be prevented through reflection on our performance and through developing self-awareness as discussed later.

Secondly, self-awareness enables us to make what Heron (1977b) calls 'conscious use of the self'. Without awareness we will tend to feel that any counselling interventions we make are spontaneous and not offered consciously. Now, the point of conscious use of the self is that we learn to reflect on what is happening during the counselling relationship and we choose the interventions we make. In other words, the words and phrases that we use are intended and chosen consciously, rather than their just happening. Initially, such conscious use of the self can seem awkward and clumsy. We tend to be socialised into dividing human action up into natural (and, therefore, presumably sincere) and contrived (and, therefore, presumably, insincere). The suggestion that we choose particular types of words or expressions smacks of unnaturalness and therefore tends to sound disagreeable.

On reflection, however, it may be noted that all other human skills, apart from listening and talking to others, are learned through the process of consciously considering what we are doing. If we are to become skilled as nurses, doctors or social workers, we must concentrate on what we do and observe the outcomes of our actions. The verbal skills of counselling can also be learned in a similar way, and the concept of 'conscious use of self' has a variety of applications.

As we have already noted, in the first place, such use of the self can enable us to choose the right sort of counselling intervention for the right occasion. It can bring clarity and precision to the counselling relationship. If, for example, we use the category analysis identified in Chapter 1, we can choose to vary our repertoire of verbal interventions in a way that helps this particular person at this particular time. In this sense, then, the conscious use of the self enhances sensitivity to the other person's needs.

Next, conscious use of the self can help us to distinguish between the client's problems and our own. In this way it serves to maintain and clarify the ego boundaries alluded to at the beginning of this chapter. In the process of developing conscious use of the self, we learn to notice ourselves and to pay attention to how we are reacting to the unfolding, counselling session. Such self-noticing can enable us, again, to make more sensitive use of our counselling interventions, to be more tactful and truly meet the arising needs of the client. This process also has other connotations, for as Rollo May (1983) notes, what the counsellor is feeling is often a direct reflection of what the client is feeling, once the counselling relationship deepens and becomes more intense. Thus, attention by the counsellor to her own changing feelings can help in the process of understanding and empathising with the client.

The process of developing conscious use of self can be an uncomfortable one. Three stages in its development may be noted and these are described as follows:

First stage

In this stage, the person is unaware of the range of possible skills and interventions that is available to her. This is the stage of being natural or spontaneous. There is a tendency, in this stage, for the person to believe that people are 'born counsellors' and that the skills of counselling either come naturally to the individual or they cannot be developed at all. This may be called the unskilled stage.

Second stage

In the second stage of the process, the person becomes aware of the possible range of interventions available to her and feels clumsy as a result. It may be compared to the process of learning to drive a car. In the first place, we do not know how to drive the car at all. As we learn to drive, we have to pay attention to a wide range of different actions, and the net result is that we are awkward and clumsy. So it is with the process of learning counselling through conscious use of the self. This may be called the clumsy stage.

Third stage

In the final stage of learning, the skills and interventions involved in counselling are absorbed by the person and she becomes skilled in counselling. Conscious use of the self has become a normal part of her repertoire of behaviour and no longer feels awkward or clumsy. Interestingly, too, the naturalness returns. The skills having been learned, emerge without forethought: the counsellor no longer has to consider what to say or what not to say but readily responds in the counselling situation out of the wide range of skills that have become her own. What remains conscious, however, is the ability to notice what is happening as the relationship unfolds. What has changed is the ability to act in an appropriate and sensitive manner whilst being guided by the observations made during this process of noticing. This may be called the skilled stage of counselling development.

NOTICING IN THE DEVELOPMENT OF COUNSELLING SKILLS

It will be noted that frequent reference will be made to the notion of *noticing*, of paying close attention to what is happening both in the counselling relationship and in the counsellor herself. This notion is a key one in the whole of the process of learning to become, and learning to remain, a skilful and effective counsellor. It is also a central concept in the idea of self-awareness and one that will be referred to again in this context. Clearly, unless we notice what is happening to us, we cannot become self-aware. In exploring the notion of self-awareness as it applies to counselling, it will be useful, first, to consider the concept of the self.

The action of noticing can be readily used in any health care setting. It is useful and instructive merely to notice our reactions to certain situations that occur. For instance, what do we notice about our own reactions to any of the following:

- attempted suicide;
- severe incontinence in a young adult;
- severe and disfiguring handicap;
- the psychiatric patient admitted to a general ward.

We may want to argue that, as professionals, we do not react to such human problems but we take action to help them. If this sort of argument is offered, it is worth listening a little closer to what is going on inside! It is easy for us to delude ourselves that we do not react to extreme aspects of human suffering as do other non-professionals. Again, it is salutary to question this stance and vital to do so if we are to become effective counsellors. We can never afford to become 'case-hardened' as carers or as counsellors.

THE SELF

The idea of what it means to have a self has been discussed down through the ages by philosophers, theologians, psychologists, sociologists, psychiatrists and political theorists. Psychologists have approached the concept from a variety of points of view. Some have tried to analyse out the factors that go to make up the self rather as a chemist might try to discover the chemicals that are present in a particular solution. Others have argued that there are certain consistent aspects of the self that determine, to some extent, the way in which we live our lives. Psychoanalytical theory, as we have seen, argues that early childhood experiences profoundly affect and shape the self, determining how, as adults, we react to the world. Childhood experiences, in this theoretical construction, lay the foundations of the self that may be modified by life experience but, nevertheless, stay with us throughout life. Such a view, as we noted on p.39, is deterministic in that it argues that our present sense of self is determined by earlier life experiences and we are shaped, to a greater or lesser extent, by our childhoods.

Other psychological theorists argue that there are problems with reductionist theories – theories that attempt to analyse the self into discrete parts. Such theorists prefer to view the self from a holistic or gestalt perspective. This approach argues that the whole or totality of the self is always something more than the sum of the parts that go to make it up. Just as we cannot discover exactly what we like about a piece of music by examining it note by note, neither can we fully understand the self by compartmentalising it. In this sense, then, the self can never completely be defined, for the subject of our study – the self – is always evolving and is always more than the sum of the parts.

It is worth noting, too, that we do not exist as selves-in-isolation. What we are and who we are depends, to a very considerable extent, on the other people with whom we live, work and relate. Our sense of self also depends upon how those other people define us, too. In this sense, other people are frequently telling us who we are. As health professionals, we rely on other colleagues, on clients and on friends offering us both positive and negative feedback on our performance as people. Such feedback is slowly absorbed by the individual, modifying and (hopefully) enhancing the sense of self.

A note of caution is important. The idea of the self is an *abstraction*. It is a way of talking about inner aspects of the person. To this end, it cannot be said to 'exist' in the way that a table or a book exists. We should, therefore, be careful of at least two things. The first is the temptation to *reify* the self. Reification is the mistake of treating an abstraction as though it does have concrete reality and therefore making more dogmatic claims about it than are reasonable to make. The second is to have an awareness of the fact that when we talk about abstractions we are basing our discourse on *belief* rather than on *fact*. You cannot, in the end, *demonstrate* aspects of the self. The following debate, then, is necessarily a tentative one and one that you may or may not agree with. What is probably more important, as a person using counselling skills, is for you to consider what *your* beliefs are about the nature of the self.

It may be useful, then, to consider the range of aspects that may go to make up a sense of self. As with any such analysis of self, it cannot hope to be exhaustive of all aspects of the self but it may serve to highlight the complex and multifaceted nature of the subject. Five aspects of self are considered here:

- the physical self;
- the private self;
- the social self;
- the spiritual self;
- the self-as-defined-by-others.

Clearly, this is not an exhaustive account of ways of looking at the self. The self remains an abstraction, a way of talking. It seems to me that it would be impossible to capture all of the facets connoted by the term 'self'. The account that follows is something of a 'shorthand' way of considering aspects of the self as they apply to the field of counselling.

The physical self

The physical self refers to the bodily or 'felt' sense of self. We are all (like it or not!) contained within a body and our perception of what we and other people think we look like contributes to how we see ourselves as a person. Further, there is an intimate link between how we feel psychologically and how we feel physically. To argue otherwise is to invoke the famous Cartesian split – the notion (propounded by the French philosopher Descartes) that the body and the mind could be considered separately. The acknowledgement that the mind and body are so closely linked (and, arguably, the body 'produces' the mind) has considerable implications for counselling as we shall see in a later chapter. Suffice to say, here, that in noticing our 'body self' we may learn much about how we perceive ourselves generally. Noticing changing bodily sensations can be one route towards developing self-awareness.

The private self

The private self alludes to that part of us that we live inside – the hidden part of us that we reveal slowly – if at all – to other people. R. D. Laing has written a considerable amount on this concept (Laing, 1959) and suggested that it is quite possible for the 'private' self to watch the 'public' self in action! Certainly from the point of view of developing self-awareness, it is useful to become aware of this inner, private self and to notice to what degree and with whom that private sense of self is shared. Again, from the counselling point of view, such a notion of private self has considerable relevance, for it is that private self that is often shared in the counselling relationship.

It is sometimes worth thinking about the degree to which there is a *gap* between private and public aspects of self. When you are particularly upset, disturbed or preoccupied, it may become 'safer' to present quite a different 'public' self from the self that is churning away beneath the surface. The question remains, however, to what degree a person with a completely 'hidden' sense of self can make an effective counsellor. After all, in counselling, the counsellor is inviting the client to share something of his or her private self with the counsellor. If, for her part, the counsellor is unable to share something of *her* private self, then the relationship becomes particularly unbalanced. Another view, of course, is that the counselling relationship is *always* unbalanced, for it is always the client who is expected to disclose aspects of him- or herself and no such expectation is necessarily levelled at the counsellor.

The social self

The social self is that aspect of the person that is shared openly with others. It may be contrasted with the private self. It is the self that we choose to show to other people. The degree to which there is congruence between our private self and our social self may indicate our level of emotional and interpersonal security. Both Rogers (1951) and Laing (1959) have argued that when there is a close correspondence between the inner experience of self and the outer presentation of it, emotional security and stability *tend* to be present also. It is interesting and salutary to reflect on the degree to which this is true for us at the moment of reading this! As we have just noted, a great discrepancy between the one and the other may indicate personal problems of a magnitude that make functioning as a counsellor difficult.

The spiritual self

The spiritual self refers to the aspect that is concerned with a search for personal meaning. As we noted in the first chapter, personal meaning may be framed within a variety of contexts: religious, philosophical, political, sociological, psychological and so forth. It is the spiritual aspect of the self that makes sense of what is happening to the person. It is that aspect of self concerned with belief and value systems. It may also be that part of the self that is concerned with the *transpersonal* aspects of being – that which unites all persons. Rogers (1967) has alluded to such a dimension when he concludes that what is most personal in the counselling relationship is, almost paradoxically, most universal.

Developing this notion of the transpersonal further, Jung (1978) argued for the existence of a 'collective unconscious' – a domain that contains all human experience, both past and present, to which we all have access. Supporting arguments for the existence of this collective unconscious include the fact of what Jung called synchronicity or meaningful coincidence. We may, for example, be thinking of someone and she phones us or we are about to say something and the person we are with says exactly the same thing. These are examples of synchronous events. The appearance of symbols in dreams is also offered as evidence for the collective unconscious: Jung maintained that certain types of symbols (crosses and circles, for example) occur through the ages in all parts of the world and in many contexts and cultures. Further, these symbols often appear in our dreams, and Jung argues that such appearances were made possible through our tapping the collective unconscious. Jung did not offer the concept dogmatically but suggested that it may be a useful one in order to try to make sense of those aspects of self that seem to be shared by all persons.

The self-as-defined-by-others

The self-as-defined-by-others refers to the way in which others see us. This is a particularly complicated issue in that how others see us will depend upon so many variables. Their perception of us will be coloured by at least the following factors – their relationship to us, their previous experiences of people who are like us and different from us, how they think we view them, their views on sexuality, race and roles, their own view of themselves. The matter is further complicated by the fact that other people's perception of us is, presumably, not static. It changes according to the aforementioned variables and in accordance with our relationship with them. This issue of the self-as-defined-by-others is of particular importance in counselling. The client's view of the counsellor at any given time in the relationship may serve as a useful barometer for measuring the nature and depth of the relationship. At times, the view of the counsellor will be unequivocally positive; at others it will be far less so. All of these changes reflect, to a greater or lesser degree, the amount of dependence and independence that the client is maintaining at that particular time. This changing concept of the counsellor in the eyes of the client has been called *transference* and is explored further in Chapter 11.

These, then, are some of the many facets that go to make up a sense of self. Another way of making sense of the concept of self is to view it in terms of different types of knowledge.

The self defined through types of knowledge

Three types of knowledge that go to make up an individual may be described: propositional knowledge, practical knowledge and experiential knowledge (Heron, 1981). Whilst each of these types is different, each is interrelated with the other. Thus, whilst propositional knowledge may be considered as qualitatively different from, say, practical knowledge, it is possible, and probably better, to use propositional knowledge in the application of practical knowledge.

Propositional knowledge

Propositional knowledge is knowledge that is contained in theories or models. It may be described as textbook knowledge and is synonymous with Ryle's (1949) concept of 'knowing that', which was developed further in an educational context by Pring (1976). Thus, a person may build up a considerable bank of facts, theories or ideas about a subject, person or thing, without necessarily having any direct experience of that subject, person or thing. A person may, for example, develop a considerable propositional knowledge about, say, midwifery, without ever necessarily having been anywhere near a woman who is having a baby! Presumably, it would be more useful to combine that knowledge with some practical experience, but this does not necessarily have to be the case. This, then, is the domain of propositional knowledge. Obviously it is possible to have propositional knowledge about a great number of subject areas ranging from mathematics to literature or from counselling to social work. Any information contained in books (including this one!) must necessarily be of the propositional sort.

Practical knowledge

Practical knowledge is knowledge that is developed through the acquisition of skills. Thus, driving a car or giving an injection demonstrates practical knowledge, though equally, so does the use of counselling skills that involve the use of specific verbal and non-verbal behaviours and intentional use of counselling interventions as described in later chapters. Practical knowledge is synonymous with Ryle's (1949) concept of 'knowing how', which was developed further in an educational context by Pring (1976). Usually more than a mere knack, practical knowledge is the substance of a smooth performance of a practical or interpersonal skill. A considerable amount of a health professional's time is taken up with the demonstration of practical knowledge – often, but not always, of the interpersonal sort.

Traditionally, most educational programmes in schools and colleges have concerned themselves primarily with both propositional and practical knowledge, particularly the former. Thus the propositional knowledge aspect of a person is the aspect that is often held in highest regard. Practical knowledge, although respected, is usually seen as slightly less important than the propositional sort. In this way, the self can become highly developed in one sense – the propositional knowledge aspect – at the expense of being skilled in a practical sense.

Experiential knowledge

The domain of experiential knowledge is knowledge gained through direct encounter with a subject, person or thing. It is the subjective and affective nature of that encounter that contributes to this sort of knowledge. Experiential knowledge is knowledge through relationship. Such knowledge is synonymous with Rogers' (1983) description of experiential learning and with Polanyi's concept of 'personal' knowledge and 'tacit' knowledge (Polanyi, 1958). If we reflect for a moment, we may discover that most of the things that are really important to us belong in this domain. If, for example, we consider our personal relationships with other people, we discover that what we like or love about them cannot be reduced to a series of propositional statements, and yet the feelings we have for them are vital and part of what is most important in our lives. Most encounters with others contain the possible seeds of experiential knowledge. It is only when we are so detached from other people that we treat them as objects that no experiential learning can occur.

Not that all experiential learning is tied exclusively to relationships with other people. For example, I had considerable propositional knowledge about the US before I went there. When I went there, all that propositional knowledge was changed considerably. What I had known was changed by my direct experience of the country. I had developed experiential knowledge of the place. Experiential knowledge is not of the same type or order as propositional or practical knowledge. It is, nevertheless, important knowledge, in that it affects everything else we think about or do.

Experiential knowledge is necessarily personal and idiosyncratic. Indeed, as Rogers (1985) points out, it may be difficult to convey to another person in words. Words tend to be loaded with personal (often experiential) meanings and thus to understand each other we need to understand the nature of the way in which the people with whom we converse use words. It is arguable, however, that such experiential knowledge is sometimes conveyed to others through gesture, eye contact, tone of voice, inflection and all the other non-verbal and paralinguistic aspects of communication (Argyle, 1975). Indeed, it may be experiential knowledge that is passed on when two people (for example, a counsellor and her client) become very involved with each other in a conversation, a learning encounter or counselling. Counselling, then, may be concerned very much with the discussion of experiential knowledge: certainly it is more about this domain than it is about the domains of propositional or practical knowledge.

These three domains of knowledge are important aspects of a sense of self. What we know in these three domains is what we are. Thus, a balanced sense of self within this framework is achieved by a balance between our theoretical knowledge, what we can do with it in terms of practical and interpersonal skill and what we have in terms of personal experience. All three domains grow and increase throughout the life cycle, though they are not always equally recognised. As we have seen, propositional knowledge tends to take precedence over the other two and, in academic terms, experiential knowledge often counts for very little.

From the points of view of counselling and of self-awareness, it may be useful to keep all three aspects in balance. The skilled counsellor, then, is one who combines theoretical knowledge about counselling with well-developed interpersonal competence and considerable life experience.

THE CONCEPT OF PERSONHOOD

Yet another way of considering the self is via the notion of *personhood*: what it means to be a person. If we can identify those basic criteria that distinguish persons from all other sorts of things, we may be clearer about what it means to talk of the self. Bannister and Fransella offer a list of criteria for personhood that may be helpful in clarifying such a notion.

It is argued you consider yourself a person in that:

- You entertain a notion of your own separateness from others; you rely on the privacy of your own consciousness.
- You entertain a notion of the integrality or completeness of your experience, so that you believe all parts of it are relatable because you are the experiencer.
- You entertain a notion of your own continuity over time; you possess your own biography and live in relation to it.
- You entertain a notion of the causality of your actions: you have purposes, you intend, you accept a partial responsibility for the effects of what you do.
- You entertain a notion of other persons by analogy with yourself; you assume a comparability of subjective experience (Bannister and Fransella, 1986).

Such a notion of personhood can do much to clarify what it means to entertain a notion of self and may also serve as a framework for understanding the personal factors that we are addressing in the process of counselling. For if we accept Bannister and Fransella's idea of personhood, then we necessarily accept that idea as applying to the person who is in front of us in the counselling relationship. The notion of personhood addresses the concepts of separateness from others, completeness of human experience, personal biography, at least partial responsibility for actions, and appreciation of other persons as being similar to ourselves. All of these concepts are addressed when one person sets out to counsel another.

AN INTEGRATED MODEL OF THE SELF

What is needed now is a model that brings together the notions of self so far described. Figure 3.1 offers a fairly comprehensive model of the self through which to understand the idea of self-awareness. It incorporates Jung's work on the four functions of the mind: thinking, feeling, sensing and intuiting (Jung, 1978) and also an adaptation of Laing's (1959) concept of an inner and outer self. The outer, public self is what others see of us and is compatible with the notion of the self-as-defined-by-others, described on p.36. The inner, private aspect is what goes on in our heads and bodies. In one sense, the outer experience is what other people are most familiar with. We communicate the inner experience through the outer. Our thoughts, feelings and experiences are all communicated through this outer experience of behaviour. Of what does it consist?

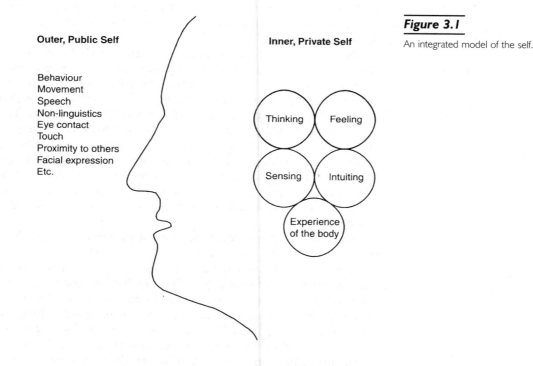

Outer, Public Self

Behaviour
Movement
Speech
Non-linguistics
Eye contact
Touch
Proximity to others
Facial expression
Etc.

Inner, Private Self

Thinking
Feeling
Sensing
Intuiting
Experience of the body

Figure 3.1

An integrated model of the self.

The outer experience of the self

At its most simple, behaviour consists of body movements, the crossing of arms and legs, walking, running and so forth. At a more subtle level, however, the issue becomes more complicated. There is a whole variety of more subtle behaviours that convey the inner sense of self through the outer. First, there is speech. What we say – the words, phrases, metaphors, expressions we use – is a potent means by which we convey feelings, thoughts and experiences to others. How we come to choose these particular words, phrases and expressions, however, depends upon a wide range of variables including our past experiences, education, cultural inheritance, knowledge of the language, attitudes, belief systems, social positions and the company we are in. Alongside those words and phrases is a wide range of non-linguistic aspects of speech, including timing, pitch, pacing, silences and so on. The use of such non-linguistic aspects of communication is a subtle way of communicating aspects of our inner selves to others.

When we talk to other people, we usually look at them. Heron (1970) notes that there can be a wide variation in the intensity, amount and quality of eye contact. Our emotional status and our relationship with the person with whom we are speaking tend to govern the amount of eye contact we allow ourselves to make with him or her and the amount we expect in return. In the context of counselling, it is important to remain sensitive to aspects of eye contact and to monitor consciously the amount we use in relation to the client. Such monitoring of eye contact is in line with the notion of conscious use of the self, described on p.58.

The amount of physical contact or touch that we have with others is also a potent means of conveying our inner experience to others. Typically, we touch more those people to whom we are close: members of the family, people we love and very close friends. Some people, it would seem, are 'high touchers' and others 'low touchers'. There are also cultural factors governing the use of touch between people of different races, between sexes and between people of different relative status. Again, in the context of counselling we need to be careful that our use of touch is unambiguous, acceptable to the client and never viewed by that person as an intrusion. If we are a high toucher, for example, we cannot assume that all of our clients are also high touchers!

When we relate to others, the fact of communicating verbally with them means that we necessarily are near them. How we sit or stand in relation to others is determined, again, by a number of factors, including the level of intimacy we have with them, our relationship with them, certain cultural factors, personal preferences for closeness or lack of it and whether or not we occupy a dominant or subordinate position *vis-à-vis* the other person (Brown, 1986). In the counselling relationship it is easy for the counsellor not to realise that she is occupying a dominant position in that relationship by the very nature of being the counsellor! As a result, the temptation is sometimes to sit closer to the client than is comfortable for him. An easy, practical solution to this is to allow the client to draw up the chair and thus to define the personal space between counsellor and client.

Another indicator of our inner experience is our facial expression. Raised eyebrows, grins and sneers can do much to convey to others our internal status. An important concept, here, is that of *congruence* in communication. Bandler and Grinder (1975) identify three aspects of congruence. A person is said to be congruent when:

1 what they say, matches
2 how they say it and
3 both are matched by the appropriate facial expression.

If one or more of these factors mismatch, then communication is likely to be unclear. Sometimes these mismatches are caused by internal conflicts or by our not saying what we really mean. In terms of counselling, it is important that we learn to be congruent in our dealings with others. We must be seen to mean what we say: just saying it is not sufficient! Such congruence needs careful attention and a considerable amount of self-awareness. It is surprising how easily ambiguous thoughts 'leak out' through our facial expressions! External congruence in terms of words, tone of voice and facial expression also calls for internal congruence in terms of our being clear about what we think and feel about what we are saying. It is rare that we can completely disguise our internal thoughts and feelings and anyway, if we are to be genuine in our counselling, it is important that we be clear, honest and unambiguous.

These, then, are aspects of the outer self – that part of ourselves that others see and through which we communicate our inner experience. Not that such outer, visible behaviour is read by others entirely accurately. When other people perceive us, they do so through their own particular frame of reference and tend to interpret what they see in terms of that frame. No one views another objectively. Everyone's perception of others is more or less coloured by his or her own history and experience. All the more reason, then, as counsellors to ensure that our external behaviour is as clear and as genuine as it can be. It *will* be misread by the client at times, but less so if our initial intentions are clear.

The inner experience of the self

The inner, private experience of the self may be divided into (a) aspects of mental function according to Jung's typography: thinking, feeling, sensing and intuiting and (b) the experience of the body. As we have already noted, this division will necessarily be artificial as both mental and physical events are inextricably linked. As Searle (1983) acknowledges, a mental event is also a physical one. Physical status also affects mental and psychological performance and a person's self-concept. It is interesting to note the growing interest in healing this apparent split between the mind and the body. Increasingly, the move is towards a holistic approach in health care that emphasises the interrelatedness between mind, body and (sometimes) spirit. Any concept of self must take into account the mind and body as a totality.

Thinking

Thinking refers to all the aspects of our mental processes, both logical and illogical. If we reflect on thinking we will realise that it is not a linear process. We do not think in sentences or even in logical sequences of phrases. The whole process is much more haphazard than that and has much in common with the technique known as *free association*, used in psychoanalysis. Free association asks of the client that he repeats whatever comes into his mind. The result is usually a string of not obviously related statements, ideas and expressions of feelings. Such, perhaps, is the nature of thinking.

Nor can we be sure that our thinking is accurate or realistic. As we noted in the last chapter, Kelly (1955) argued that we are continually creating hypotheses about how the world is and then testing those hypotheses in the light of our experience. In this sense, then, thinking may be concerned with the creation of a number of theories about the world. Guy Claxton suggests an important pair of principles on this issue. He argues that:

1 What I do depends on what my theory tells me about the world, not on how the world really is ... and
2 What happens next depends on how the world really is, not how I believe it to be (Claxton, 1984).

Thus, if our theory about the world is very distorted, there will be a sense of jarring as we progress though it. If our theory about the world is grounded in some sort of reality, then our perception of the world and our place in it will be that much more congruent. This, again, has implications for counselling. The thing that causes many people discomfort in their lives is, arguably, that they hold in their heads a particular view or set of beliefs about the world that does not match reality. This, in turn, may lead to the sort of thinking that is prefaced by expressions such as, 'If only ...', 'Things would be much easier if ...', 'I know there's no point in thinking like this, but ...'. All such thoughts tend to lead to a distorted picture of what is actually happening in a person's life. Part of the process of counselling may be to enable people to identify these false perceptions and to clarify them. This is not to argue that there is one sure way of looking at the world, but to note that people need to be happy for themselves that what goes on in their heads bears a reasonable resemblance to how things actually are in the world.

So, too, must the counsellor work at the process of clarifying her thoughts in line with what she actually perceives about the world. This can be done in a variety of ways – through talking things through with a colleague or a friend, through reading and continuing education and through introspection – the process of looking inward and exploring what the poet Gerard Manley Hopkins called the 'inscape' (Hopkins, 1953).

Feelings

Feeling refers to the emotional aspect of the person: joy, love, anger, disappointment and so forth. Heron (1977a) argues that in our present society we have learned to hold on to or to repress many of our feelings because the cultural norm dictates that we do not overtly express them

– particularly the stronger expressions of anger, tears, fear and embarrassment. He argues, also, that such repression leads to people carrying through with them a great deal of unexpressed feeling that acts as a block to rational thinking, creativity and general enjoyment of life.

Counselling is frequently concerned with allowing people to express such pent-up emotions and there seems to be a direct link between the degree to which a counsellor can freely and appropriately express her own emotions and the degree to which she can *allow* the client to express his. It seems as though, if we block off a lot of our own stronger feelings, when we are faced with another person who wants to express feelings we feel reticent about allowing them to do so. Very often this is because the other person's emotion stirs up memories of our own feelings. As we have hung on to them for so long, a mechanism seems to come into play that encourages us to disallow that expression in others and thus allows us to carry on holding on to our own.

A simple experiment may serve to demonstrate the degree to which we carry around bottled-up emotion. Next time you feel moved to tears by something that you see on television, switch off the set and allow yourself to cry. Then listen inwardly to what you are crying about. The chances are that it will be something to do with your own personal history rather than being related directly to what you saw on the screen.

The health professional who is concerned with counselling many people who wish to express pent-up feelings should seriously consider exploring her own emotional status. This can be done through the medium of counselling supervision, in which the counsellor meets regularly with another trained counsellor and talks through and explores her work load. It can also be achieved through the process known as co-counselling, which is described in Chapter 11. It can also help to join a peer-support group (Ernst and Goodison, 1981) in which feelings can be explored in a safe and supportive atmosphere. Such support groups can be instituted and facilitated by a number of like-thinking colleagues and can do much to relieve the pressure of working with the emotionally stressed. Without such support, the health professional can easily slip into a position where she can no longer help the person who wants to express feelings because her own emotional needs are not catered for. The net result, as we noted earlier, can be burnout – a feeling of profound physical and emotional exhaustion caused by job-related stress. Self-awareness, then, must concern itself not only with the thinking side of the person but also with the feelings or emotional side.

Sensing

Sensing refers to inputs through the five special senses: touch, taste, smell, hearing, sight and also to proprioceptive and kinaesthetic sense. Proprioception refers to our ability to know the position of our bodies and thus to know where we are in space. We may note, for instance, that we do not have to think whether or not we are sitting down or standing up: we know that – through our proprioceptive sense, through bundles of nerve fibres which constantly feed the information back to our brains. Kinaesthetic sense refers to our sense of body movement. Again, this is a sense that we do not normally have to think about – we just move!

Much of the time, we are not aware of the potential stimulation that exists for our senses: we filter out many of the stimuli. A short experiment will illustrate how this filtering process works. Stop reading this book for a moment and pay attention to everything coming in through your senses. What can you hear? What can you see? What can you smell? What can you taste? What can you feel? In recognising these various inputs through the senses, it becomes apparent just how much is normally not noticed in the course of a day. Now, for much of the time, such filtering out is useful in that it allows us to concentrate on a particular task in hand. In terms of counselling, however, it is vital that we learn to develop an acute awareness of the inputs coming in through the senses, particularly those of hearing and of sight. When counselling, we are not only hearing what clients are saying but also paying attention to how they say it – their tone of voice, the inflection, the volume of their voice and so on. Further, we need to pay attention also to clients' appearance in terms of how they are dressed, how they sit and how they use non-verbal communication: eye contact, body movement, touch, proximity to the counsellor and so forth. Without an awareness of these points of communication, we stand to lose a lot of important information that can help to guide us in deciding how best to intervene in the counselling relationship.

Fortunately, the process of developing such awareness is, in one sense, easy – we just have to do it! If an amount of time is set aside each day just to notice what is going on around us, we can quickly learn to extend this period until we are much more acutely aware of sensory input. Such noticing can become a way of life. The process of noticing is often blocked, however, by internal distraction – recurrent thoughts and worries. Clearly, it is less easy to pay such close attention to what is going on around us when our lives are particularly stressful and we are preoccupied for much of the time with some sort of 'internal dialogue'. Certainly we cannot be effective counsellors unless we can give almost total attention to the client and therefore, at times of personal emotional stress, the health professional is likely to function less well in the capacity of counsellor. This, perhaps, is another reason why the person regularly acting in a counselling role should seriously consider peer support of some sort. Such support is not only useful in talking through difficult issues in counselling, but it may also serve as a means of the counsellor working through some of her own problems in living.

Intuiting

The intuitive aspect of the person is perhaps the most undervalued. Intuiting refers to knowledge and insight that arrives independently of the senses. Ornstein (1975), in a study of the two sides of the brain, came to the conclusion that the intuitive function is associated with the right side of the brain, whilst the more cognitive process is associated with the left. If Ornstein is right, the implication is that, if the intuitive aspect is developed further, then both sides of the brain will function optimally. Certainly Ornstein sees the two processes as complementary and argues, with Jung, that the intuitive side of the person should be developed alongside the more cognitive aspect. Western culture tends to be dominated by the left brain approach to education and development – certainly rationality is usually viewed as more important than intuition. Ornstein places intuition beyond mere intellectual understanding in terms of importance and suggests the use of metaphors, allegories, music and Sufi fables as the means by which intuition can be developed.

It may be the case that the intuitive aspect of the person is neglected through fear that it may not be trusted. It is probably true that most of us have intended to act at some time from an intuitive feeling but have held back at the last minute because we could not be sure that our intuition was right. On the other hand, many aspects of the counselling process demand an intuitive approach. In order to empathise with another person, we are required to grasp intuitively what it is to be like them. Certainly, very sensitive issues require an intuitive approach – mere logic or rationality is somehow not enough. Carl Rogers noted that whenever he felt a hunch about something that was happening in the counselling relationship, it invariably helped if he verbalised it (Rogers, 1967), although he acknowledged, too, that he often also doubted his own intuitive ability and took the rational approach, only to find out later that his hunch had been accurate! Using intuition consciously and openly takes courage, but used alongside more rational approaches it can enhance the counselling relationship in a way that logic never can.

On the other hand, once again it is necessary to note that intuition is an *abstraction* – it does not have concrete reality that we can point to. Some of the situations in which we posit intuition as having played a part *may* be explained in other ways. For example, it may sometimes be the case that I think I have discovered something 'intuitively' simply because I have forgotten that I had learned the fact before. Sometimes, it may be possible that I anticipate what someone else will say 'intuitively' because I have got to know them quite well and have knowledge of the sorts of things that this person *does* say. Not everything we think of as 'intuitive' may be so. Alternatively, of course, there are still plenty of things that happen that we cannot give a better name to than 'intuition'.

These four aspects of the internal part of the person – thinking, feeling, sensing and intuiting need to be developed in combination. Jung argued that many people rely heavily on a one-sided approach – particularly the thinking/sensing approach. Such people, he argued, prefer rational argument, backed up by evidence through the senses of a fairly concrete nature. In other words, such people dismiss what they cannot directly see, hear, taste, smell or touch or which cannot be rationally argued about. Such a position, whilst clearly safe, arguably dismisses some of the more subtle and even metaphysical aspects of life. Certainly it tends to denigrate emotional experience and, presumably, dismisses intuition on the grounds of its not being rational! In terms of the counselling relationship, it would seem valuable to develop all four aspects of the self for it is those four aspects that the client very often has problems with. Life problems are not always of the rational, thinking sort. Nor are they concerned only with what can be directly sensed. Many problems in living are directly related to emotions, feelings and sometimes 'un-nameable' problems – problems concerned with the intuitive domain. Herman Hesse sums up the problems of these sorts of issues, our tendency to ignore the feeling and intuitive domains and our temptation to seek too readily clarification through rationality:

> *... each of us paints and misrepresents every day and every hour the jungle of mysteries, transforming it into a pretty garden or a flat, neatly drawn map, the moralist with the help of his maxims, the man of religion with the help of his faith, the engineer with the help of his slide-rule, the painter with the help of his palette, and the poet with the help of his examples and ideals. And each one of us lives completely and content and assured in his pseudo-world and on his map, just so long as he does not feel, through some breach in the dam or some frightful flash of lightning, reality, the monster, the terrifying beauty, the appalling horror, falling upon him, inescapably embracing him and lethally taking him prisoner.*

(Hesse, 1979)

The experience of the body

Another aspect of this integrated model of the self is the experience of the body. If, as has been argued, the mind and body are inextricably linked, then any mental activity will manifest itself as some sort of bodily change and vice versa. It is notable, however, how often we divide the two up. Expressions such as, 'My mind is OK; it's my body that's the problem' and 'I'm not happy with my body' indicate how easy it is to make this artificial distinction. A moment's reflection, however, will reveal how artificial this distinction really is. In fact, we do not have a mind and body, we are our mind and body. When we speak of the self, we are speaking of both aspects – mind and body.

Coming to notice the sometimes small changes that take place in the mind–body takes time and patience. Stop reading for a moment and notice your own body. What do you notice? Do you have areas of muscle tension – in the shoulders or neck, for example? What parts of the body are you not aware of? Have any bodily sensations changed since you started noticing? What is your breathing like? Fast, slow, deep or shallow? Many of these small changes in the body tempo can help us to locate changes in mood. Often the first symptom of a mood or state of mind is a bodily change. In learning to notice the body, we can learn to make valuable observations about ourselves and thus further develop self-awareness. Such noticing is also of value in the counselling relationship, for a client's emotions are also often expressed in physical terms. A sudden change of breathing rate can indicate rising anxiety, for example. Psychological tension is often expressed in the form of tightened muscles.

Learning to listen to the body in this way can help us more accurately to assess our true feelings about ourselves and others. Wilhelm Reich (1949), a contemporary of Freud and a psychoanalyst who was particularly interested in the mind–body relationship, argued that many of us carry around with us unexpressed emotion that is somehow 'stored' in our musculature. Emotions, then, could become trapped in sets of muscles. He maintained that direct manipulation of those sets of muscles could release the emotion trapped within them. Such therapy applied directly to the body has become known as Reichian bodywork and can be a powerful means of releasing pent-up emotion and gaining self-awareness through a very direct method.

Similar but different versions of this physical approach to psychological issues may be found in Rolfing (Rolf, 1973), bioenergetics (Lowen, 1967), Feldenkrais (Feldenkrais, 1972) and the Alexander technique (Alexander, 1969). Other examples of the approach to self-awareness through the mind–body include massage, yoga, the martial arts, certain types of meditation, dance and certain sorts of sports and exercise.

All of these methods can enhance self-awareness through attention to changes in the body and thus create insight into psychological states. They can also aid development of awareness of body image. If we notice people in everyday life, we may observe how many people walk in a lopsided manner or stoop their shoulders and may even have different sorts of expressions on either side of their face! Bodywork methods may help in balancing the person and may lead to a greater sense of physical (and, therefore, psychological) symmetry. It would seem reasonable to argue that it would be strange to concentrate on developing awareness of the mind whilst totally ignoring the body. Similarly, it is perhaps odd to concentrate on physical fitness or balance without paying attention to psychological status. This joint focus also applies to the process of counselling. Effective counselling involves paying attention to both what the client says and what he does. Thus the mind–body is attended to as a totality.

This, then, is an integrated model of the self, focusing on the outer, public expression of self, through our behaviour and an inner, more private aspect of self. Clearly this is only one way of discussing the self, and, as we noted earlier, the self has many facets, including the self-as-perceived-by-others. The model offered here, however, may allow us to make a start at developing self-awareness as an important tool in the process of skilful counselling. For self-awareness can never be developed purely for its own sake, but as a means of enhancing our caring and helping skills.

SELF-AWARENESS

What is self-awareness? First, the point needs to be made that it is not self-consciousness in the sense of becoming painfully aware of how we imagine other people see us. Sartre (1956) describes this condition well when he says that when we come under the scrutinising gaze of another person, we perceive ourselves as being turned into objects by that other person. It is as though we become a thing rather than a person. Such a notion of treating people as things and the resultant self-consciousness is a valuable concept in the context of counselling, for it is important that we do not become interested in the problems of the people we are counselling to the extent that they merely become interesting cases. Once we do this, we have made them into things and as a result they may feel distinctly uncared for and uncomfortable.

Self-awareness is the evolving and expanding sense of noticing and taking account of a wide range of aspects of self. As we explore our psychological and physical make-up we get to know ourselves better. Chapman and Gale (1982) notice a curious paradox about this process. They note that to gain knowledge of something does not normally change that thing. If, for instance, I learn an equation, that equation does not change as a result of my having learnt it. With self-awareness, however, the subject of the learning – the self – changes as more is learnt about it. In this sense, then, the process of developing self-awareness is a continuous process because we are continuously changing. Self-awareness, curiously, may speed up that change.

Two different and complementary methods of developing self-awareness may be described. One is through the process of introspection or looking inward. The other is through receiving feedback about ourselves from other people. The two used in balance can lead to a reasonable and hopefully accurate picture of the self. One without the other can lead to a curiously skewed sense of self. Thus, introspection on its own can lead to either an unnecessarily harsh judgement of the self or a narcissistic and self-centred view. Relying only on feedback from others can lead us to concentrate only on the external or public aspect of the self. Again, there is no guarantee that another person's assessment of us is any more or any less accurate than our own but it is important to hear it! To be able to hear it undefensively is yet another skill. Often, when other people tell us what they think of us, for good or bad, we react to it. The skill here may be to accept it, in much the same way as it has been suggested that we accept what the client says to us in counselling. If we can free others to tell us easily their impression of us, we are slightly more likely to get an honest view from them on other occasions. This has implications for work in peer-support groups used as vehicles for self-awareness development. Just as we must be prepared to listen fully to the client in counselling, so we must be prepared to listen fully to our peers in such a group.

Figure 3.2 offers a variety of practical methods for developing self-awareness that may be used by the individual working on her own or by

Aspects of self-awareness	Methods of developing self-awareness

1. *Thinking, including*
  – stream of consciousness
  – belief systems
  – ideas
  – fantasies
    etc.
	Discussion/conversation
	Group work
	Introspection
	Brainstorming
	Meditation
	Writing
	Use of problem-solving cycle, etc.

2. *Feeling, including:*
  – anger
  – fear
  – grief
  – embarrassment
  – joy/happiness
  – mood swings
    etc.
	Discussion/conversation
	Group work
	Introspection
	Gestalt exercise
	Meditation
	Co-counselling
	Supervision
	Analysis
	Cathartic work
	Sensitivity training
	Encounter group work
	Role play, etc.

3. *Sensations, including*
  – taste
  – touch
  – hearing
  – smell
  – sight
    etc.
	Focusing attention on one or more sensations
	    at a time
	Group exercises
	Use of sensory stimulation/deprivation
	    exercises, gestalt exercises
	Noticing in everyday life, etc.

4. *Sexuality, including*
  – orientation (heterosexual/homosexual/
    bisexual)
  – expression of sexuality
    etc.
	Discussion/conversation
	Counselling/co-counselling
	Values, clarification exercises, etc.

5. *Spirituality, including*
  – belief systems
  – life philosophy
  – awareness of choice
  – varieties of religious experience
  – atheism and agnosticism
    etc.
	Discussion/conversation
	Group work
	Meditation
	Prayer
	Reading
	Aesthetic experience (art, music, poetry, etc.)
	Life planning, goal setting

6. *Physical status, including*
  – the body system
  – health status
    etc.
	Self-examination
	Medical examination
	Exercise
	Sport
	Martial arts
	Meditation
	Massage
	Bodywork, etc.

7. *Appearance, including*
  – dress
  – personal style
  – height, weight
    etc.
	Discussion/conversation
	Self- and peer assessment
	Self-monitoring
	Use of video, etc.

	Continued

Figure 3.2

Methods of developing self-awareness.

Aspects of self-awareness	Methods of developing self-awareness

8. *Knowledge, including*
  – level of propositional knowledge
  – level of practical knowledge
  – level of experiential knowledge
	Discussion/conversation
	Group work
	Examination/testing/quizzing
	Study
	Use of distance-learning packages
	Enrolment on courses
	Self- and peer assessment, etc.

9. *Needs and wants, including:*
  – financial/material
  – physical
  – love and belonging
  – achievement
  – knowledge
  – aesthetic
  – spiritual
  – self-actualization
    etc.
	Discussion/conversation
	Group work
	Values clarification work
	Assertiveness training
	Lifestyle evaluation etc.

10. *Spirituality, including:*
  – verbal and non-verbal skills
  – values
  – unknown/undiscovered aspects of the self
	Discussion/conversation
	Counselling/ co-counselling
	Self-analysis
	Social skills training

groups of peers working together in a group. It is not suggested that it represents an exhaustive list of self-awareness methods, but it can serve as a starting point. In practice, the individual will often identify particular preferences for certain methods of self-awareness development. It is important, however, to occasionally 'freshen the act' and try new methods!

It is important to note that self-awareness development should be an enjoyable process. It should neither be too earnest nor too concentrated. A sense of perspective and a sense of humour are essential to the process as is keeping a sense of the 'larger picture' – the social situation in which the individual exists. A political and social awareness is vital to the development of counselling skills as is a sense of self-awareness.

AGAINST THE SELF

The concept of 'self' is not universal. In the Buddhist culture, the teaching is that the idea of 'self' is a delusion – a development of an abstraction. The aim is to lose attachment to an idea of 'self'. Just as all life is changing, at all times, so the person is changing all the time and it cannot be argued that any sort of concrete, unmovable sense of self exists. Harvey (1990) offers a useful explanation of this idea:

> *The not-self teaching can easily be misunderstood and misdescribed; so it is important to see what it is saying. The Buddha accepted many conventional uses of the word 'self' ... as in 'yourself and 'myself'. These he saw simply as a convenient way of referring to a*

particular collection of mental and physical states. But within such a conventional, empirical self, he taught that no permanent, substantial, independent, metaphysical self could be found ... The not-self teaching does not deny that there is a continuity of character in life ... but while character traits may be long-lasting, they can and do change, and are thus impermanent and so 'not-self', insubstantial.

(Harvey, 1990)

One of the points of Buddhism is to accept things as they are: forever changing and to note those changes and to move on. For Buddhists, then, the concept of 'self' as a set of constructs is not particularly useful.

This non-self concept can, of course, be valuable in helping a person to face life problems. For if everything is subject to constant change, the present, uncomfortable, situation a person finds themselves in, is also subject to change. Helping a person accept things as they are and to accept that, like all other things, *this* situation is fleeting, can be to help relieve certain existential fears and anxieties. This approach of 'no-self' is not for everyone but it is a view held by many people in the world – particularly in south-east Asia. As we shall see in the chapter on culture, it is vital to have an understanding of views and beliefs that are, sometimes, different to our own.

Perhaps, sometimes, we cling to a view of 'self' because it gives our lives shape and purpose. We feel, if we entertain a notion of 'self', that there is something to work on, to modify and, at the same time, an inner core that is relatively unchanging. However, to live without a sense of self can also be liberating: the person who has no self is caught up, like all other objects and beings in the world, in the constant flux of life. Rather than attempting to hold back the flow of change (in the end, an impossibility) we can, rather, choose to accept the impermanent nature of life and the world and, by extension, of 'ourselves'.

Communication quotes

Knowing others is wisdom, knowing yourself is Enlightenment.

Tao Tzu

Blessed are those who can laugh at themselves, for they shall never cease to be amused.

Anonymous

The most basic of all human needs is the need to understand and be understood. The best way to understand people is to listen to them.

Ralph Nicholl

Communication leads to community, that is, to understanding, intimacy and mutual valuing.

Rollo May

> *They may forget what you said, but they will never forget how you made them feel.*
>
> Carl W. Buechner

SELF-AWARENESS AND THE HEALTH PROFESSIONAL

As we have seen, self-awareness underlies almost every aspect of the counselling relationship. In all of the health professions, the fact that the professional forms close and personal relationships with her clients emphasises this need for understanding of the self. When other people are physically, emotionally, socially or spiritually distressed, that distress cannot but affect us too. We need not only professional knowledge and know-how, related to our particular speciality and an awareness of how our work fits in with the work of others in the caring team, but also personal awareness that can inform our practice in the health field. Such self-awareness can help us to develop an understanding of the basic principles of counselling discussed in Chapter 5. On the other hand, we might also reflect on whether or not 'the self' exists or whether, rather, it is a convenient way of talking about aspects of what it is to be human. Another view, as we have noted, is that there is no self, but, rather, that like all other aspects of life, we are caught up in constant and inevitable change.

4

CULTURE AND COMMUNICATION

We all live within and are influenced by our culture. Most of the time, our own is taken for granted. We only 'notice culture' when we see someone else's and when it is markedly different from our own. We are probably hardly aware of our own culture, until faced with another. This chapter explores the notion of culture and relates it to international differences in interpersonal communication and counselling. For we cannot take a person out of his or her culture and we cannot counsel him or her in cultural isolation. As we shall see, people in some cultures are more likely to benefit from counselling than people from others. Indeed, it is important to note that, in some cultures, counselling is not likely to be something that is used for helping solve the problems of living.

The chapter draws on the author's work on culture and communication in Thailand and makes comparisons between 'Western' and Thai cultures as a way of illustrating some cultural differences (Burnard and Naiyapatana, 2004). All of these elements are important for anyone who counsels people from other cultures.

CULTURE

Sapir (1948) defines culture as embodying any socially inherited element in the life of man, material and spiritual. In Linton's (1945) terms, the culture of society is the way of life of its members: the collection of ideas and habits which they learn, share and transmit from generation to generation. Harris (1999) asserts that a culture is the socially learned ways of living found in human societies and that it embraces all aspects of social life, including both thought and behaviour. In the field of nursing and health care, Leininger (1991) provides a more concise definition for the concept of culture as the 'learned, shared and transmitted values, beliefs, norms, and lifeways of a particular group that guides their thinking, decisions, and actions in patterned ways'.

Bodley (2000) offers the following examples of different approaches to defining culture:

- Topical: culture consists of everything on a list of topics, or categories, such as social organization, religion, or economy.
- Historical: culture is social heritage, or tradition, that is passed on to future generations.
- Behavioural: culture is shared, learned human behaviour, a way of life.
- Normative: culture is ideals, values, or rules for living.
- Functional: culture is the way humans solve problems of adapting to the environment or living together.

- Mental: culture is a complex of ideas, or learned habits, that inhibit impulses and distinguish people from animals.
- Structural: culture consists of patterned and interrelated ideas, symbols, or behaviours.
- Symbolic: culture is based on arbitrarily assigned meanings that are shared by a society.

He goes on to suggest that:

> *Culture involves at least three components: what people think, what they do, and the material products they produce. Thus, mental processes, beliefs, knowledge, and values are parts of culture. Some anthropologists would define culture entirely as mental rules guiding behaviour, although often wide divergence exists between the acknowledged rules for correct behaviour and what people actually do. Consequently, some researchers pay most attention to human behaviour and its material products. Culture also has several properties: it is shared, learned, symbolic, transmitted cross–generationally, adaptive, and integrated.*
>
> (Bodley, 2000)

Kluckhohn (1969) offers a similar breakdown of possible definitions, as follows:

- the total way of life of a people;
- the social legacy the individual acquires from his group;
- a way of thinking, feeling, and believing;
- an abstraction from behaviour;
- a theory on the part of the anthropologist about the way in which a group of people in fact behave;
- a storehouse of pooled learning;
- a set of standardized orientations to recurrent problems;
- learned behaviour;
- a mechanism for the normative regulation of behaviour;
- a set of techniques for adjusting both to the external environment and to other men (or women);
- a precipitate of history;
- a behavioural map, sieve, or matrix.

Culture is often described as that which includes knowledge, belief, morals, laws, customs and any other attributes acquired by a person as a member of society (McLaren, 1998). Nemetz Robinson (1985) made the following distinction about definitions of culture:

- The categories of behaviours and products reflect a notion of culture as observable phenomena.
- The category of ideas reflects a notion of culture as not observable: something which is internal but which can also be explicitly described.

Thus culture may involve observable behaviours but also a felt sense – a sense, perhaps, of identity, of who we are. When we communicate, interculturally, we not only communicate words and ideas but, also, something of ourselves and of our roots.

Triandis summarises some of the more specific elements of culture and indicates how it affects and directs behaviour:

> *Cultures include more than customs. They develop characteristic ways of categorising experience, linguistic terms that correspond to these categories, widely shared associations among the categories, beliefs about how the categories are linked to each other, beliefs about correct action in specific situations (norms), beliefs about actions that are appropriate for persons who hold specific positions in social structures (roles), and guiding principles that direct the lives of individuals (values). These entities constitute some of the elements of subjective culture ... that are widely shared and transmitted from generation to generation.*
>
> (Triandis, 1994)

Triandis goes on to discuss the distinctions between what are called individualist cultures and collectivist cultures. Triandis places the emphasis on culture as a determinant of behaviour and on how it informs the way in which people live in any given society. He pays special attention to the ways in which language shapes cultural behaviour and perception.

Clearly, culture is a changing thing. No society or community is static. Just as language evolves, so do all of the other aspects of culture. Cultures continue to modify themselves in the light of things like technology, research-based evidence, political change and even fashion. Communication patterns also change in this way. Sometimes, too, aspects of culture are manufactured – either as a means of attempting to shore up a government or ruling body and sometimes for the purposes of tourism. As global tourists move away from 'beach holidays' they tend to look for holidays which will allow them to sample other cultures. In response, tourist boards and governments attempt to supply something 'unique' for those tourists. What cannot always be guaranteed is the authenticity of that experience. It seems unlikely that tourist-aimed 'culture shows' will offer a real glimpse into the culture of a country.

Clarity and misunderstanding in communication are key issues. Those coming to this country, or going to another, not only have to learn a language but also a set of what might be called 'communication rules'. This is often an acute problem for the person coming to work as a student or as a nurse. However, all parties can learn from this anxiety. We can learn a considerable amount about our own communication patterns by observing 'different' ones in students, colleagues or friends coming from another culture.

How well we communicate depends on how we behave. After language, non-verbal communication seems to be the key factor that enhances or detracts from the way we communicate with others. The behaviours involved in non-verbal communication need to be clear and unambiguous. But, further, when we use non-verbal behaviour, we need to be confident that the other person or persons will understand it. Berger put it this way:

> *To interact in a relatively smooth, co-ordinated, and understandable manner, one must both be able to predict how one's interaction partner is likely to behave, and, based on those predictions, to select from one's own repertoires those responses that will optimize outcomes in the encounter.*

(Berger, 1992)

So the newcomer to a culture not only has to learn a set of non-verbal behaviours but also has to learn the 'right' ones to use at any given time:

> *Knowledge about another person's culture – its language, dominant values, beliefs and prevailing ideology – often permits predictions of the person's possible responses to certain messages ... Upon first encountering a stranger, cultural information provides the only grounds for communicative predictions. This fact explains the uneasiness and perceived lack of control most people experience when thrust into an alien culture: they not only lack information about the individuals with whom they must communicate, they are bereft of information concerning shared cultural norms and values.*

(Miller and Sunnafrank, 1982)

A familiar problem with anyone entering a different culture is the sudden or gradual realisation of 'difference'. Those behaviours and ways of communicating that we take for granted are, suddenly, not those being used around us. This jarring in meeting another culture is sometimes termed 'culture shock' (Dodd, 1991). Gudykunst and Kim sum up the problems surrounding non-verbal, cultural differences as follows:

> *When strangers violate our nonverbal expectations we tend to interpret those violations negatively. These negative interpretations decrease the effectiveness of our communication with strangers. To communicate effectively with strangers we must learn to accurately interpret their nonverbal behaviour and their violations of our expectations.*

(Gudykunst and Kim, 1992)

There are huge numbers of cultural variables to be considered when thinking about verbal and non-verbal communication. This chapter can only consider a few. What follows are some examples of the sorts of things that health care professionals and counsellors might consider when thinking about cultural aspects of communication. In them, we see the 'taken for granted' questioned by cultural practice.

Individualist and collectivist cultures

The distinction has been made between individualist societies, in which 'I' comes before 'we' and collectivist societies in which 'we' comes before 'I' (McLaren, 1998). Hofstede describes these differences as follows:

Individualism pertains to societies in which the ties between individuals are loose: everyone is expected to look after himself or herself and his or her immediate family. Collectivism as its opposite pertains to societies in which people from birth onwards are integrated into strong, cohesive in-groups, which throughout people's lifetime continue to protect them in exchange for unquestioning loyalty.

(Hofstede, 1994)

Triandis offers a more detailed list of factors that help to shape individualist and collectivist cultures:

- The individualist pattern stresses that the views, needs and goals of the self are most important, whereas the collectivist emphasises the views, needs and goals of some collective.
- Behaviour can be explained by the pleasure principle and the computation of personal profits and losses, whereas the collectivist stresses that behaviour is a function of norms and duties imposed by the collective.
- Beliefs distinguish the individual from the in-group, allowing the individual to be an autonomous entity, whereas the collectivist pattern emphasises shared beliefs, that is, what the individual and the collective have in common.
- Social behaviour is independent of and emotionally detached from the collective, whereas, in the collectivist pattern, it is dependent, emotionally attached and involved with the collective. Furthermore, social behaviour in collectivist cultures is co-operative and even self-sacrificing towards in-group members, but indifferent, even hostile toward out-group members (Triandis, 1994).

It may be hypothesized, then, that students from an individualist culture, with its emphasis on values such as self-motivation and self-development, may express higher levels of self-esteem than students from collectivist cultures in which emphases are on values such as working together, respect for others and the fulfilment of others' needs (Triandis, 1972).

There is an important issue for counselling in this distinction between individualist and collectivist cultures. In the individualist culture, with its strong emphasis on 'self', a person is encouraged to talk about his or her problems and to discuss them with others. Thus the role of the counsellor is usually well established in individualist cultures. In the collectivist culture, with the emphasis on dismissal of self as a concept (especially in Buddhist cultures), the tendency will be for people with problems to be 'jollied along' and not encouraged to discuss problems – for to worry other people with your problems is often seen as an imposition and a lack of respect for other people's feelings. Thus, in collectivist cultures, the idea of employing counsellors to help people with their problems in living is likely to be rarely subscribed to – if at all. It is quite common, however, for more 'directive' counselling (for example, AIDS or genetic counselling) to be in place in these countries. In Muslim cultures, it is usual for people with problems to go to a religious advisor, who can advise on a Quranic prescription for working on problems.

It is interesting to note Hofstede's (1994) findings from a survey of various countries. Hofstede suggests that the vast majority of people in the world live in collectivist societies in which the interest of the group prevails over the interest of the individual. The first group, in the collectivist society, is the family into which a person is born. In most collectivist societies, the 'family' within which the child grows up consists of people living closely together and not just the parents and other children but also grandparents, aunts, servants or other house-mates – the extended family. When children grow up they learn to consider themselves as part of the we group, a relationship that is not voluntary but given. The we group is usually distinct from other people in society, who belong to a they group of which there are many. The we group is the major source of identity for the person in a collectivist culture and often the only security one has against the hardships of life. A strong practical and psychological bond forms between the person and the we group to which he or she belongs.

Again, in the collectivist culture, problems are more likely to be discussed within families – if at all – rather than being taken to a counsellor. In individualist cultures, with the tendency for nuclear family living, people with problems are likely to feel less concerned about talking things over with a counsellor than would be the case in the collectivist culture.

If Hofstede's findings were accurate, then, we may assume that the UK is a more individualistic, and Thailand a more collectivist, culture. However, as Triandis et al. note, we need to be cautious about such distinctions and use them, perhaps, as a general guide:

> *It is not enough to know the culture or the other person. It is also necessary to know something about demographic and biographic information, because individuals from urban, industrialised, mobile, migrating, affluent environments with much exposure to the media are likely to be idiocentric, even if they come from collectivist cultures.*
>
> (Triandis *et al.*, 1991)

Hofstede (1994) also noted that almost everyone belongs to a range of different groups and categories at the same time. He offers the following examples:

- a national level according to one's country (or countries, for people who migrated during their lifetime);
- a regional and/or ethnic and/or religious and/or linguistic affiliation level, as most nations are composed of culturally different regions and/or ethnic and/or religious and/or language groups;

- a gender level, according to whether a person was born as a girl or as a boy;
- a social class level, which separates grandparents from parents and children;
- for those who are employed, an organizational or corporate level, according to the way employees have been socialized by their work organization (Hofstede, 1994).

Perhaps, however, the notions of 'individuality' and of 'the individual' are beginning to wane. Frie notes the impact of postmodernity on the self and the individual:

> *In contrast to the modernist emphasis on the autonomy of the individual mind, postmodernism asserts that the person, or subject, is not only shaped but also subverted by the contexts in which it exists. More radical versions of postmodernism deny the very existence of a person with the capacity for reflexive thought and self-determining action. In place of the person as an active, responsible being, they herald the so-called death of the subject.*
>
> (Frie, 2003)

Postmodernists usually claim that the world around us is something of a construct. We do not 'discover reality' but invent it (Watzlawick, 1984). We cannot apprehend the world directly or objectively, but only through language and the notions and concepts we have invented. We are not able to measure our thoughts against any objective reality as we cannot transcend or stand outside of our own concepts or language. It is impossible, then, for us to achieve any sort of undistorted view of the world (Frederickson, 2003). All of this applies, equally, to our attempting to understand other cultures and other peoples. We do not have any way of knowing that what we are observing reflects any sort of verifiable 'truth'. Just as the postmodernists suggest that 'the reader writes the text' so we might say that the cultural observer or ethnographer 'invents the culture' that he or she observes from his own, subjective and unverifiable viewpoint.

Perhaps, in the end, as is often the case, much depends on how the notions of 'individual' and 'individualist' are defined. Also, we must, I suppose, be careful that the postmodern position does not subvert cross-cultural research projects to the point where they become so difficult to verify in any sense that they cease to be worthwhile as projects. Even if we cannot look at the world 'as it really is', our reflections on that world are sometimes of value to those who read our work and compare what they read with what they see for themselves. If the thought is provoked, 'I don't agree with that!' then something has been achieved. Conversely, if what a person reads sometimes corresponds to his or her own experience of the world, then that, too, is of value.

ETHNOCENTRISM

The idea of ethnocentrism is thought to have started with the sociologist William Sumner. He suggested that it was:

> *the technical name for the view of things in which one's own group is the centre of everything, and all others are scaled and rated with reference to it.*

> (Sumner, 1906)

Sumner's choice of language may seem quaint today, with its reference to the 'technical name' for a concept, but the idea is still a recognisable and valid one.

Ethnocentrism is inevitable: as we have noted, we are all bound by our own culture and our immersion and upbringing within it. Research has supported the idea that similarity of culture will be a determining factor in our attitude towards others. Wanguri (1996) notes, 'We tend to like people who are similar to us and dislike those who are dissimilar'. This is perhaps too strong a position. We are, after all, often attracted, also, to the 'difference' in other people. The point, is, perhaps, that ethnocentrism becomes a problem when we are unconscious of it. Hellweg *et al.* make the following point:

> *What makes ethnocentrism such a powerful and insidious force in communication is that it often exists invisibly (for example, when we only study western philosophers) and is usually invisible in its manifestations (for example, we approach problems with a western orientation) ... Other cultures may also demonstrate these feelings of conscious or unconscious superiority.*

> (Hellweg *et al.*, 1991)

It is ethnocentric to imagine that 'Counselling is for everyone'. Not all cultures and not all people value talking about their problems. In Thailand, for example, the task of friends and family is more to 'jolly people along' and reassure them that things will be OK. It is not a cultural norm to 'work through' problems of living. The important thing, rather, is to be distracted from them.

The concept of ethnocentrism is further compounded by the ways in which society views expressions of it. Describing this 'tangle', Korzenny suggests:

> *We are most likely to attribute positive traits to those similar to us, but because to do so is, paradoxically, a societal taboo, we deny it. The denial of ethnocentrism is one of the most crucial barriers to intercultural communication because such denial prevents confrontation, clarification and acceptance.*

> (Korzenny, 1991)

We may attempt to show our lack of ethnocentrism by denying difference and by proclaiming that 'We are all the same under the skin', in a similar way to those who would hold that 'All religions have some truth in them'. These blandishments do little to help us understand both the similarities and differences of people in other cultures. While most people have a similar physiological make-up (although differences exist there too), the way our culture shapes us does make us different from those who live in other cultures. A useful meeting point between the extremes of, 'We are all different' and 'We are all the same', lies with the often quoted triplet: people are in certain respects:

- like no other persons (idiosyncratic norms);
- like some other persons (group norms);
- like all other persons (universal norms) (Kluckholm, Murray and Schiener, 1953).

Writing of the difficulties of facing both our own ethnocentrism and our own ignorance of other cultures, Said wrote as follows:

> *For if it is true that no production of knowledge in the human sciences can ever ignore or disclaim its author's involvement as a human subject in his own circumstances, then it must also be true that for a European or American studying the Orient there can be no disclaiming the main circumstances of his actuality: that he comes up against the Orient as a European or American first, as an individual second.*
>
> (Said, 1979)

In a 'foreign' culture, one is first of all aware of one's cultural difference rather than of one's personal difference. The most notable experience of this is described in the concept of 'culture shock'. McLaren (1998) describes this experience as follows:

> *Culture shock is the disorientation that comes from being plunged into an unfamiliar setting. Everything people do is different: travelling, ordering meals, telephoning – all can be exhausting in an unfamiliar culture. Add to this the loneliness, unfamiliar attitudes towards time, towards women and family, dress, customs, finance, food, accommodation, and different ideas about cleanliness, medicine, transport, privacy, tips and levels of formality. No wonder sojourners feel tired, incompetent, confused and worried about seeming stupid to the hosts.*
>
> (McLaren, 1998)

Sometimes it is liberating to know that other people's customs are not the same as ours and that other people's languages are not gibberish (or even substitutes for English!). The author recalls telling a university lecturer, in an Eastern European university, that he was leaning Thai. The lecturer replied: 'Do they have a language or do they just make sounds?' It is good, also, to know that other people's perceptions of reality and life are just as valid as our own and that their value systems are as appropriate as our own, even though they are different. Much can be learned by seeing the way other people live.

It seems reasonable to claim that the perceptive visitor has a 'clearer' and 'newer' view of what he or she is seeing and experiencing. He or she 'sees' things in another culture that the resident has grown familiar with to the point of filtering it out of his or her sensory perception mechanisms. Keeping that 'freshness' may be an important factor in working at the development of ethnography. However, it is soon lost. Most people want to 'fit in' to a culture and, in the process of doing this, they tend to lose some of their sense of difference and some of their observational powers. In wanting to make the unfamiliar, familiar, they begin, quite quickly, to stop 'noticing' – at least in terms of the little differences.

Before we get carried away by culture, we should bear in mind that it is only one of a number of factors that impinge on people's lives. Or is it? Writing on factors that affect health, Helman writes as follows:

> ... *the culture into which you are born, or in which you live, is by no means the only such influence. It is only one of a number of influences which includes individual factors (such as age, gender, size, appearance, personality, intelligence and experience), educational factors (both formal and informal and including education into a religious, ethnic or professional subculture), and socioeconomic factors (such as social class, economic status, and the networks of social support from other people).*
>
> (Helman, 1990)

On the other hand, some of the factors that Helman mentions are also aspects of culture too!

The challenge, for the ethnographer, appears to be that of attempting to transcend his or her own ethnocentrism: clearly a gargantuan task. As we have noted, we bring to any other culture, the inbred and socialised 'baggage' that comes from the culture into which we were born. The author acknowledges many periods of personal frustration and misunderstanding in trying to throw off his own ethnocentric views in order to, at least minimally, understand another.

Cultural sensitivity is a concept related to ethnocentrism and culture shock. It is the ability to appreciate that, while I will never understand another culture fully, I have an appreciation of some of its aspects. Hanvey identifies four stages in this process:

1 The stage of stereotypes, of awareness of superficial or very visible cultural traits: this limited awareness usually comes from brief travel and from reading popular magazines. The differences noted seem exotic and bizarre.
2 The stage when a person notices unfamiliar significant and subtle cultural traits: this often comes from cultural conflict situations and seems frustrating and irrational.
3 The stage when a person notices unfamiliar significant and subtle cultural traits but analyses them intellectually, accepting them and trying to understand them.
4 Finally the stage where the person is aware what it is like to belong

in another culture. This comes from cultural immersion, from living the culture. The person not only understands, as at stage 3, but personally empathises with the culture (Hanvey, 1979).

The issues, for counselling, are clear. If we come from a 'Western' cultlure (and the concept of 'West' and 'East' is problematic), we are likely to think that the 'normal' thing for a concerned person to do is to talk over his or her problems. Further, we might believe that it is the right thing to do. However, to adopt these positions is to adopt ethno-centric views. The rest of the world may not live according to these beliefs about problems and their resolution.

The issue of cultural integration is a complex one. While, on the surface, it would seem preferable to encourage those of different cultures, living in a given society, to integrate freely and for the community to absorb some of those cultural mores, in practice, many people from many cultures prefer to maintain their cultural 'difference'. However, it also seems likely that cultural non-integration might be encouraged by having ethnic 'experts', who, like everyone else, will have their own particular view on the culture they represent.

'Culture', then, is multifaceted and complex. It is neither static nor easily bounded and described. For every 'cultural rule' there would seem to be exceptions, and an attempt to pinpoint a given moment in culture seems problematic. At best, perhaps, anthropologists and ethno-graphers offer a slightly romanticised (and sometimes even fictional) 'snapshot' of what a culture appeared to be like to them, viewed through a particular lens, in poor lighting conditions.

Tatar and Bekerman offer the following definitions of the field of culture as it relates to counselling:

> *Reviewing counselling literature we can extract at least two distinct approaches to the concept of culture as it relates to counselling. The first approach, in trying to partially overcome a solipsistic perspective of human experience, points at the need to account for context in our attempts to better understand human behaviour. More specifically, the setting becomes the larger context within which the counselling activity is constituted and must be realised. In this case organisational culture is what counsellors are asked to identify so as to adapt their counselling interventions to the culture of the setting or institution in which they work. The second approach emerges from what has come to be known as a multicultural approach that calls for the recognition of the variety of ethnic cultural backgrounds of those involved in the counselling situation and the need to account for this variety in our efforts to better counselling practice. We refer to this as the multicultural approach in counselling.*

> (Tatar and Bekerman, 2002)

What follows are some examples of how cultural differences vary in different cultural settings. Again, they should be read and reflected upon with caution. It is easy to create cultural stereotypes that sometimes are and sometimes are not reflections of the case (e.g. 'All English people drink tea', 'All Americans chew gum and wear baseball hats', 'All south-east Asians are polite'). One example of the problem of identifying cultural aspects of communication is as follows. As we shall see, Thai people use the wai to greet others, to show apologies, to thank, and so on (the wai is a prayer-like gesture of the hands, discussed later). The temptation is to say and write that 'Thai people do not shake hands, but wai'. In practice, of course – and particularly in business circles, some Thai people do shake hands – particularly when meeting Westerners. However, other examples of differences are less tangible and less obviously noticeable than the wai or the handshake. As we shall see, there are wide variations in other aspects of communication.

This complicated web of behaviours highlights a tension between, on the one hand, *individual behaviours* (what a person does because he or she is a 'one off') and *cultural behaviours* (what a person does because he or she is part of a culture). The wise counsellor is one who notes a person's culture and then also notes the individual. For, despite varying degrees of importance placed on 'the self' in different cultures, it is quite clear that everyone experiences him- or herself as 'a person'.

Given that we live in multicultural societies, as counsellors we need to have a fairly detailed understanding of the ways in which culture impinges upon people, in different parts of the globe. Simply believing that what we do is 'right' is a particular form of ethnocentrism that is unlikely to be helpful to those whom we attempt to counsel from other cultural settings.

Greetings and partings

In the UK and US, greeting behaviour can be elaborate. It may involve a greeting, a handshake and an enquiry about each other's health. This question about health is not a 'real' enquiry but part of what is termed 'phatic communication' (Malinowski, 1923). Phatic communication refers to the ordinary 'chit-chat' that helps to cement relationships. It can be compared and contrasted with 'information giving and receiving'. The aim of phatic communication is not to collect or give information and, to this extent, it is 'content free'. What is being said is not important. What is important is that the two people are being friendly with each other.

In some south-east Asian cultures, handshaking does not occur so frequently and, in some cases, it is replaced by the 'wai': the bringing together of the palms of the hands, in front of the body. There is a considerable protocol surrounding who initiates the wai process. Thus it is not sufficient merely to know how to execute a wai but also to know when to use it and with whom. Further, the wai varies considerably from country to country. In Nepal it is sometimes a sweeping gesture; in Thailand it is a very neat, precise one. There is an elaborate protocol surrounding the use of the wai. A foreign visitor would rarely initiate a wai and an older foreign visitor would normally simply return the wai but not bow his or her head. Children are not waied and their wais are not returned. Some Thai people believe that to wai a child is to reduce his or her lifespan.

There are different 'heights' of wai. The lowest is the putting together of the palms at just above waist level. Travellers on the national Thai airline will be offered these on entering the plane. The next level is just below the chin and a third is at the level of the nose. There is also a 'high wai', in which the hands are pressed together above the head and this is reserved for certain religious and royal ceremonies. Each wai may or may not be accompanied by a gentle bowing of the head. The less senior person of a pair initiates the wai and usually bows his or her head. The more senior person returns the wai but without bowing the head. Wais given by service staff, including waiters and shop assistants, are never returned. Very senior people will receive both a wai and a small curtsy or 'bob'. Monks are always waied as a greeting and for thanks but never return a wai.

An appropriately given wai, by a foreign visitor, is something that is appreciated by many Thai people. The excessive and incorrect use of the wai is not appreciated. Most visitors to the country are advised to observe the use of this gesture, over time, before attempting to use it or return it. It should never be thought of as an all-purpose form of greeting. A nod of the head (as an acknowledgement), if in doubt, is mostly all that is required of a foreigner.

Also, south-east Asian greetings are often brief and sometimes, between friends, barely noticeable. In our study it was noted that between close friends, greetings and partings were not 'notable' events and the various players did not appear either to acknowledge each other's arrival or say goodbye to them (Burnard and Naiyapatana 2004). Cooper and Cooper (1991) comment as follows:

> *Almost as rare [as saying 'thank you', in Thailand] is saying hello to people. 'Hello, how are you' would be an appropriate greeting for somebody you have not seen for some time, but is unnecessary for people you see everyday. The English 'good morning' is expressed quite adequately in Thai with a smile. Thai goodbyes can be equally brief.*

> (Cooper and Cooper, 1991)

Parting behaviour varies. Once a phone conversation or a meeting terminates in Thailand, the two parties may just stop talking and leave. Again, UK and US styles of communication tend to favour lengthier partings with often a number of 'false starts' at finishing the conversation and leaving. A mobile phone conversation, in Thailand, will start with an (English) 'Hello' and end with a seemingly abrupt 'OK na'. There is no direct translation of the syllable 'na'. It is a word added to the end of a sentence to soften it, make it polite, indicate pleading, ordering, surprise or emphasis. It is similar, in use, to the Chinese 'la' – often heard at the ends of questions and statements between friends.

Not appreciating differences of greeting and parting behaviours may lead people from various cultures to believe that what they are experiencing is rudeness on the part of the other person. It is essential to try to observe these differences in colleagues, patients and friends. For the Thai person, UK greetings and partings sometimes seem excessive.

Another example of leaving differences can be observed in restaurants. In a UK restaurant, the time to leave is usually negotiated and 'flagged up' in various ways. One of the party may, for example, say, 'It's quite late, I must be going soon'. In some Chinese and south-east Asian cultures, all parties leave as soon as the last person has finished eating. If this does not occur, then the act of getting up to leave appears almost to be a joint but spontaneous act.

Please and thank you

Another cultural variable is the degree to which people use the terms 'please' and 'thank you' – or their appropriate, linguistic equivalents. Although Indonesia and Thailand are very 'polite' cultures, the terms are not widely used. In the UK, not using them tends to be viewed as an example of 'bad manners'. However, in some cultures, overuse of these terms may be deemed examples of brashness or servility or felt to be just plain unnecessary. The Thai response is noted as follows:

> *Thais still say thank you less than the average well-bred farang ... Whereas we believe that 'please' and 'thank you' are basic provisions of a good upbringing, high-born Thais view the matter quite differently ... For them, such expressions are rarely necessary because social position already indicates which way gratitude is due – from the bottom up. If you help them, that counts as recognition of the nature of things.*
>
> (Redmond, 1998)

The problem for the unaware counsellor is that he or she may encounter these variations in the use of please and thank you as rudeness. Exploring cultural differences is vital for those who would counsel the culturally different.

Compliments

Cultures vary in the ways in which they treat or give compliments. Within UK culture, it is common to belittle a compliment once it is given. It is not unusual for the hearer to dismiss the compliment with a phrase such as 'not really'. In other cultures, it is not uncommon for compliments to be returned. Valdes (1986) gives the following example of a conversation between two Iranian friends:

> *Your shoes are nice.*
> *It is your eyes which can see them that are nice.*

As a rule, Thai people seem to enjoy paying each other, and other people, compliments. This is part of the more general principle (of kreng jai) that we should put others before ourselves and help to make sure that they feel comfortable and at ease.

Answering questions

In a UK or US context, people expect others to answer questions clearly and unambiguously. In some cultures, however, it is considered rude to say 'no' as an answer to a question. The Japanese 'no', for example, if given at all, will be given with a sigh – indicating the speaker's reluctance to use it. The Chinese 'no' is more likely to be worded 'that may be difficult' to avoid the problem (Varner and Beamer, 1995).

Similarly, in some cultures, giving very direct answers to questions, if those questions are posed by persons of senior status, is frowned upon. Again, 'no' answers are often given only very reluctantly. Further, students may worry about offering a 'challenging' response to a teacher's question in class. Someone from a south-east Asian background is likely to be loath to force a teacher to question his own statements. To do this would mean 'loss of face' on the part of both the student and the teacher. This goes some way to meet the criticism, often heard in UK nursing colleges, that 'Overseas students won't criticise or debate issues in class'.

Turn taking

In any conversation between two or more people, there is a time for a person to speak and a time to be silent or to listen. This is known as 'turn taking'. In many so-called Western cultures, this happens in a fairly formal way. One person speaks while the others listen. If someone interrupts, he or she may well apologise for the fact and withdraw. However, in other cultures, the timing of such turn taking varies considerably and it may not be considered 'bad manners' to speak at the same time as another person. To the unfamiliar, this can be confusing. The current writer recalls many phone conversations with a Thai friend that the writer used to punctuate with 'sorry', because both parties seemed to be speaking at once! Learning that this can be a cultural norm can help smooth out misunderstandings of this sort.

Similarities in communication

Despite cultural differences, there are some behaviours and ways of communicating that seem to be universal. Almost all cultures appreciate politeness and respect between communicators (Brown and Levinson, 1987). Most languages have an equivalent of 'hello' as a form of greeting and have rules about the freedom with which people can use forms of other people's names. Using given names is usually the prerogative of friends and seniors (however, in Thailand, for example, given names are used routinely but may be prefaced by a title: 'Mr David' or 'Professor Sarah').

In most cultural groups, it is appreciated if the visitor or foreigner attempts to use the local language. British and American people have probably become lazy about learning other languages because of the seeming universality of the use of English. If the visitor moves out of large cities and into rural environments, however, it quickly becomes clear that English is not so 'universally' spoken.

The process of learning cultural differences – both in communication and more generally – is not always without pain and a certain sense of loss. The 'enculturation process' (a process of cultural adaptation) can also involve a loss of one's own sense of culture, as Hoffman so graphically illustrates in this description by a Polish student living in England:

> *My mother says I'm becoming English. This hurts me, because I know she means I'm becoming cold. I'm no colder than I've ever been, but I'm learning to be less demonstrative. I learn this from a teacher who, after contemplating the gesticulations with which I help myself describe the digestive system of a frog, tells me to 'sit on my hands and then try talking'. I learn my new reserve from people who take a step back when we talk because I'm standing too close, crowding them. Cultural distances are different, I learn in a sociology class, but I know it already.*
>
> (Hoffman, 1989)

Although the examples in this chapter, which have been used to highlight some of the cultural differences in communication, have often been drawn from what traditionally have been called 'East' and 'West', it is not particularly helpful or accurate to think in these terms, especially as most societies, including the UK, are now multi-cultural. Therefore, most counsellors are likely to come into contact with patients from other societies or cultures who may, on occasions or in certain circumstances, communicate differently.

Although differences between cultures are often most noticeable between those physically distanced from each other, this need not be the case (the French, for example, usually shake hands on meeting friends: British people tend not to with the same frequency).

PHATIC COMMUNICATION

Phatic communication is an everyday feature of interaction. First used by the anthropologist Malinowski (1922, 1923) – although he used the phrase 'phatic communion' – the term is used to refer to 'language used in free, aimless, social intercourse' (Malinowski, 1922). Brown and Levinson (1987) observed that for such talk, 'The subject of talk is not as important as the fact of carrying on a conversation that is amply loaded with ... markers of emotional agreement'. The *Hutchinson Encyclopaedia* (2000) defines phatic communication as, 'Denoting speech as a means of sharing feelings or establishing sociability rather than for the communication of information and ideas'. Discussing, on the Internet, speech in organisations, Prusak notes:

> *There's a wonderful phrase used by anthropologists called phatic speech. It's not emphatic, but phatic. And that is speech in which it's*

not the content that matters, but the fact that you're saying it to bond with another person, or doing it as a ritual. It's like saying, 'How are you?' to someone. It's a phatic statement. You may not really give a damn. It's sort of ritualistic. And it's saying, 'I acknowledge your presence'. A lot of that sort of speech you're talking about is phatic speech. It means, 'Let's get together. We all trust each other. Here's who we are.'

(Prusak, 2003)

We might think of phatic communication as 'ordinary chat' or 'small talk'.

Examples of phatic communication are scattered throughout most conversations. Most greetings and acknowledgements are phatic. An obvious example of a phatic exchange is as follows:

Hi! How are you getting on?
I'm OK thanks. How about you?
Yes, fine, thanks.
Good. I'm not doing so badly!

Note that, in such an exchange, the point is not to establish the health status of the other person but simply to acknowledge his or her presence and to establish that 'we are friends'. In this way, phatic communication can be compared and contrasted with information requesting and receiving. In the phatic exchange, the content of the conversation is not important. The point of such communication is to establish or re-establish social relationships.

The degree of phatic communication used in any culture probably varies. Cooper and Cooper (1991) acknowledge that, without learning Thai, the visitor to Thailand is unlikely to get into a 'meaningful conversation' and that they are likely to remain at the superficial level. However, they also comment on one form of conversation that comes under the heading of phatic:

One of the most pleasant aspects of Thai small talk is the Thai zest for flattery. Try to keep your ego within limits when everything about you is being praised. Height, hair, eyes and skin colour are all acceptable subjects for praise. Having admitted to being over 40, you will be told you look 30. Such flattery can cross the sex line (within limits), but try to remember it is only small talk!

(Cooper and Cooper, 1991)

However, such small talk can backfire. The author recalls a Thai colleague noting that, 'You look much better than you did last time you were here!' Sometimes, too, Thai people can appear 'blunt' to Europeans. A Thai friend remarked to the author that 'The difference between you and me is that you are fat and I am not!' At the risk of sounding defensive, the author is not fat by Western standards but might well be by Thai! Topics that are out of bounds for Western visitors may not be for Thais. Salary, weight and age are all topics that may be queried as part of small talk.

Content

Sometimes, phatic communication is almost completely devoid of content or formal meaning. Consider, for example, the use of language by young people. It is not uncommon, at present, for younger people to insert the word 'like' into their conversation in a way that has little formal meaning. An example of such use, in a phatic sense, would be the following statement, 'I mean, I was like "wow"!'.

The statement has little formal content but is used, perhaps, to indicate a certain emotional tone to the listener. Also, the adoption of a language style that includes the fairly random use of the word 'like', may be used by younger people to exclude older people. In this sense, the phatic communication becomes almost a private language or a means of indicating solidarity between people of the same age. It may also be the language of songs, poetry and rapping.

It seems possible that there is sometimes a 'private language' at work in certain forms of mental illness. Certain types of psychotic states are sometimes characterised by unusual use of language. However, it is important to distinguish, perhaps, between the 'modern' or 'popular' use of language as used by young people, and the evidence of some cognitive or emotional disturbance displayed by people with problems in living.

Phatic communication is important. Without it and with only 'informative' communication taking place between two people, conversations would be stark affairs. Consider, for example, the following exchange:

Do you want to talk?
Yes.
When?
Later.
Where?
In private.

This, more normally, is 'padded' with a little phatic communication, perhaps as follows:

Do you want to talk about how you are feeling, at all?
Yes, I do, I think ...
When is the best time for you to sit down and talk, do you think?
Not at the moment, thanks. I want to be quiet for a bit. Later on this afternoon?
Where would you feel most comfortable talking?
In private, I think. In your office, perhaps?

Much of this exchange is redundant as far as understanding and the passing on of information are concerned. However, we are social animals and we do not communicate simply to pass on information but also to develop relationships.

In counselling, the slope at which we move from phatic talk to therapeutic talk is important. On the one hand, it is probably too abrupt simply to ask our clients very direct 'counselling' questions as soon as they arrive. We need a bit of small talk to help both parties settle down. On the other hand, if our counselling conversations remain at the level of the phatic, it seems unlikely that they will be particularly therapeutic.

This chapter has considered the cultural aspects of counselling through some comparisons between UK (or 'Western') cultural forms and those from Thailand. The importance of culture in counselling cannot easily be overstated. To attempt to understand someone's problems is also to have an understanding of his or her cultural background. The problem, perhaps, for both parties (counsellor and client) is that they are likely to take their own cultures for granted. As we saw at the beginning of this chapter, we do not readily reflect on our own cultural influences. Further – and from an ethnocentric point of view – we are likely to believe that what we do is 'right' and that other people in the world are, by and large, like us. However, in studying culture and by exploring cultural differences, we can grow in our awareness of how others live, gain insights into their problems and explore ways in which we may or may not help them. We should never assume that counselling is a universal activity nor should we assume that, if only they had access to it, most people would benefit from it. Much depends on beliefs about (a) self, (b) what it means to have problems and (c) how problems should be resolved. Indeed, even the idea of 'problem resolution' is not a universal one. In the Buddhist culture, for example, the aim is normally to 'accept' rather then to 'resolve' issues. All life is problematic and it is not necessarily the case that there are always answers to problems.

It is, perhaps, worth reflecting on the degree to which these varieties of cultural experience challenge our own views of what it means to be a counsellor and what it means to counsel. Nelson-Jones (2002) offers the following useful comments about the need for counsellors to consider their own cultural assumptions, values and biases:

> *The beliefs held by culturally skilled counsellors and therapists include being sensitive to their own cultural heritage, being comfortable with the differences of clients from other cultures and races, and recognising the limitations of their own competence and expertise. Counsellors and therapist should know about their cultural and racial heritage and how this affects the therapeutic process, understand how oppression, racism and discrimination may affect them personally and in their work and know about the impact of how they communicate on culturally different clients. Skills include seeking out relevant education and training experiences, actively understanding oneself as a cultural and racial being, and seeking a non-racial identity.*

(Nelson-Jones, 2002)

Perhaps the most difficult thing of all is likely to be our own cultural 'blindness'. Because we take for granted our own cultural place, we may find it almost impossible to tease out what is 'cultural' in our belief system and what is learned from other sources. Much of what we do and think occurs without too much thought as to whether or not others applaud those actions or believe what we think to be the case. Without thinking, then, we assume that we 'share' our beliefs and thoughts with millions of others. Clearly, we do not. Cultural differences can be immense and it is only by carefully considering those differences, giving them real thought and, ideally, experiencing the differences at first hand, that we are likely to make the unconscious, conscious. It is only by experiencing a different cultural perspective that we truly illuminate our own. Travel may not always broaden the mind but it certainly helps – at least if we can move away from the usual safety of the well-worn tourist tracks and attempt to engage, directly in a local culture different from our own.

BASIC PRINCIPLES AND CONSIDERATIONS

5

In order to function effectively as a counsellor, it is necessary to consider some principles that can enhance or detract from the relationship. First, it may be useful to look at what may be considered the ideal counselling relationship. Fiedler, in 1950, asked a wide variety of counsellors what they considered to be the ingredients of an ideal therapeutic relationship. The list that was generated by his research included:

- an empathic relationship;
- the therapist and patient relate well;
- the therapist sticks closely to the patient's problems;
- the patient feels free to say what he likes;
- an atmosphere of mutual trust and confidence exists;
- rapport is excellent (Fiedler, 1950).

Note, again, that many of these points are abstractions. What, for example, does it mean to 'relate well' and what does is mean to say that 'rapport is excellent' and who decides?

In 1957, Carl Rogers developed Fiedler's work and identified what he called the six necessary and sufficient conditions for therapeutic change via the counselling relationship. He argued that the following conditions had to exist and continue for a period if counselling was to be effective:

1 Two persons are in psychological contact.
2 The first, whom we shall term the client, is in a state of incongruence – vulnerable or anxious.
3 The second person, whom we shall term the therapist, is congruent and integrated in the relationship.
4 The therapist experiences unconditional regard for the client.
5 The therapist experiences an empathic understanding of the client's internal frame of reference and endeavours to communicate this experience to the client.
6 The communication to the client of the therapist's empathic understanding and unconditional positive regard is to a minimal degree achieved (Rogers, 1957).

There are various problems that we may identify with Rogers' list. First, it is not clear what it means to be 'in psychological contact'. Secondly, we cannot assume, perhaps, that all clients are necessarily 'incongruent' (and, indeed, it is possible to question what this might mean). Thirdly, we might question what it is for the therapist to be 'congruent and integrated in the relationship'.

Whether or not Rogers' claim that these conditions are necessary and sufficient is completely accurate in the philosophical sense of those terms, need not concern us here. What is particularly useful is that the list identifies certain personal qualities that must exist in the person in order for he or she to function as an effective counsellor. The particular personal qualities that Rogers discusses frequently in his writing about counselling are unconditional positive regard, empathic understanding, warmth and genuineness (Rogers, 1967). The need for these qualities is also borne out by the research conducted by Truax and Carkuff (1967), and the characteristics of empathy, warmth and genuineness are often referred to as the 'Truax Triad' (Schulman, 1982). To these qualities may be added those of concreteness and immediacy, also suggested by Carkuff (1969). All of these qualities are worth exploring further as they can lay the foundations for effective counselling in any context.

NECESSARY PERSONAL QUALITIES OF THE EFFECTIVE COUNSELLOR

Unconditional positive regard

Rogers' rather clumsy phrase conveys a particularly important predisposition towards the client, by the counsellor. It is also called *prizing* or even just *accepting*. It means that the client is viewed with dignity and valued as a worthwhile and positive human being. The 'unconditional' prefix refers to the idea that such regard is offered without any preconditions. Often in relationships, some sort of reciprocity is demanded: I will like you (or love you) as long as you return that liking or loving. Rogers is asking that the feelings that the counsellor holds for the client should be undemanding and not requiring reciprocation. Also, there is a suggestion of an inherent goodness within the client. This notion of persons as essentially good can be traced back at least to Rousseau's *Emile*, and is possibly philosophically problematic. Arguably, notions such as goodness and badness are social constructions, and to argue that a person is born good or bad is fraught. However, as a practical starting point in the counselling relationship, it seems to be a good idea that we assume an inherent, positive and life-asserting characteristic in the client. It seems difficult to argue otherwise. It would be odd, for instance, to engage in the process of counselling with the view that the person was essentially bad, negative and unlikely to grow or develop! Thus, unconditional positive regard offers a baseline from which to start the counselling relationship. In order to further grasp this concept, it may be useful to refer directly to Rogers' definition of the notion:

> *I hypothesize that growth and change are more likely to occur the more that the counsellor is experiencing a warm, positive, acceptant attitude towards what* is *the client. It means that he prizes the client, as a person, with the same quality of feeling that a parent feels for his child, prizing him as a person regardless of his particular behaviour at the moment. It means that he cares for his client in a non-possessive way, as a person with potentialities. It involves an open willingness for the client to be whatever feelings*

are real in him at the moment – hostility or tenderness, rebellion or submissiveness, assurance or self-depreciation. It means a kind of love for the client as he is, providing we understand the word love as equivalent to the theologian's term agape, *and not in its usual romantic and possessive meanings. What I am describing is a feeling which is not paternalistic, nor sentimental, nor superficially social and agreeable. It respects the other person as a separate individual and does not possess him. It is a kind of liking which has strength, and which is not demanding. We have termed it positive regard.*

(Rogers and Stevens, 1967)

Unconditional positive regard, then, involves a deep and positive feeling for the other person, perhaps equivalent in the health professions to what Alistair Campbell has called 'moderated love' (Campbell, 1984b). He talks of 'lovers and professors', suggesting that certain professionals profess to love, thus claiming both the ability to be professional and to express altruistic love or disinterested love for others. The suggestion is also that the health professional has a positive and warm confidence in her own skills and abilities in the counselling relationship. Halmos sums this up when he writes:

'You are worthwhile!' and 'I am not put off by your illness!' This moral stance of not admitting defeat is possible for those who have faith or a kind of stubborn confidence in the rightness of what they are doing.

(Halmos, 1965)

For Halmos, the counselling relationship is something of an act of faith. There can be no guarantee that the counselling offered will be effective but the counsellor enters the relationship with the belief that it will be. It is this positive outlook in the counsellor and this positive belief in the ability of the client to change for the better that is summarised in Rogers' notion of unconditional positive regard (Rogers and Stevens, 1967). Such an outlook is also supported by Egan who, in his 'portrait of a helper' says:

They respect their clients and express this respect by being available to them, working with them, not judging them, trusting the constructive forces found in them, and ultimately placing the expectation on them that they will do whatever is necessary to handle their problems in living more effectively.

(Egan, 1982)

Empathic understanding

Empathy is the ability to enter the perceptual world of the other person: to see the world as they see it. It also suggests an ability to convey this identification of feelings to the other person. Kalisch (1971) defines empathy as 'the ability to perceive accurately the feelings of another person and to communicate this understanding to him', whilst Mayeroff

(1972), in a classic book on caring, describes empathic understanding from this point of view of caring for another person:

> *To care for another person I must be able to understand him and his world as if I were inside it. I must be able to see, as it were, with his eyes what his world is like to him and how he sees himself. Instead of merely looking at him in a detached way from outside, as if he were a specimen I must be able to be with him in his world, 'going' into his world in order to sense from 'inside' what life is like for him, what he is striving to be, and what he requires to grow.*
>
> (Mayeroff, 1972)

Gislason offers another perspective on empathy:

> *Empathy is the ability to recognize the sentience and suffering in another being. Empathy is the basis of high-level altruism that does not depend on the barter principle. The ethic of empathy is the Golden Rule: do unto others, as you would have them do to you.*
>
> *Empathy depends on knowing that the other person feels pain as much as you do or will feel happiness as much as you do if they are well treated. If another human is grieving, you feel their suffering and offer help. If another human is injured, you stop everything to help them and you treat their injured body with care to avoid increasing their pain. This ability to feel the experience of others in your own consciousness is one of the great accomplishments of brain evolution.*
>
> (Gislason, 2004)

Empathy is clearly different from sympathy. Sympathy suggests feeling sorry for the other person or, perhaps, identifying with how he feels. If I sympathise, I imagine myself as being in the other person's position and imagine how I would feel. If I empathise, however, I try to imagine how it is to be the other person – feeling sorry for him does not really come into the issue.

As with unconditional positive regard, the process of developing empathy involves something of an act of faith. When we empathise with another person, we cannot know what the outcome of that empathising will be. If we pre-empt the outcome of our empathising, we are already not empathising – we are thinking of solutions and of ways of influencing the client towards a particular goal that we have in mind. The process of empathising involves entering into the perceptual world of the other person without necessarily knowing where that process will lead to. Martin Buber, the Hassidic philosopher, mystic and writer on psychotherapy, summed up well this mixture of willingness to explore the world of the other without presupposing the outcome, when he wrote:

> *A man lost his way in a great forest. After a while another lost his way and chanced on the first. Without knowing what had happened to him, he asked the way out of the woods. 'I don't know,' said the*

first. 'But I can point out the ways that lead further into the thicket, and after that let us try to find the way together.'

(Buber, 1948)

The process of developing empathic understanding is the process of exploring the client's world, with the client neither judging nor suggesting. It can be achieved best through the process of careful attending and listening to the other person and, perhaps, by use of the skills known as *reflection* discussed in a later chapter of this book (p.154). Essentially, though, it is also a way of being, a disposition towards the client, a willingness to explore and intuitively allow the other person to express himself fully. Again, as with unconditional positive regard and with all aspects of the client-centred approach to counselling, the empathic approach is underpinned by the idea that it is the client in the end who will find his own way through and will find his own, idiosyncratic answers to his problems in living. To be empathic is to be a fellow traveller, a friend to the person as he undertakes the search. Empathic understanding, then, involves the notion of befriending alluded to in Chapter 1. Just as a friend can (usually!) accept another friend 'warts and all', so the counsellor, in being empathic, is offering such acceptance.

There are, of course, limitations to the degree to which we can truly empathise. Because we all live in different worlds based on our particular culture, education, physiology, belief systems and so forth, we all view that world slightly differently. Thus, to truly empathise with another person would involve actually becoming that other person! Clearly impossible! We can, however, strive to get as close to the perceptual world of the other by listening and attending and by suspending judgement. We can also learn to forget ourselves temporarily and give ourselves as completely as we can to the other person.

In the following dialogue, a young girl, Rebecca, is talking to her social worker about the situation at home. The dialogue illustrates something of the nature of developing empathy:

Rebecca: I don't know, I just don't seem to be getting on with people.
Social worker: When you say people?
Rebecca: I mean my parents. They don't have any idea.
Social worker: They don't have any idea about you?
Rebecca: No, they think that I want to stay at school and go to university and everything. Well, I do, in a way. But I wish they wouldn't push me all the time! They think they have to tell me how to do things all the time.
Social worker: It's as if they want to push you in a certain direction and you're not sure whether or not you want to go that way.
Rebecca: That's exactly it! I don't know what I want to do any more! They push me so much that I don't know what I want!
Social worker: And that's upsetting you?
Rebecca: Yeah, a lot ... I get upset easily these days and I'm sure it's got a lot to do with what's happening at home.

In this example, the two people become closely involved in the conversation, and the social worker, rather than directing the conversation in a particular way, follows the thoughts and feelings that Rebecca expresses. Empathy is developed through this following process and through a willingness to listen to both what is said and what is implied in what is being said. An intuitive ability is just as important in empathy as is technical skill.

Barrett-Lennard (1981, 1993) writes of the *empathy cycle model* and viewed empathy as an intentional, purposeful activity, developed by the counsellor. He envisaged the empathy cycle as comprising five stages, as follows:

Stage one: *Empathic set of the counsellor*. The client is actively expressing some aspect of his or her experiencing. The counsellor is actively attending and receptive.

Stage two: *Empathic resonation*. The counsellor resonates to the directly or indirectly expressed aspects of the client's experiencing.

Stage three: *Expressed empathy*. The counsellor expresses or communicates his or her felt awareness of the client's experiencing.

Stage four: *Received empathy*. The client is attending to the counsellor sufficiently to form a sense of perception of the counsellor's immediate personal understanding.

Stage five: *The empathy cycle continues*. The client then continues or resumes self-expression in a way that provides feedback to the counsellor concerning the accuracy of the empathic response and the quality of the therapeutic relationship (Barrett-Lennard, 1981).

Although it might be argued that Barrett-Lennard's representation of empathy is a little wordy, what *is* highlighted in this cycle is the *process* aspect of empathy and the need, not only for the counsellor to express empathy, but also for the client to be able to *experience* it.

Warmth and genuineness

Warmth in the counselling relationship refers to a certain approachability and willingness to be open with the client. Schulman (1982) notes that the following characteristics are included in the concept of warmth – equal worth, absence of blame, nondefensiveness and closeness. Warmth is a frame of mind rather than a skill and perhaps one developed through being honest with oneself and being prepared to be open with others. It is also about treating the other person as an equal human being. Martin Buber (1958) distinguishes between the I–it relationship and the I–thou (or I–you) relationship. In the I–it relationship, one person treats the other as an object, a thing. In the I–thou relationship, there occurs a meeting of persons, despite any differences there may be in terms of status, background, lifestyle, belief or value systems. In the I–thou relationship there is a sense of mutuality, a sense that can be contagious and is of particular value in the counselling relationship:

In a meaningful friendship, caring is mutual, each cares for the other; caring becomes contagious. My caring for the other helps activate his caring for me; and similarly his caring for me helps activate my caring for him, it 'strengthens' me to care for him.

(Mayeroff, 1972)

What is less clear, however, is the degree to which a counselling relationship can be a mutual relationship. Rogers (1967) argues that the counselling relationship can be a mutual relationship but Buber acknowledges that, because it is always the client who seeks out the counsellor and comes to that counsellor with problems, the relationship is, necessarily, unequal and lacking in mutuality:

He comes for help to you. You don't come for help to him. And not only this, but you are able, *more or less to help him. He can do different things to you, but not help you ... You are, of course, a very important person for him. But not a person whom he wants to see and to know and is able to. He is floundering around, he comes to you. He is, may I say, entangled in your life, in your thoughts, in your being, your communication, and so on. But he is not interested in you as you. It cannot be.*

(Buber, 1966)

Thus warmth must be offered by the counsellor but the feeling cannot necessarily be reciprocated by the client. There is, as well, another problem with the notion of warmth. We each perceive personal qualities in different sorts of ways. One person's warmth is another person's patronage or sentimentality. We cannot guarantee how our presentation of self will be perceived by the other person. In a more general way, however, warmth may be compared to coldness. It is clear that the cold person would not be the ideal person to undertake counselling! Further, our relationships with others tend to be self-monitoring to a degree: we anticipate, as we go, the effect we are having on others and modify our presentation of self accordingly. Thus, we soon get to know if our warmth is suffocating the client or is being perceived by him in a negative way. Certainly this ability to constantly monitor ourselves and our relationships is an important part of the process of developing counselling skills.

Genuineness, too, is an important facet of the relationship. We either care for the person in front of us or we do not. We cannot fake professional interest. We must be interested. Now, clearly, some people will interest us more than others. Often, those clients who remind us at some level of our own problems or our own personalities will interest us most of all. This is not so important as our having a genuine interest in the fact that the relationship is happening at all. The strength of interest is not the important issue, but the commitment to involvement is.

There may appear to be a conflict between the concept of genuineness and the self-monitoring previously alluded to. Self-monitoring may be viewed as artificial or contrived and therefore not genuine. The genuineness discussed here relates to the counsellor's interest in the human relationship that is developing between the two people. Any ways in which that relationship can be enhanced must serve a valuable purpose. It is quite possible to be genuine and yet aware of what is happening: genuine and yet committed to increasing interpersonal competence.

Genuineness starts with self-awareness. This is summed up in Shakespeare's observation:

> *This above all – to thine own self be true;*
> *And it must follow, as the night the day,*
> *Thou canst not then be false to any man.*

(Hamlet, Act 1, Scene 3)

Egan sums up the notion of genuineness in the context of counselling when he identifies the following aspects of it:

> *You are genuine in your relationship with your clients when you:*
> * *do not overemphasise your professional role and avoid stereotyped role behaviours;*
> * *are spontaneous but not uncontrolled or haphazard in your relationships;*
> * *remain open and non-defensive even when you feel threatened;*
> * *are consistent and avoid discrepancies – between your values and your behaviour, and between your thoughts and your words in interactions with clients – while remaining respectful and reasonably tactful. Are willing to share yourself and your experience with clients if it seems helpful.*

(Egan, 1990)

Reflecting on counselling

The discussion about personal qualities of the counsellor hinges on the idea that we are all in agreement about what constitutes 'warmth', 'empathy' and so on. Is this assumption sound? It might be argued that one person's 'warmth' is another person's 'sickliness'. It is worth considering to what degree there is general agreement about the use of these terms.

Concreteness

Concreteness refers to the idea that the counsellor should be clear and explicit in her dealings with the client and should help the client to express himself clearly. This is essential if communication between the two parties is to be successful. Concreteness involves helping the client to put into words those things that are only being hinted at in order that both client and counsellor are understanding what the client is perceiving at any given time. The following conversation demonstrates the counsellor attempting to develop this sense of concreteness:

Client: I don't know, I feel sort of disinterested a lot of the time ... as if no one cared much about what was going on.
Counsellor: You seem to be saying two things: you feel disinterested and you feel that no one cares for you.
Client: They're not interested in what I do.
Counsellor: Other people aren't interested in you?
Client: Yes, that's right. I'm OK ... it's just that other people don't want to know about me.
Counsellor: When you say other people, who do you mean?
Client: You know ... my family ... my wife especially.

In this way, the counsellor helps the client to clarify what he is saying and enables him to be more specific. Without such clarification it is possible for both parties to be talking to each other without either really understanding the other. Whenever the counsellor senses that she is losing the client it is useful for her to return to this concrete approach.

It is important, too, that the counsellor does not mystify the client by overpowering him with technique or with unasked-for interpretations. This is another sense of the notion of being concrete. The client should at no time feel threatened by the counselling relationship nor feel that the counsellor is 'doing something strange'. Sometimes, the person new to counselling will feel more comfortable hiding behind a mystique and a sense of being a therapist. Such behaviour cuts across the notions of remaining warm and empathic. The counselling relationship should remain clear and unmysterious to the client. Rogers (1967) has used the word 'transparent' to describe this sense of openness and clarity.

Immediacy

When people are distressed by the life situation in which they find themselves when they talk in a counselling relationship, there is a temptation for them to spend a considerable amount of time reminiscing about the past. Somehow, it seems safer to talk of the past rather than face feelings in the here and now. One of the tasks of the counsellor is to help the client to identify present thoughts and feelings. In this way, current issues are addressed and problem-solving can relate directly to those present-day issues. This is not to say that the client should never be allowed to talk about the past but to note that the counsellor may function more effectively if she keeps a check on the degree to which such reminiscing occurs. In a sense the present is all there is: the past is past and the future has not yet arrived. The client who talks excessively about how things were avoids the reality of the present.

'DON'TS' IN THE COUNSELLING RELATIONSHIP

Having identified some of the qualities and characteristics that go to make up an effective counselling relationship, it is time to turn to some things that do not enhance it. These can be discussed most easily in the form of a list of 'don'ts'. Like any such list, there will be occasions on which any one of these items may be helpful in the counselling relationship: that is an illustration of how such relationships are unique and unpredictable! As a general rule, however, the following issues run contrary to the qualities identified previously and are best avoided.

Don't ask 'why' questions

(Example: Why do you feel depressed?)

The word 'why' suggests interrogation, probing and a sense of disapproval. Further, the 'why' question can encourage the client to discuss his feelings in a theoretical way. In other words, when the counsellor asks the client why he is depressed, she is inviting him to offer a theory about why he feels that way. In the following example of dialogue between a community psychiatric nurse and her patient, we see this shift from feelings to theory:

Nurse: Tell me a bit more about how you're feeling at the moment.
Patient: It's difficult to say ... I feel depressed, really.
Nurse: Why do you feel like that?
Patient: My mother was depressive ... perhaps I take after her ...

The 'why' question in this example does nothing to help the patient expand on his expression of feeling but leads him immediately to offer a theoretical explanation of his feelings. 'Why' questions are best avoided altogether in the context of counselling, although a considerable effort may have to be exerted on the part of the new counsellor to drop them from her repertoire! 'Why' questions tend to be very frequent ones in everyday conversation, and the temptation to ask them can be very strong. Perhaps, too, they derive from an almost inherent sense of nosiness that most of us feel at some time or another!

Don't use 'shoulds' and 'oughts'

(Example: You realise that what you should do is ...)

Moralising rarely helps. When the counsellor suggests what the other person should do, she forces her own frame of reference, her own value system, on the client. It is difficult to imagine many situations in which a counsellor can really advise another person about what he should do. Possible exceptions to this rule are those situations in which concrete facts are under discussion. For example, a doctor may suggest that a patient should finish a course of medicine. In counselling, however, the issues under discussion are usually the client's problems in living. The counsellor's value system is rarely of use in helping the client to untangle his life and find a solution to his problem.

Don't blame

(Example: I'm not surprised, you've been very stupid.)

As with the question of 'oughts' and 'shoulds', trying to suggest or apportion blame is not constructive. In a sense, it doesn't matter who is to blame in any particular situation. The point is that a situation has occurred and the client is trying to find ways of dealing with it.

Don't *automatically* compare the client's experience with your own experience

(Example: I know exactly what you mean ... I'm like that too ...)

The key word, here, is automatically. Sometimes, shared experience can be helpful to the client. Often, however, it can lead to an exchange of experiences that is neither helpful nor progressive. Luft (1969) uses the descriptor *parallaction* to describe the sorts of parallel conversations that can occur as a result of such comparison. In the following example, two friends are discussing the previous evening:

> *I had a good night, last night. Went to the cinema.*
> *Yes, we went out to a restaurant.*
> *I hadn't seen a film for months.*
> *We don't get out for meals very often.*
> *I saw* Gone With the Wind ... *it must be 30 years old!*
> *Have you seen David in the last few weeks?*

In the conversation, neither person is really listening to the other. Each wants to talk about himself and neither is prepared to hear the other. Clearly, such an exaggerated situation is unlikely to occur in counselling, but it is surprising how such comparisons of experience can lead down blind alleys. An example of how this can occur is as follows. The conversation is between a social worker and her client:

> *Client:* I get very anxious, sometimes ... especially when I've got exams coming up.
> *Social worker:* I suppose everybody does ... I know I do ...
> *Client:* I get to think that I won't make it ... that I'm not good enough.
> *Social worker:* I know what you mean. I thought I wouldn't get my social-work exams ... I got really upset.

The counselling relationship belongs to the client: it is his time to explore his problems. If the counsellor constantly compares her own experience with that of the client, she is taking away some of that time from the client. More importantly, perhaps, she is saying to the client, 'Your problems are my problems'. And yet, it is the client who is coming to see the counsellor and not vice versa! It is likely that, if the counsellor expresses such similarity of experience to the client, the latter will resent it, for how can it be that both have similar problems and yet one has to sort out the other to help solve those problems? Such a contradiction can confuse and irritate the client and spoil the counselling relationship.

Don't invalidate the client's feelings

(Example: Of course you're not angry/depressed/in love ... you just think you are ...)

This sort of judgement is a curious one. It suggests a number of possibilities: (a) the client is not telling the truth, (b) the client doesn't use words appropriately (presumably in accordance with the counsellor's definitions!), or (c) the counsellor is better able to judge the client's feelings than the client himself. Yet such interventions are by no means rare. Rarely are they therapeutic. A more appropriate approach may be to explore the expressed feeling in order to understand more fully the way in which the client is using words to describe feelings.

These, then, are some 'don'ts'. They are approaches to counselling interventions that are best avoided in that they are either heavily prescriptive, judgemental or inappropriate. As we have noted, there will be times when each is appropriate with this client at this point in time – particularly, perhaps, as the counselling relationship develops and both counsellor and client get to know each other better.

QUESTIONS TO CONSIDER PRIOR TO COUNSELLING

Prior to commencing counselling, there are some questions that may usefully be considered in order to establish whether or not I am the appropriate person to counsel this person at this time.

Am I the appropriate person to counsel?

Sometimes we are too close to the person who comes to us for counselling. The concept of *therapeutic distance* is useful here. If we are emotionally too involved with the other person, we are probably too close to him to be able to stand back from him and assess his situation with reasonable objectivity. On the other hand, it is possible to stand too far back and be so detached from the other person that we are unable to appreciate his problems with any sensitivity at all. There would appear to be an optimum position in which to stand in relation to the client so that we are both disinterested and involved. Examples of people with whom we may be too involved include members of our family and close friends. Examples of people from whom we may be too distanced include (paradoxically) those people who present us with a number of problems that are very similar to our own, and those people who are so different to us that we fail basically to even empathise with them.

Have I the time to counsel?

Counselling takes time. It is tempting to think that, at the outset, we may easily be able to afford the time we offer the client. This seems to be no problem when the client is initially depressed and it does not seem unreasonable to offer time. Once the client has begun to unravel some of his problems, the time factor becomes more pressing and it is remarkably easy to find that we are no longer sure that we have the time! It is important that we decide at the outset of the counselling relationship that we will be able to apportion adequate time for the other person. If we cannot, we should consider referring him to someone else.

On the other hand, there is much to be said for structuring the amount of time spent in counselling. It is useful to lay down clear time parameters as to the start and finish of the counselling session. It is often true that real client disclosure occurs towards the end of a counselling session – the important things are said last. If the client has no idea of when the session will end, he will clearly be unable to make these late and important disclosures. This issue of time will be discussed further in the next chapter.

Have I the client's permission to counsel?

It would seem to be a curious notion that counselling is voluntary: no one can be forced to disclose things that he is not ready or willing to disclose. On the other hand, it is easy to pressurise people into thinking that they should be counselled! When this happens, it is arguable that the counselling relationship is no longer a voluntary one: subtle coercion has taken place. It would seem better that it is always the client who seeks out the counsellor and never the counsellor who seeks out the client!

The term 'permission', as it is used here, is nearly always tacit permission: the fact that the client comes to the counsellor at all suggests that he gives permission for counselling to take place. Even when this initial, tacit contract has been established, however, it is important that the counsellor does not become intrusive and attempt to force disclosure where it is not freely offered. It is tempting, at times, for us to believe that disclosure will 'do the other person good'. This is an interesting value judgement but one that may say more about the counsellor's needs than those of the client!

Where will the counselling take place?

In an ideal world, counselling takes place on neutral territory: neither in the client's home nor in the office of the counsellor. Ideally, too, it is conducted in a room that free from distractions, including other people who may knock on the door, telephones that may ring and surroundings that are so overstimulating that they distract the client's or counsellor's attention away from the task in hand. In practice, however, the environment is usually far removed from meeting these ideal criteria. Very often, counselling takes place wherever it occurs. Few people who work in the health professions can engineer the situation to such a degree that they can set up a particularly appropriate environment.

Having said that, there are environmental factors that may be borne in mind in almost all counselling settings. First, the chairs that both people sit in can be of the same height. This helps to create a certain equality in the relationship. If the counsellor sits at a higher or lower level than the client, it will be difficult for the relationship to develop. When the counsellor is sitting on a higher chair than the client, it puts her in a dominant position. When she is sitting on a lower chair, the relationship is such that the client is placed in a dominant position and may find this counterproductive to the telling of his story and to disclosing himself to the counsellor.

A further consideration is a seemingly odd one. It refers to where the counsellor and client sit in relation to the nearest window! It is difficult if either person sits with the window behind them (unless the lights are on!). If the counsellor sits with her back to the window, she will appear as a rather shadowy form because the client will be unable to see her properly. If the client sits in that position, the counsellor will not be able to see him properly and may miss vital aspects of non-verbal communication that can do much to convey particular thoughts and feelings. More suitable positions are well away from windows or ones in which both counsellor and client sit with the window to one side of them.

These are some important practical considerations that the health professional needs to consider prior to setting out as a counsellor. All of these things need to be borne in mind before the specific skills of counselling are considered. Before such skills are discussed in detail, it may be useful to consider some basic principles of counselling that arise out of the literature and out of the discussion raised so far. These may be enumerated as follows:

1 The client knows what is best for him or her.
2 Interpretation by the counsellor is likely to be inaccurate and is best avoided.
3 Advice is rarely helpful.
4 The client occupies a different personal world from that of the counsellor and vice versa.
5 Listening is the basis of the counselling relationship.
6 Counselling techniques should not be overused; however,
7 Counselling can be learned.

BASIC PRINCIPLES OF COUNSELLING

The client knows what is best for him or her

We all perceive the world differently as we have all had different personal histories that colour our views. Throughout our lives we develop a variety of coping strategies and ways of managing that we use when beset by personal problems. Central to client-centred counselling, particularly, is the notion that, given the space and time, we are the best arbiters of what is and what is not right for us. We can listen to other people but in the end we, as individuals, have to decide upon our own courses of action.

Belief in the essential ability of all persons to make worthwhile decisions for themselves arises from the philosophical tradition known as existentialism (Macquarrie, 1973; Pakta, 1972). Existentialists argue, amongst other things, that we are born free and that we 'create' ourselves as we go through life. For the existentialist, nothing is predetermined: there is no blueprint for how any given person's life will turn out. Responsibility and choice lie squarely with the individual: we choose what we will become. Sartre sums up this position when he argues that:

> *Man first of all exists, encounters himself and surges up in the world and defines himself afterwards. If man, as the existentialists see him, is not definable, it is because to begin with he is nothing. He will not be anything until later and then he will be what he makes of himself.*

> (Sartre, 1973)

No one is free in all respects. We are born into a particular society, culture, family and body. On the other hand, our psychological make-up is much more fluid and arguably not predetermined. We are free to think and feel. One of the aims of the counselling relationship is to enable the client to realise this freedom to think and feel and, therefore, to act.

Once a person has to some extent recognised this freedom, he begins to realise that he can change his life. This is a central issue in the humanistic approach to counselling: that people can change (Shaffer, 1978). They do not have to be weighed down by the past or by their conditioning: they are more or less free to choose their own future. And no one can choose that future for them. Hence the overriding principle that clients know what is best for them.

Interpretation by the counsellor is likely to be inaccurate and is best avoided

To interpret, in this sense, is to offer the client an explanation of his thinking, feeling or action. Interpretations are useful in that they can help us to clarify and offer a framework on which the client may make future decisions. However, they are best left to the client to make.

As we have seen, we all live in different perceptual worlds. Because of this, another person's interpretation of my thinking, feeling or action will be based on that person's experience, not mine. That interpretation is, therefore, more pertinent to the person offering it than it is to me, coloured as it is bound to be by the perceptions of the other person. Such colouring is usually more of a hindrance than a help. Often, too, interpretations are laced with moral injunctions – oughts and shoulds. Thus, an interpretation can quickly degenerate into moralistic advice that may lead to the client feeling guilty or rejecting the advice because it does not fit in with his own belief or value system.

Advice is rarely helpful

Attempts to help 'put people's lives right' is fraught with pitfalls. Advice is rarely directly asked for and rarely appropriate. If it is taken, the client tends to assume that 'That's the course of action I would have taken anyway', or he becomes dependent on the counsellor. The counsellor who offers a lot of advice is asking for the client to become dependent. Eventually, of course, some of the advice turns out to be wrong and the spell is broken: the counsellor is seen to be 'only human' and no longer the necessary lifeline perceived by the client in the past. Disenchantment quickly follows and the client–counsellor relationship tends to degenerate rapidly. It is better, then, not to become an advice-giver in the first place.

There are exceptions to this principle where giving advice is appropriate – advice about caring for wounds, taking medication and health education, for example. In the sphere of personal problems, however, giving advice is rarely appropriate. Sartre (1973) notes with some irony, that we tend to seek out people who we think will give us a certain sort of advice, the sort that we would tend to give ourselves! A further indication, perhaps, that it is better to enable the client to formulate his or her own advice rather than our supplying it.

The client and counsellor live in different 'personal worlds'

The fact that we have had varied experiences, have different physiologies and differing belief and value systems means that we perceive the world through different frames of reference. We tend to act according to our particular belief about how the world is. What happens next, however, is dependent upon how the world really is. If there is a considerable gap between our personal theory of the world and how the world actually is, we may be disappointed or shocked by the outcome of our actions. We may experience dissonance between what we believe to be the cause and what actually is.

It is important for the counsellor to realise that her own belief system may not be shared by the client and that the client may not see the world as she does. This is a basic starting point for the development of empathy in the relationship. To try to enter the frame of reference of the client accurately is one of the most important aspects of the relationship. It may also be one of the hardest, for we are always being invaded by our own thoughts, feelings, beliefs and values as we counsel.

A useful starting point is for the counsellor to explore her own belief and value systems before she starts. Simon *et al.* (1978) offer a series of useful exercises in the clarification of values. It is often surprising how contradictory and inconsistent our belief and value systems are! Once we are able to face some of these contradictions, we may be better able to face the contradictions in the client.

The counsellor's task is to attempt to enter and share the personal world of the client. That view usually changes as counselling progresses (Rogers and Dymond, 1978), after which the client may no longer feel the need for the counsellor. When this happens, the counsellor must develop her own strategies for coping with the separation that usually follows. Counselling is a two-way process. While the client's personal world usually changes, so may the counsellor's. The counselling relationship can, then, be an opportunity for growth and change for the counsellor as well as for the client.

Listening is the basis of the counselling relationship

To really listen to another person is the most caring act of all and takes skill and practice. Often when we claim to be listening, we are busy rehearing our next verbal response, losing attention and failing to hear the other person. Listening involves giving ourselves up completely to the other person in order to fully understand him or her.

We cannot listen properly if we are constantly judging or categorising what we hear. We must learn to set aside our own beliefs and values and to suspend judgement. We must also learn to develop *free-floating attention* – the ability to listen to the changing ebb and flow of the client's verbalisations and not to rush to pull them back to a particular topic. In this sense, what the client is talking about now is what is important. It is a process of offering free attention; of accepting, totally, the other person's story and accepting that his or her version of how the world is may be different but just as valid as our own.

We need to listen to the metaphors, the descriptions, the value judgements and the words that the client uses: they are all indicators of his or her personal world. So too, are facial expressions, body movements, eye contact (or lack of it) and other aspects of non-verbal communication.

Counselling techniques should not be overused

If we can arm ourselves with a whole battery of counselling techniques, perhaps learned through workshops and courses, we stand to run into problems. The counsellor who uses too many techniques may be perceived by the client as artificial, cold and even uncaring. Perhaps we have all encountered the neophyte counsellor whose determined eye contact and stilted questions make us feel distinctly uncomfortable! It is possible to pay so much attention to techniques that they impede listening and communication.

Some techniques, such as the use of questions, reflections, summary, probing and so forth, are very valuable. They must, however, be used discreetly, and the human side of the counsellor must show through the techniques at all times. In the end, it is the quality of the relationship that is more important than any techniques that may be used.

Counselling can be learned

Counselling, arguably, is not something that comes naturally to some and not to others. We can all develop listening skills and the ability to communicate clearly with other people, which is the basis of effective counselling. The skills can be learned through personal experience and lots of practice, which may be gained in experiential-learning workshops for the development of counselling skills and through the actual process of doing counselling.

The list of principles offered here is not claimed to be exhaustive. It attempts to identify some of the important principles involved and to explain them. The next task will be to consider the process of the counselling relationship and to identify some of the stages that the relationship passes through as the client explores his or her world.

BASIC PRINCIPLES AND CONSIDERATIONS IN COUNSELLING IN THE HEALTH PROFESSIONS

The degree to which the issues identified previously will fit with a particular health profession will vary according to the nature of the role of those professionals. For the physiotherapist, for example, the need to give clear and exact information may often be more of a priority than talking through emotional problems. For the nurse working with elderly people, the role of listening and of listening to relatives may play a large part in the overall caring role. Given the different sorts of professional relationships that abound in the professions, it is important to modify the principles discussed in this chapter accordingly. Having said that, the principles apply fairly broadly to almost all relationships in one way or another. They need to be linked, also, to the maps of the counselling relationship discussed in the next chapter and the counselling skills outlined in the following chapters.

MAPS OF THE COUNSELLING RELATIONSHIP 6

Two counselling relationships can never be the same. As we have noted, we all come to counselling, whether as counsellor or as client, from different backgrounds and life experiences. Having said that, it may be helpful to sketch out in broad detail the possible nature of a typical counselling relationship. To this end, we need a *map* that can help us to explore the changing course of what happens between counsellor and client. Like any map, it is never the same as the territory itself. If we consider, for instance, the map of the London underground system, it bears no geographical relationship to the actual layout of the rail network. More importantly, though, it gets us around London! So it may be with a map of the counselling process. It may never match exactly what happens in counselling, but it can help us to move through the relationship with greater ease.

Three different sorts of maps are offered here. The first is an eight-stage model that considers the changing and developing nature of the relationship. The second offers a very practical method of structuring the counselling process. The third considers three dimensions of counselling as a means of evaluating the relationship as it develops. The three can be used in various ways. First, one can be chosen as a way of working in counselling – the map chosen by the counsellor as the preferred one to be used in everyday practice, rather in the way that a person may use an AA map in preference to an Ordnance Survey map. Alternatively, any combination of the three may be used to highlight different aspects of counselling. The first, for example, may give a general overview of the whole relationship. The second may offer a practical set of steps that can be worked through. The third may highlight various aspects of counselling work that must be considered at various points throughout the relationship. The maps are not mutually exclusive: they all relate to the same thing and can be used together.

AN EIGHT-STAGE MAP OF THE COUNSELLING RELATIONSHIP

The stages in the model are enumerated as follows. It is suggested that this model offers a broad overview of how the relationship, typically, will unfold. Now not all relationships will necessarily pass through each of the stages: some will reach certain stages and not others. Other relationships will by-pass certain of the stages. The aim of the map is to offer a broad overview of the sorts of potential stages that many relationships will move through:

Stage one: meeting the client;
Stage two: discussion of surface issues;
Stage three: revelation of deeper issues;

Stage four: ownership of feelings and possibly, emotional release;

Stage five: generation of insight: the client's life is viewed by him in a different light;

Stage six: problem-solving/future planning;

Stage seven: action by the client;

Stage eight: disengagement from the counselling relationship by the client.

Stage one: meeting the client

In this first stage, the client meets the counsellor for the first time. Each is sounding out the other and setting tacit ground rules for the relationship. In a sense, both client and counsellor are 'on their best behaviour'. This is an important part of the larger counselling relationship in that it sets the tone for the whole dialogue. The skilled counsellor will set the client at ease in this stage and encourage him to gently spell out his reasons for talking to the counsellor. It is likely that both parties will experience some anxiety in this phase of the relationship: the client will want to be seen in a good light by the counsellor and the counsellor will be keen to ensure that the client feels comfortable in her company.

Stage two: discussion of surface issues

As the relationship slowly unfolds, the client will begin to tell his story or identify his problems in living. These will usually start with 'safe' disclosures: the deeper issues will reveal themselves later. Murray Cox (1978) offers a useful device for identifying the level of disclosure in the counselling relationship. He distinguishes between three levels of self-disclosure by the client: first, second and third levels. First-level disclosures are safe and relatively unimportant disclosures. Examples of first-level disclosures will vary according to the context but examples may be:

> *It took me a long time to get here today.*
> *It took me a long time to find your office.*
> *I haven't been to this part of the town before.*

These are usually fairly polite statements that act as 'feelers' in the relationship. They serve to test out the relationship in terms of trust and confidence. As the relationship deepens, so the level of self-disclosure increases. Level two and three of Cox's model are in the following stage.

Stage three: revelation of deeper issues

Level two of Cox's (1978) model refers to the disclosure of feelings. Again, such disclosures will depend on the individual and the context but examples of such second-level disclosures may be:

> *I feel really angry about that.*
> *I find it very difficult to feel positive about anything.*
> *I'm not happy when I'm at home.*

Second-level disclosures will not occur until the relationship between counsellor and client is sufficiently developed to the point where the client feels confident and trusting with the counsellor. It is a significant indicator that the relationship has deepened when the client begins to offer disclosure of how he is feeling.

Third-level disclosures are those that indicate the really deep, existential concerns of the client – the sorts of things that he may not have disclosed to any other person or has disclosed to very few people. If you stop reading for a moment and think of two things that very few people know about you, those would be third-level disclosures if you revealed them to another person. A clear principle emerges here: the client's potential third-level issues are not necessarily the same as the counsellor's third-level issues and vice versa. There is considerable danger in being misunderstood and in misunderstanding if we forget this. There is a temptation to believe that what troubles us is what troubles most people.

On the other hand, there is a certain paradox arising at this point, for as Rogers (1967) notes, 'What is most personal is most general'. Some of the most difficult things to talk about turn out to be difficult for all of us. There is a certain commonality of human experience that makes it the case that we all share certain fundamental difficulties. However, we would be wrong to assume that it is necessarily true that what I as a counsellor worry about, my clients worry about. Identification with the client is perhaps the most difficult issue here. We must be careful to draw the boundaries between ourselves and the client himself if we are to allow the latter to express his own third-level issues in his own time. It is arguable, too, that we will not allow the client to make third-level disclosures until we are accepting enough and comfortable with ourselves. We can easily and unconsciously put the client in the position of not being able to make these profound disclosures by our being defensive. To really listen to another person talking of his deeper human concerns is often a difficult business. This is yet another reason why we should, as counsellors, develop self-awareness: it may be only when we have faced some of our own third-level problems that we will allow the client to discuss his.

Third-level disclosures are often heralded by certain changes in the client. He may become quieter, his facial expression may change and eye contact may be less sustained. If the person is disclosing something that has taken him considerable courage to disclose, that disclosure is bound to be accompanied by considerable anxiety. Often, if the counsellor sits quietly and attentively, the client will make the disclosure. If the counsellor is too talkative or questioning, the disclosure may be avoided all together. The timing of third-level disclosures by the client is fairly critical, and, if the circumstances of the relationship are not optimal and the disclosure *has* been made, all that is often necessary is for the counsellor to sit and listen to the client as he struggles to make sense of what has happened. Little intervention is needed at this point, and the counsellor should avoid the temptation to 'overtalk' the client because of her own anxiety at being offered the disclosure (Heron, 1986).

Examples of typical third-level disclosures are difficult to describe. More than any other sort, they tend to be idiosyncratic and defined by the context of the relationship. Many are metaphorical in nature. For example, the client may say, 'I never really had a childhood' or 'I realise that I have never felt anything really'. Others are more direct:

> *I've never loved my wife.*
> *I hated my parents more than anything else.*
> *I'm a transvestite.*

Third-level disclosures do not occur all together: they tend to be made at various points throughout the counselling relationship. Figure 6.1 demonstrates what may be termed the *rhythm of counselling* – the cycle of disclosures that starts with level one, deepens to level two and deepens still further to level three. It then, typically, lightens again and the client gradually returns to less difficult topics. Then the cycle restarts and the relationship deepens again. It may be important that this changing of level from deeper to lighter occurs. Too much disclosure, too quickly, can lead to the client feeling embarrassed, and very deep disclosure made much too quickly can lead to the client returning only to first-level disclosures, never to return to the more profound issues. Indeed, such sudden deep disclosure may lead to the client's subsequent withdrawal from the relationship altogether. Having made this very sudden disclosure, the client leaves feeling embarrassed and finds it difficult to return to face the counsellor again.

If such sudden, deep disclosure seems imminent at the beginning of a counselling relationship, it is sometimes sensible to lighten the conver-

Figure 6.1

The rhythm of counselling (based on Cox, 1978).

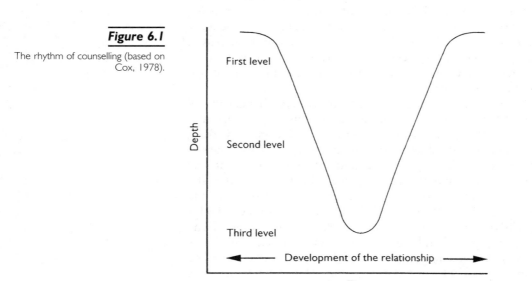

sation and allow the disclosure rate to slow down. In this way, the client discloses more gently and stands to feel more comfortable in the following sessions.

Third-level disclosures would seem to be an important part of the counselling process. The very fact that a client can articulate some of his deeper fears, anxieties and problems means that the possibility of resolving them is more likely. Also, the process of self-disclosure can often serve to change the client's perceptions of his problems. A considerable amount of energy is taken up with holding onto these more profound problems. The disclosure of them is often accompanied by a great sense of relief.

Clearly, third-level disclosures need to be received and heard by the counsellor with great tact. It is important that the client does not feel patronised or judged after such a disclosure. The very process of disclosure, itself, has been difficult enough, without the counsellor making the person feel more uncomfortable. As we have seen, the counsellor is often required to do nothing but listen. Also, too, the disclosure may be followed by a period of silence on the part of the client as he pieces together his thoughts on what he has said.

It is important to note that *another person's third-level disclose would not, necessarily, be our own third-level disclosure.* In other words, what one person finds difficult to disclose, another person does not – and, conversely, what *we* find difficult to disclose, other people may not. We need to listen to the tone of the disclosure, observe the non-verbal behaviours that accompany it and note the context in which the third-level disclosure is made. Very often, third-level disclosures are made after a pause or, conversely, very quickly – as if it might be easier to get the thing said. Sometimes, too, third-level disclosures come out of the blue: the client drops what is obviously an important statement into the middle of a more 'chatty' piece of dialogue. The skill, for the counsellor, remains the *recognition* of third-level and important personal disclosures. There is further discussion of Cox's model later in the chapter.

Stage four: ownership of feelings and possible emotional release

When the client has begun to talk about the very profound problems of his life, the tone of the dialogue will often change in a very significant way. The client stops talking about the feelings that he has in a general or detached sort of way and begins to experience the feelings themselves. In other words, the feelings begin to accompany the conversation. This can be described as *ownership* of those feelings. An example of the change in emotional state is illustrated in the following passage, 'Sometimes ... sometimes when I'm at home, I get quite angry with various members of the family ...' and 'Something odd is happening ... I'm feeling angry now ... I'm really furious! I won't be treated like that! It's my son, David ... I'm really mad with him ...'. The change can be quite dramatic as the client begins to thaw out and experience the feelings that he may have been bottling up for a considerable period. Sometimes the switch to experiencing the feelings as they are talked about is only transitory and the client quickly switches back to the safety of talking in the abstract. Sometimes, however, the sense of experiencing the feeling leads to more profound release of emotion. Thus, as the feelings are experienced, the person expresses those emotions through tears, anger or fear – cathartic release. Sometimes, too, the embarrassment of the sudden realisation of feeling leads to expression of that feeling in the form of laughter (Heron, 1989). This embarrassed laughter may quickly tip over into tears, anger or fear. Again, the counsellor's role, here, is to allow the expression of feelings, the cathartic release. The tears, anger or fear may last for a few moments or may be sustained. The longer the counsellor can refrain from jumping to rescue the client from his feelings, the more likely it is that the client will benefit from the release.

Stage five: generation of insight: the client's life is viewed by him in a different light

It would seem that cathartic release generates insight (Heron, 1977b). If we can allow the expression of pent-up feeling and not interrupt the expression or attempt to interpret it, the client will come to view his life situation differently. It is as though the expression of pent-up feeling releases in the client a natural ability to think more rationally and see things more clearly. Often all that is required in this stage is to sit quietly as the client experiences that insight and verbalises it. There is, of course, no reason to suppose that clients will necessarily verbalise the insights gained through cathartic release but their non-verbal behaviour will usually indicate that they are piecing the insights together. Often they will sit looking away from the counsellor, clearly thinking deeply. The temptation is often to interrupt that process with a series of questions but, as a general rule, the process is best left undisturbed. The gain in insight is usually greater if the client can be allowed the time and space to appreciate it.

Stage six: problem-solving/future planning

The expression of pent-up emotions and the insight gained through its release are not enough in themselves. The client still has to consider ways in which he is going to use that insight to change certain aspects of his life. Thus, once the tears have been shed and the perceptual shift has occurred, the client is often helped by the use of a practical problem-solving cycle (Burnard, 1985). Figure 6.2 offers one such cycle. In phase one, the problem is clearly defined. This comes about through talking through the client's situation carefully and helping him to express what he sees as the problem as concisely as he can. In the second phase, the client and the counsellor generate as many possible solutions to that problem as they can. This process is sometimes known as brainstorming and involves considering every possibility, both rational and sensible and the more bizarre! Such a process can open up a fruitful and creative series of possible solutions that a plainly logical approach may not.

Phase six:
problem resolution:
no further action
required

Phase one: *problem identification:*
the problem is clearly defined

Phase two: *generation of possible
solutions:* the client and
counsellor brainstorm possible
solutions, both practical and
impractical. No solutions
are rejected at this stage

Phase three: *prioritisation:* the
client draws up a short list of
possible solutions

Phase five:
action: the solution
is applied. If it works, the client
moves to phase six. If not, he
returns to phase one

Phase four:
choice of solution: one solution
is chosen and its implementation
planned

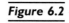

Figure 6.2

A problem-solving cycle.

In phase three, a short list of possible solutions is drawn up, and in stage four, the client makes a decision about which solution he will choose. Next, the solution is put into operation in the client's life and, if it works, the problem is resolved. If it does not, the problem-solving cycle can be worked through again, perhaps with a clearer definition of the problem.

Stage seven: action

As we noted at the outset, counselling must have a practical end. In this case, as the client comes to identify his problems of living, talk them through with the counsellor, express pent-up emotion and identify solutions, it is important that he introduces changes in his life. Indeed, if no such changes take place, the counselling is of very little use. This action stage of the relationship takes place away from the counsellor–client meetings and consists of the client trying new ways of living. During this stage, the client will obviously need a considerable amount of support from the counsellor but essentially, this will be the client's independent aspect of the relationship. It will also involve a growing independence on the part of the client who comes to realise that he can live without the counsellor and can make life choices without the counsellor's help. This stage shades into the next.

Stage eight: disengagement from the counselling process

This is what it says. Gradually, or sometimes abruptly, the client feels more and more able to cope on his own. Thus, the counselling relationship comes to an end. This may create considerable anxieties in both counsellor and client. The relationship has developed into a close one and, to some degree, both people have become dependent on each other. The skilled counsellor is one who can effectively help in the disengagement process and not require the client to remain attached to her. This is the ultimate act of altruism, perhaps. It is the process of saying goodbye, with no strings attached. The goodbye must be unequivocal and without regret or remorse. The counsellor has completed her task and the client has learned to live for himself and with himself. Often, old issues of separation come to the fore, here. Bowlby (1975) wrote of 'separation anxiety' – the anxiety some people feel when they find a relationship coming to an end. Bowlby hypothesised that such people had experienced difficulties in early separations – in childhood or even in early infancy. Here, again, we find the need for the counsellor's developing self-awareness and the need for her to explore any identified difficulties with separations and with the ends of counselling relationships. It is important that such partings are smooth and that both parties are comfortable with the ending.

Reflecting on counselling

Can you be a counsellor and a personal friend to the client? Should you know the client 'outside' of the professional relationship? This issue involves a considerable number of ethical issues which anybody setting out in counselling should consider.

A THREE-STAGE MODEL OF THE COUNSELLING RELATIONSHIP

The second map for guidance in the process of counselling is Egan's (1990, 2002) three-stage model of the helping relationship. His three stages are:

1 identifying and clarifying problem situations;
2 goal-setting: developing and choosing preferred scenarios;
3 action: moving towards the preferred scenario.

In stage one, the counsellor helps the client to tell his story – to explore his present life situation as he sees it now. Out of that story emerges the specific problems of living that could not have been identified prior to this exploratory process. It is as if the very telling of the story brings out the problems and puts a name to them. Egan notes also, that this stage is useful for exploring 'blind spots' – aspects of the client's life that he had not considered.

In stage two, the client is helped to imagine a possible future situation that would be preferable to the present one. Initially, this often means imagining a variety of possible future scenarios, out of which the client slowly homes in on one. Once this realistic scenario has been discussed, the client and counsellor can identify goals that can help in the achievement of the proposed future state.

In stage three, the client and counsellor devise ways in which the proposed future scenario is achieved. In the first instance, this can be aided by the process of brainstorming, previously described. All possible methods of achieving the desired outcome are identified and then, gradually, a particular approach is chosen out of all the possibilities. Then, an action plan is drawn up in order to aid the achievement of the desired scenario further. The final substage of stage three is action on the part of the client – the time when the client makes the discussion concrete and puts the plan into action, supported by the counsellor.

Egan's (1990, 2002) three-stage model can serve as a useful and practical map in counselling and a means of bringing structure to the process of counselling. The three stages, although interrelated, can be dealt with as separate aspects of counselling and thus the relationship takes shape and has specific goals. Keeping the three stages in mind can help the counsellor to assess where the relationship is going and how it is developing. Obviously, no time limit can be put on how long each of the stages may take to work through with any given person, but using them can ensure that the relationship remains dynamic and forward-moving.

Egan's model in practice

June is an occupational therapist working with a group of young patients in a small psychiatric day hospital. She is approached by one patient, Alice, a girl recently discharged from hospital where she was treated for anorexia nervosa. Alice says that she wants to talk but is unclear about what her problems are. June uses Egan's three-stage model and allows Alice to describe everything that is happening to her at the present time. Thus, a picture of Alice's life emerges. Out of this picture, Alice identifies two problem areas: her overdependent relationship with her mother and her lack of self-confidence. June asks her to clarify how she would like the future to be. Alice talks of greater independence from her mother and an enhanced ability to socialise and mix more easily.

Out of their discussion, June and Alice draw up a list of practical, manageable tasks for the immediate future, including:

1 Alice to set aside time to talk to her mother
2 Alice to consider the practicality of finding a flat or bedsitter near her parents' home
3 Alice and June to work out a social skills training programme for Alice to follow with a group of other day hospital clients
4 Alice to attend a weekend workshop on assertiveness training at a local college.

THREE DIMENSIONS OF THE COUNSELLING RELATIONSHIP

Yet another way of mapping the relationship is in terms of three dimensions: time, depth and mutuality (Cox, 1978). Again, although each dimension overlaps with the other and is dependent on the other, each may be considered separately.

Time

The concept of time in the counselling relationship can be understood in at least two ways. First, there is the logical structuring of the counselling relationship itself. It makes sense for the counsellor to suggest a well-defined period of time for the counsellor–client meeting. Setting a boundary in this way has many advantages: once set, it can be forgotten about by both counsellor and client. Both know how long they will be together and when the session will finish. In an open-ended session, both may be confused about how long the session will last. A stated contract of an hour, for example, overcomes this problem. The contract also means that the client will tend to use the time available constructively. As we have already noted, the client will often disclose important information towards the end of the meeting. If he does not know when that end will come, he may never make the disclosure. Also, an unstructured session may be fine when the counsellor is not busy, but when constraints of work mean that the counselling session has to be truncated, the client may feel rejected. On balance, then, it seems better to structure the time more formally at the outset.

A second, more subtle aspect of time structuring relates to the focus of the counselling in terms of past, present and future. These three aspects may be considered as follows:

1 past – the client's past, personal history;
2 present – the client's present situation and the present situation for the client and counsellor together;
3 future – the client's aspirations, plans and hopes for what is to come.

In counselling those with emotional or psychological problems, it may be useful to consider spending roughly equal time in discussing all three time zones.

Our past experience has much to do with how we view the present. Indeed, what we are in the present may be seen as having grown out of past experience. Both past and present experience will determine, to a greater or lesser extent, how we make use of the future. Some people seem to want to live in the past; perhaps it was more comfortable or acceptable. Others look forward to what may happen in the future and dismiss the past as irrelevant – so much 'water under the bridge'. Tomorrow will always be better than today. Both living in the past and living for the future are, perhaps, unrealistic. To live in the present, with a strong sense of both past and future may be more useful and constructive.

A balanced counselling relationship may take into account all three of these aspects of time. The counsellor may want to ask how the present situation is affected by past events and how the client views the future, given the present climate. If past, present and future are addressed in roughly equal amounts, then the momentum of the relationship remains continuous. There is a sense of continuity running through the relationship.

Depth

The second dimension in this map is depth. This refers to the aspects of intimacy and personal disclosure in the relationship and it depends on the amount of time invested in it. Depth cannot be hurried. It evolves out of the feeling of trust engendered by the client–counsellor process, but it does seem to develop in a cyclical manner. At the beginning of the relationship (and at the beginning of each counselling hour), there is usually a discussion of superficial things (first-level disclosures). As the relationship and the hour develop, so the depth of the relationship increases (through second- and third-level disclosures). The client slowly reveals himself to the counsellor and discloses more and more. Towards the end of the relationship (and the hour), the atmosphere lightens and the counselling relationship moves once again to a more superficial note. Thus, Cox's (1978) three levels of disclosure may be used to assess the depth of the relationship, both on a session-to-session basis and from the point of a longer-term relationship. The three levels that Cox describes are illustrated in Figure 6.3.

First-level disclosures	'Lightweight' and easy disclosures	Example: 'It's warm today and I seem to be in a bit of a hurry about things.'
Second-level disclosures	Disclosures of feelings accompanied by the affect	Example: 'I feel really angry. I mean, I feel angry now!'
Third-level disclosures	Deepest, existential disclosures, perhaps never made before	Example: 'I feel as though I have never really been loved or loved anyone in my life . . . '

Figure 6.3

Three levels of disclosure.

Many factors determine the depth of the relationship. A short list would include the counsellor's ability to empathise with the client, the counsellor's range of skills, the personalities and temperaments of counsellor and client, the degree of 'match' between the two people and the prevailing moods of both people.

First-level disclosures are clearly the easiest to make: they may sometimes merely be conversation. At other times, they signal the move towards greater trust in the counsellor and greater depth in the relationship. Second-level disclosures usually indicate that the client is able to express him or herself more fully at the level of *feelings* and, thus, also indicate a further level of trust in the counselling relationship. Third-level disclosures occur once a considerable amount of work has been done in the counselling relationship and once the client feels able to trust the counsellor with his or her deepest fears or feelings. Paradoxically, though, they may also occur, spontaneously, at *any* stage in the counselling relationship and may cause surprise to both the client and the counsellor. It is also vital that the counsellor *hears* third-level disclosures and does not miss them. Sometimes, they occur so quickly and so spontaneously, that the counsellor is caught unawares and does not really take in the importance of what has been disclosed. Sometimes, though, such disclosures are heralded by the client clearly building up towards 'saying something important'. There may be non-verbal signs. The client's tone of voice may drop, eye contact may be lessened as the client builds up the courage to say what he or she may not yet have said to anyone else. We can, perhaps, take it as something of a compliment that another person trusts us sufficiently to share his or her thoughts and feelings with us at this level. Such disclosure does not, of course, happen in all counselling relationships nor with all people. There are those who find disclosure easier than others. While the three-stage model of disclosure is not foolproof, it does offer some guidance as to the depth that is being experienced in the counselling relationship. A more detailed discussion of the Cox disclosure model is found within the aforementioned debate about the eight-stage counselling model.

Mutuality

The third dimension of structure is mutuality. This refers to the client's and counsellor's shared relationship with each other. As we noted earlier (p.106), Martin Buber referred to the 'I–thou' relationship – the natural unfolding of relationship between two people who know each other on a reasonably equal and intimate level. Carl Rogers (1967) described the process of emerging from what resembled a hypnotic trance at the end of the counselling session. This trancelike state reflects the close nature of the truly mutual client-counselling relationship. Everything outside the relationship is forgotten while the client and counsellor are together – a close bonding occurs.

How does such mutuality develop? Arguably, it arises out of shared experiences and self-disclosure (although limits to this have been discussed). The counselling relationship, far from being a one-way traffic of disclosure from the client to the counsellor, becomes a time when human experiences are pooled. This is not to say that the counsellor should burden the client with her own problems, but to acknowledge that 'disclosure begets disclosure' (Jourard, 1964). I feel more understood when the person to whom I am talking shares something of his or her own experience with me.

To develop mutuality, counsellors have to develop an open, non-defensive and transparent presentation of self. Rather than hiding behind a professional mask, they allow themselves to be seen as they are, warts and all! It is worth noting that professionals who allow themselves to make mistakes occasionally are generally sensed as far more approachable and human than are their highly skilled perfect counterparts. It would seem that affability is a necessary prerequisite of good counselling.

If this mutuality is missing, then the counselling process will remain superficial. If the counsellor always presents a professional facade and never allows the client to know her, then mutuality cannot develop. Mutuality is a measure both of the depth of the relationship and of the counsellor's commitment to the relationship. It develops out of the counsellor's life experience, ability to empathise, skill and genuine commitment to the task.

These, then, are three ways of mapping out the counselling relationship. They differ in approach and degree of detail and perhaps they will appeal to different sorts of counsellors. Whilst no map is essential to counselling, some structure can help the unfamiliar to look a little less frightening. It can also suggest the direction forward and, at best, counselling should always be a dynamic and evolving process, though, at times – like life itself – it will become stuck! Often, it is these periods of being stuck that are some of the most important. If we can stand to stay with the stuckness and even to abandon the map, the result for the client in the long term can be much more rewarding.

MAPS OF THE COUNSELLING RELATIONSHIP AND THE HEALTH PROFESSIONAL

What map a particular health professional chooses in order to bring structure to his or her counselling will depend to a degree on the time available and the nature of the relationship. Where time is limited and a reasonable amount of resolution of a problem must be achieved, Egan's (1990) three-stage model is excellent. It is practical, structured and allows both health professional and client to see where the relationship is going and how it is progressing. Those professionals concerned with longer-term relationships may choose the first and third models described in this chapter, for they emphasise, more, the processes that occur in the development of the counselling relationship. None of the maps, however, is mutually exclusive. Any of the maps may be used in conjunction with any of the others and combined with the use of effective counselling skills described in the following chapters.

7 COUNSELLING SKILLS I: LISTENING AND ATTENDING

Listening and attending are by far the most important aspects of the counselling process. Often, the best counselling is that which involves the counsellor solely listening to the other person. Unfortunately, most of us feel that we are obliged to talk! Unfortunately, too, it is 'overtalking' by the counsellor that is least productive. If we can train ourselves to give our full attention to and really listen to other people, we can do much to help them. First, we need to discriminate between the two processes: attending and listening.

ATTENDING

Attending is the act of truly focusing on the other person. It involves consciously making ourselves aware of what the other person is saying and of what he or she is trying to communicate to us. Figure 7.1 demonstrates three hypothetical zones of attention. The zones may help to further clarify this concept of attending and have implications for improving the quality of attention offered to the client.

Figure 7.1

Three possible zones of attention.

ZONE ONE: *attention out* When attention is focused in this zone, the counsellor is fully listening to the client and paying attention to all verbal and non-verbal cues.	ZONE TWO: *attention in* When attention is focused in this zone, the counsellor is caught up with his/her own thoughts and feelings. Attention to the client is only partial.
	ZONE THREE: *attention focused on fantasy* When attention is focused in this zone, the counsellor is busy trying to work out *theories* about the client. Rather than giving full attention, he/she is *interpreting* what is going on.

Zone one, in the diagram, represents the zone of having our attention fully focused 'outside' of ourselves and on the environment around us or, in the context of counselling, on the client. When we have our attention fully focused 'out' in this way, we are fully aware of the other person and not distracted by our own thoughts and feelings.

There are some simple activities, borrowed from meditation practice, that can help and enhance our ability to offer this sort of attention. Here is a particularly straightforward one. Stop reading this book for a moment and allow your attention to focus on an object in the room that you are in: it may be a clock, or a picture or a piece of furniture – anything. Focus your attention on the object and notice every aspect of it: its shape, its colour, its size and so forth. Continue to do this for at least one minute. Notice as you do this, how your attention becomes fully absorbed by the object. You have focused your attention 'out'. Then discontinue your close observation. Notice what is going on in your mind. What are your thoughts and feelings at the moment? When you do this, you shift your attention to zone two: the 'internal' domain of thoughts and feelings. Now shift the focus of your attention out again and onto another object. Study every aspect of it for about a minute. Notice, as you do this, how it is possible to consciously and awarely shift the focus of your attention in this way. You can will yourself to focus your attention outside of yourself. Practice at this conscious process will improve your ability to fully focus attention outside of yourself and onto the client.

Clearly, if we are to pay close attention to every aspect of the client, it is important to be able to move freely between zones one and two. In practice, what probably happens in a counselling session is that we spend some time in zone one, paying full attention to the client and then we shuttle back into zone two and notice our reactions, feelings and beliefs about what they are saying, before we shift our attention back out. The important thing is that we learn to gain control over this process. It is no longer a haphazard, hit-and-miss affair but we can learn to focus attention with some precision. It is not until we train ourselves to consciously focus attention 'out' in this way that we can really notice what the other person is saying and doing.

Zone three in the diagram involves fantasy: ideas and beliefs that we have that bear no direct relation to what is going on at the moment but concern what we think or believe is going on. When we listen to another person, it is quite possible to think and believe all sorts of things about him. We may, for example, think, 'I know what he's really trying to tell me. He's trying to say that he doesn't want to go back to work, only he won't admit it – even to himself!' When we engage in this sort of 'internal dialogue' we are working within the domain of fantasy. We cannot 'know' other things about people, unless we ask them, or as Epting puts it, 'If you want to know what another person is about, ask them, they might just tell you!' (Epting, 1984). We often think that we do know what other people think or feel, without checking with them first. If we do this, it is because we are focusing on the zone of fantasy: we are engaged in the processes of attribution or interpretation. The problem with these sorts of processes is that, if they are wrong, we stand to develop a very distorted picture of the other person! Our assumptions naturally lead us to other assumptions, and if we begin to ask questions directly generated by those assumptions, our counselling will lack clarity and our client will end up very confused!

A useful rule, then, is that, if we find ourselves within the domain of fantasy and we are 'inventing' things about the person in front of us, we stop and if necessary check those inventions with the client to test the validity of them. If the client confirms them, all well and good: we have intuitively picked up something about the client that he was, perhaps, not consciously or overtly telling us. If, on the other hand, we are wrong, it is probably best to abandon the fantasy all together. The fantasy, invention or assumption probably tells us more about our own mental make-up than it does about that of our client! In fact, these 'wrong' assumptions can serve to help us gain more self-awareness. In noticing the wrong assumptions we make about others, we can reflect on what those assumptions tell us about ourselves.

Awareness of focus of attention and its shift between the three zones has implications for all aspects of counselling. The counsellor who is able to keep attention directed out for long periods is likely to be more observant and more accurate than the counsellor who is not. The counsellor who can discriminate between the zone of thinking and the zone of fantasy is less likely to jump to conclusions about her observations or to make value judgements based on interpretation rather than on fact.

What is being suggested here is that we learn to focus directly on the other person (zone one) with occasional moves to the domain of our own thoughts and feelings (zone two) but that we learn, also, to attempt to avoid the domain of fantasy (zone three). It is almost as though we learn to meet the client as a 'blank slate': we know little about clients until they tell us who they are. To work in this way in counselling is, almost paradoxically, a much more empathic way of working. We learn, rapidly, not to assume things about the other person but to listen to him and to check out any hunches or intuitions we may have about him.

Being able to focus on zone one and have our attention focused out has other advantages. In focusing in this way, we can learn to maintain the 'therapeutic distance' referred to in a previous chapter. We can learn to distinguish clearly between what are the client's problems and what are our own. It is only when we become mixed up by having our attention partly focused on the client, partly on our own thoughts and feelings and partly on our fantasies and interpretations that we begin to get confused about what the client is telling us and what we are 'saying to ourselves'. We easily confuse our own problems with those of the client.

Secondly, we can use the concept of the three domains of attention to develop self awareness. By noticing the times when we have great difficulty in focusing attention 'out', we can learn to notice points of stress and difficulty in our own lives. Typically, we will find it difficult to focus attention out when we are tired, under pressure or emotionally distressed. The lack of attention that we experience can come to serve as a signal that we need to stop and take stock of our own life situation. Further, by allowing ourselves consciously to focus 'in' on zones two and three – the process of introspection – we can examine our thoughts and feelings in order to further understand our own make-up. Indeed, this process of self-exploration seems to be essential if we are to be able to offer another person sustained attention. If we constantly 'bottle up' problems we will find ourselves distracted by what the client has to say. Typically, when he begins to talk of a problem of his that is also a problem for us, we will suddenly find our attention distracted to zone two: suddenly we will find ourselves pondering on our own problems and not those of the client! Regular self-examination can help us to clear away, at least temporarily, some of the more pressing personal problems that we experience. A case, perhaps, of 'counsellor, counsel thyself!'

Such exploration can be carried out either in isolation, in pairs or in groups. The skills exercises part of this book offers practical suggestions as to how such exploration can be developed. If done in isolation, meditative techniques can be of value. Often, however, the preference will be to conduct such exploration in pairs or groups. In this way, we gain further insight through hearing other people's thoughts, feelings and observations and we can make useful comparisons between other people's experience and our own. There are a variety of formats for running self-awareness groups, including sensitivity groups, encounter groups, group therapy and training groups. Such groups are often organised by colleges and extra-mural departments of universities but they can also be set up on a 'do-it-yourself' basis. Ernst and Goodison (1981) offer some particularly useful guidelines for setting up, running and maintaining a self-help group for self-exploration. Such a group is useful as a means of developing self-awareness, as a peer-support group for talking through counselling problems and also as a means of developing further counselling skills. Trying out new skills in a safe and trusting environment is often a better proposition than trying them out with real clients!

Attending in Practice

Elizabeth, a health visitor, finds that during a busy day, it is difficult to 'cut off' from one of her clients, before visiting another. She finds herself preoccupied with the problems of a previous visit during a visit to another person. Through practising the process of focusing 'attention out', between visits and by taking a few minutes, in her car, to 'disassociate' from the client she has just visited, she develops the skill of giving full attention to the next person she sees.

LISTENING

Listening is the process of 'hearing' the other person. This involves not only noting the things that they say but also a whole range of other aspects of communication. Figure 7.2 outlines some of the things that can be noted during listening.

Figure 7.2

Aspects of listening.

Linguistic aspects
- words
- phrases
- figures of speech
- 'personal' and idiosyncratic forms of speech
- etc.

Paralinguistic aspects
- timing
- volume
- tone
- pitch
- 'ums' and 'ers'
- fluency
- range
- etc.

Non-verbal aspects
- facial expression
- gestures
- touch
- body position
- proximity to the counsellor
- body movement
- eye contact
- etc.

Given the wide range of ways in which one person tries to communicate with another, this is further evidence of the need to develop the ability to offer close and sustained attention, as already outlined. Three aspects of listening are noted in the diagram. Linguistic aspects of speech refer to the actual words that clients use, to the phrases they choose and to the metaphors they use to convey how they are feeling. Attention to such metaphors is often useful, as metaphorical language can often convey more than can more conventional use of language (Cox, 1978). Paralinguistics refers to all those aspects of speech that are not words themselves. Thus, timing, volume, pitch, accent are all paralinguistic aspects of communication. Again, they can offer us indicators of how the other person is feeling beyond the words that he uses. Again, however, we must be careful of making assumptions and slipping into zone three, the zone of fantasy. Paralinguistics can only offer us a possible clue to how the other person is feeling. It is important that we check with the client the degree to which that clue matches with the client's own perception of the way he feels.

Non-verbal aspects of communication refer to 'body language': the way that the client expressed himself through the use of his body. Thus facial expression, use of gestures, body position and movement, proximity to the counsellor, touch in relation to the counsellor, all offer further clues about the client's internal status beyond the words he uses and can be 'listened' to by the attentive counsellor. Again, any assumptions that we make about what such body language 'means', need to be clarified with the client. There is a temptation to believe that body language can be 'read', as if we all used it in the same sort of way. This is, perhaps, encouraged by works such as Desmond Morris's (1978) *Manwatching*. Reflection on the subject, however, will reveal that body language is dependent to a large degree on a wide number of variables: the context in which it occurs, the nature of the relationship, the individual's personal style and preference, the personality of the person 'using' the body language, and so on. It is safer, therefore, not to assume that we 'know' what another person is 'saying' with his body language but to, again, treat it as a clue and to clarify with the client what he means by his use of it. Thus it is preferable, in counselling, to merely bring to the client's attention the way he is sitting, or his facial expression, rather than to offer an interpretation of it. Two examples may help here. In the first, the counsellor is offering an interpretation and an assumption:

> *I notice from the way that you have your arms folded and from your frown that you are uncomfortable with discussing things at home.*

In the second example, the counsellor merely feeds back to the client what she observes, and allows the client to clarify his situation:

> *I notice that you have your arms folded and that you're frowning. What are you feeling at the moment?*

LEVELS OF LISTENING

The skilled counsellor learns to listen to all three aspects of communication and tries to resist the temptation to interpret what she hears. Three levels of listening may be identified in Figure 7.3.

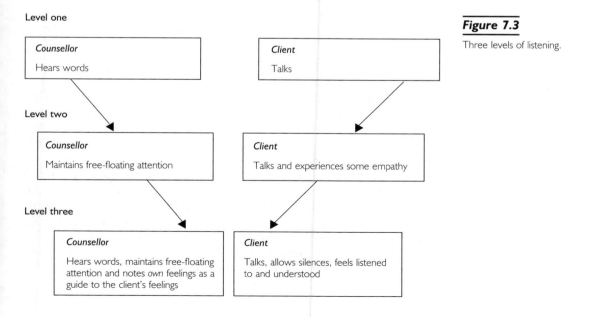

Figure 7.3

Three levels of listening.

The first level of listening refers to the idea of the counsellor merely noting what is being said. In this mode, neither client nor counsellor is psychologically very 'close' and arguably the relationship will not develop very much. In the second level of listening, the counsellor learns to develop 'free-floating' attention. That is to say that she listens 'overall' to what is being said, as opposed to trying to catch every word. Free-floating attention also refers to 'going with' the client, of not trying to keep the client to a particular theme but of following the client's conversation wherever it goes. She also 'listens' to the client's non-verbal and paralinguistic behaviour as indicators of what the client is thinking and feeling. Faced with this deeper level of listening, the client feels a greater amount of empathy being offered by the counsellor. The counsellor begins to enter the frame of reference of the client and to explore his perceptual world. She begins to see the world as the client experiences it.

In the third level of listening, the counsellor maintains free-floating attention, notices non-verbal and paralinguistic aspects of communication but also notices her own internal thoughts, feelings and body sensations. As Rollo May (1983) notes, it is frequently the case that what the counsellor is feeling, once the counselling relationship has deepened, is a direct mirror image of what the client is feeling. Thus the counsellor sensitively notices changes in her self and gently checks these with the client. It is as though the counsellor is listening both to the client and to herself and carefully using herself as a sounding board for how the relationship is developing. Watkins has described this process as 'resonance' and points out that this process is different from that of empathising:

> *Rogers says that empathy means understanding of the feelings of another. He holds that the therapist does not necessarily himself experience the feelings. If he did, according to Rogers, that would be identification, and this is not the same as empathy. Resonance is a type of identification which is temporary.*

> (Watkins, 1978)

The use of the process of resonance needs to be judged carefully. Whilst it does not involve interpreting or offering a theory about what the client is feeling, it does offer a particularly close form of listening which can make the client feel listened to and fully understood. It is notable, too, that in these circumstances, the client will often feel more comfortable with periods of silence as he struggles to verbalise his thoughts and feelings. Arguably, he allows these silences because he senses that the counsellor is 'with him' more completely than at other levels of listening. The net result of this deeper level of listening is that a truly empathic relationship develops. The client feels listened to, the counsellor feels she is understanding the client, and a level of mutuality is achieved in which both people are communicating, both rationally and intuitively.

Listening on the Internet

The most basic of all human needs is the need to understand and be understood. The best way to understand people is to listen to them.

Ralph Nichols

'Listen, learn, resubmit.'

The Write Word, on writing grants
http://www.writegrants.com/members/newfaculty/step10.html

'Look, listen, learn, lead.'

Addiction Technology Transfer Centers
http://www.nattc.org/pdf/networker01august.pdf

'Listen, learn, live.'

UNAIDS, on the World AIDS Campaign with Children and Young People
http://www.unaids.org/wac/1999/

'Listen. Learn. Prosper.'

CEOLive.com, motto
http://www.ceolive.com/content.cfm

'Look Listen Learn.'

a baby walker by Delta
http://shop.store.yahoo.com/netkidswear/looklislearw.html

Use of 'minimal prompts'

Whilst the counsellor is listening to the client, it is important that she shows that she is listening. An obvious aid to this is the use of what may be described as 'minimal prompts' – the use of head nods, 'yes', 'mm' and so on. All of these indicate that 'I am with you'. On the other hand, overuse of them can be irritating to the client: particularly, perhaps, the thoughtless and repetitive nodding of the head – the 'dog in the back of the car' phenomenon! It is important that the counsellor, at least initially, is consciously aware of her use of minimal prompts and tries to vary her repertoire. It is important to note, also, that very often such prompts are not necessary at all. Often, all the client needs is to be listened to and appreciate that the counsellor is listening, without the need for further reinforcement of the fact.

BEHAVIOURAL ASPECTS OF LISTENING

One other consideration needs to be made regarding the process of listening and that is the behaviours the counsellor adopts when listening to the client. Egan (1990) offers the acronym SOLER as a means of identifying and remembering the sorts of counsellor behaviour that encourage effective listening. The acronym is used as follows:

- sit Squarely in relation to the client;
- maintain an Open position;
- Lean slightly towards the client;
- maintain reasonable Eye contact with the client;
- Relax!

First, the counsellor is encouraged to sit squarely in relation to the client. This can be understood both literally and metaphorically. In the US and the UK it is generally acknowledged that one person listens to another more effectively if she sits opposite or nearly opposite the other person, rather than next to him. Sitting opposite allows the counsellor to see all aspects of communication, both paralinguistic and non-verbal, that might be missed if she sat next to the client. Secondly, the counsellor should consider adopting an open position in relation to the client. Again, this can be understood both literally and metaphorically. A 'closed' attitude is as much a block to effective counselling as is a closed body position. Crossed arms and legs, however, can convey a defensive feeling to the client, and counselling is often more effective if the counsellor sits without crossing either. Having said that, many people feel more comfortable sitting with their legs crossed, so perhaps some licence should be used here! What should be avoided is the position where the counsellor sits in a 'knotted' position with both arms and legs crossed.

It is helpful if the counsellor appreciates that she can lean towards the client. This can encourage the client and make him feel more understood. If this does not seem immediately clear, next time you talk to someone, try leaning away from the other person and note the result!

Eye contact with the client should be reasonably sustained, and a good rule of thumb is that the amount of eye contact that the counsellor uses should roughly match the amount the client uses. It is important, however, that the counsellor's eyes should be 'available' for the client; the counsellor is always prepared to maintain eye contact. On the other hand, it is important that the client does not feel stared at and is not intimidated by the counsellor's glare. Conscious use of eye contact can ensure that the client feels listened to and understood but not uncomfortable.

The amount of eye contact the counsellor can make will depend on a number of factors, including the topic under discussion, the degree of 'comfortableness' the counsellor feels with the client, the degree to which the counsellor feels attracted to the client, the amount of eye contact the client makes, the nature and quality of the client's eye contact and so forth. If the counsellor continually finds the maintenance of eye contact difficult it is, perhaps, useful to consider talking the issue over with a trusted colleague or with a peer-support group, for eye contact is a vital channel of communication in most interpersonal encounters (Heron, 1970).

Finally, it is important that the counsellor feels relaxed while listening. This usually means that she should refrain from 'rehearsing responses' in her head. It means that she gives herself up completely to the task of listening and trusts herself that she will make an appropriate response when she has to. This underlines the need to consider listening as the most important aspect of counselling. Everything else is secondary to it. Many people feel that they have to have a ready response when engaged in a conversation with another person. In counselling, however, the main focus of the conversation is the client. The counsellor's verbal responses, although important, must be secondary to what the client has to say. Thus all the counsellor has to do is to sit back and intently listen. Easily said but not so easily done! The temptation to 'overtalk' is often great but can lessen with more experience and with the making of a conscious decision not to make too many verbal interventions.

All of these behavioural considerations can help the listening process. In order to be effective, however, they need to be used consciously. The counsellor needs to pay attention to using them and choose to use them. As we have noted, at first this conscious use of self will feel uncomfortable and unnatural. Practice makes it easier and with that practice comes the development of the counsellor's own style of working and behaving in the counselling relationship. No such style can develop if, first, the counsellor does not consciously consider the way she sits and the way she listens.

Egan's SOLER behaviours do, of course, have limitations in certain contexts but he has recently quoted a counsellor who works for the Royal National College for the Blind (in the US) as follows – illustrating the flexibility of the general approach:

> In counselling students who are blind and visually impaired, eye contact has little or no relevance. However, attention on voice direction is extremely important and people with visual impairment will tell you how insulted they feel when sighted people are talking to them while looking somewhere else.
>
> I teach SOLER as part of listening and attending skills and can adapt each letter of the acronym (to my visually impaired students) with exception of the E ... After much thought, I would like to change your acronym to SOLAR, the A being for AIM, that is aim your head and body in the direction of your client so that when they hear your voice, be it linguistically or paralinguistically, they know that you are attending directly to what they are saying.
>
> (Egan, 2002)

In summary, it is possible to identify some of those things which act as blocks to effective listening and some aids to effective listening. No doubt the reader can add to both of these lists, and such additions will be useful in that they will be a reflection of your own strengths and limitations as a listener.

Blocks to Effective Listening

- the counsellor's own problems;
- counsellor stress and anxiety;

- awkward/uncomfortable seating;
- lack of attention to listening behaviour;
- value judgements and interpretations on the part of the counsellor;
- counsellor's attention focused 'in' rather than 'out';
- 'rehearsals' inside the counsellor's head.

While numerous conditions exist in which listening may be difficult, Egan offers a useful list of some other possibilities that can make listening to another person a problem:

- *Attraction*. You find a client either quite attractive or quite unattractive. You pay more attention to what you are feeling about the client than to what the client is saying.
- *Physical condition*. You are tired or sick. Without realising it, you tune out some of the things the client is saying.
- *Concerns*. You are preoccupied with your own concerns. For instance, you keep thinking about the argument you've just had with your spouse.
- *Overeagerness*. You are so eager to respond that you listen to only a part of what the client has to say. You become preoccupied with your responses rather than with the client's revelations.
- *Similarity of problems*. The problems the client is dealing with are quite similar to your own. As the client talks, your mind wanders to the ways in which what is being said applies to you and your situation.
- *Differences*. The client and his or her experience is very different from you and your experiences. This lack of communality is distracting (Egan, 1990).

Aids to Effective Listening

- attention focused 'out';
- suspension of judgement by the counsellor;
- attention to the behavioural aspects of listening;
- comfortable seating;
- avoidance of interpretation;
- development of 'free floating' attention;
- judicious use of minimal prompts.

LISTENING: A SKILL OR A QUALITY?

In a recent study (Burnard, 1997), I surveyed some health care students about their perceptions of the *qualities* of a good counsellor.

The term 'counsellor', in this case, was defined as 'the sort that a person might go to see to talk about personal or emotional problems'. This was to differentiate between a counsellor as helper and confidante and other sorts of counsellors such as coaches, information givers, trainers and supervisors.

Two hundred health care students, on a range of courses, were surveyed. Students could choose whether or not they completed the form. One hundred and sixty-two usable survey papers were returned – a response rate of 81%.

Respondents were asked to identify up to ten personal qualities that they might expect to find in a counsellor. They were given the following instructions:

> *I am interested in your views about what you feel are the* personal qualities *that could reasonably be expected to be found in a counsellor. A 'counsellor' in this case is the sort that a person might go to see to talk about personal or emotional problems.*
>
> *I would be grateful if you would list, below, the personal qualities that* you *would expect to find in a counsellor. There are no right or wrong suggestions but please bear in mind that this study focuses on* qualities *and not on* skills *or* qualifications. *You can list as few qualities as you like but please list no more than 10.*

Analysis of the data

Despite the request to list 'no more than 10' qualities, a number of students identified more than 10. These other qualities were included in the analysis. The range of qualities identified by individual respondents was 315.

All of the responses were listed in a word-processing file. These items were then placed in alphabetical order to facilitate frequency counting of the various items. From this list it was possible to count manually the number of occurrences, within the total sample, of various personal qualities identified by the students. Percentages were then calculated and the findings placed in rank order. Given the sampling method used, it was deemed inappropriate to use any form of inferential statistics on the data.

Findings

Among the most frequently identified qualities were those broadly in line with previous research and the literature: being non-judgemental, being empathic and understanding (Burnard, 1995; Egan, 1990; Rogers, 1967). However, other qualities, such as being approachable, sympathetic and caring rated highly, too. Often, empathy is identified in the literature as an important personal quality where sympathy is not. However, these items represent abstractions and, as such, may be difficult to define clearly. Safety and ethical qualities also appeared to be important (such as being confidential, trustworthy and honest). It should be noted, too, that some respondents addressed the issue in terms of 'negatives' (e.g. counsellors should be non-threatening, non-patronising or not forceful). The surprise 'quality', perhaps, was *good listener*. Seventy-three percent of the sample identified 'good listener' as a personal quality. As we shall see in the following discussion, this runs counter to much of the literature, which defines listening as a skill rather than as a quality. Figure 7.4 identifies the range of findings down to qualities identified by at least five respondents.

Figure 7.4

Qualities of counsellors as identified by students (n=162).

QUALITY	n	%
Good listener	119	73
Non judgemental	93	57
Empathic	56	35
Understanding	56	35
Approachable	43	27
Sympathetic	32	20
Caring	31	19
Friendly	31	19
Patient	28	17
Confidential	27	17
Supportive	22	14
Knowledgeable	19	12
Honest	18	11
Trustworthy	16	10
Experienced	12	7
Kind	12	7
Warm	12	7
Calm	11	7
Helpful	9	6
Respectful	8	5
Sense of humour	8	5
Advice giving	7	4
Considerate	7	4
Genuine	7	4
Open	7	4
Open minded	7	4
Professional	7	4
Non-patronising	6	4
Objective	6	4
Reassuring	6	4
Trusting	6	4
Broad minded	5	3
Comforting	5	3
Communicative	5	3
Relaxed	5	3

Discussion

The findings highlight an interesting ambiguity. Although the literature on counselling often identifies listening as a skill (see, for example, BAC, 1989a,b; Davis and Fallowfield, 1991; Morrison and Burnard, 1997), many of the respondents, in this study, identified it as a *personal quality*. This is all the more clearly underlined by the fact that, at the top of the response sheet, was the indication that the researcher was interested only in *personal qualities* and not in *skills*, as previously discussed.

It is made more interesting by the fact that no other skills were identified in this way. If the respondents were generally mistaking or confusing qualities for skills, it would be likely that they would identify *other* skills in this way.

Thus it would appear, for these respondents at least, the issue of skills versus qualities merges when it comes to listening. This ambiguity is hinted at, but not made explicit, in a British Association for Counselling Code of Conduct which makes an apparent demarcation between 'listening skills' and 'counselling skills':

The term 'counselling skills' does not have a single definition which is universally accepted. For the purpose of this code, 'counselling skills' are distinguished from 'listening skills' and from 'counselling'. Although the distinction is not always a clear one, because the term 'counselling skills' contains elements of these two activities, it has its own place between them. '

(BAC, 1989a)

Although the BAC is not particularly clear on the issue – partly, as it admits, because the issue, as it finds it, *is* not clear – it hints at a distinction between listening skills and counselling skills as two, possibly discrete, categories. The present findings seem to lend weight to an argument for not making such a clear distinction between 'listening', 'counselling skills' and 'personal qualities'. Listening, it would seem, may straddle a distinction between skills and personal qualities and leaves, in the air, the question, 'Is listening a skill or a quality?' For the moment, though, we should note that the BAC, in the quotation, is still considering listening as a *skill*.

The question of whether or not listening is a skill or a personal quality is not easily answered and it may be noted that at least one writer offers a definition of listening that seems to indicate something more complex – and perhaps more personal – than mere skill:

Listening is the complex, learned human process of sensing, interpreting, evaluating, storing and responding to oral messages.

(Steil, 1991)

It is notable, too, that, in the study described here, an educator who also completed one of the survey forms commented, on the form, as follows:

Qualities are very difficult to differentiate from skills because the personal qualities of a counsellor are often conveyed through competence in skills such as listening, empathic responding etc.

It would seem possible, then, that personal qualities may be mediated through the demonstration of certain skills. On the other hand, it seems quite possible to rote learn a range of skills and to *not* have the personal qualities behind those skills. The demonstration of skills does not offer conclusive evidence of particular qualities. The task of discerning under-lying qualities or intentions, from behaviour, remains problematic.

The literature on counselling training often refers to the teaching of 'listening skills' (see, for example, Ellis and McClintock, 1994; Williams, 1997). The suggestion is that, given practice and appropriate educational experiences, students can enhance their listening through rehearsing the skill. However, if listening is considered a quality or, perhaps, a quality and a skill, such an approach might have to be modified. For, it might be argued, personal qualities are not the sorts of characteristics that can so readily be honed by training.

It would seem possible that listening is more than simply a collection of behaviours to be learned. It is likely, too, that listening, in a therapeutic sense, involves more than just hearing and acknowledging the words spoken by another person. Arguably, though, many of the methods used in teaching 'listening skills' are ones which focus on behavioural elements of the process: on sitting in a certain way, on maintaining eye contact, on using minimal prompts, on paying attention to non-verbal cues and so on (Egan, 1990; Hobbs, 1992; Kagan *et al.*, 1986).

While these are likely to be valuable in helping people to focus during the listening process, they do not, perhaps, capture some of the more subtle aspects of listening. We might argue, in the light of listening being considered a personal quality, that listening also involves a more subjective, difficult-to-pin-down aspect – perhaps akin to Martin Buber's notion of the meeting of two 'subjects' in the 'I–Thou' relationship (Buber, 1958).

One possible solution to the issue of what constitutes a counselling skill and what constitutes a personal quality is to abandon the latter designation and to use the term *characteristic* in place of both. Thus we might talk of the 'characteristics of a counsellor' and that might include both skills and qualities. It is acknowledged, however, that this is, perhaps, a semantic 'fudge' and may only be a way of circumventing further debate on the importance, or otherwise, of the differences between human qualities and demonstrable skills. On the other hand, if we accept the point that 'personal qualities' may *not* play the major role in the counselling relationships and that skills are likely to be just as important, it may seem reasonable to merge the distinction between qualities and skills by the use of the term 'characteristics'.

This, in turn, may mean that some teachers of counselling skills to health care professionals may have to change their approach to such teaching. Given the emphasis in the literature on 'counselling skills', the challenge may be to find ways of presenting the characteristics of an effective counsellor in such a way as to embrace both personal qualities and previously identified skills. Further, there might be discussion about whether or not it is *possible* to 'train' health care professionals in particular personal qualities. While listening remains a skill, it seems possible to engage in skills training. If listening is more than a skill, and merges into or becomes a quality, then we may or may not be able to engage in 'qualities training'. It seems likely that many people would claim that, by definition, personal qualities are more idiosyncratic and less visible than skills. Clearly, more work needs to be done to validate or reject the particular finding of this study.

A note of caution

While the preceding paragraphs have stressed the need for the counsellor to be aware of his or her own non-verbal aspects of behaviour, while listening, it can be overdone. It is important, perhaps, not to develop a 'counsellor's face' and exercise facial expressions and eye contact to such a degree that the client is very aware that the counsellor is using such behaviours. I recall that some years ago, after I had attended a number of counselling courses, I was with a friend who, as we sat and talked, suddenly said, 'I'm being listened to!' and was clearly uncomfortable. Flannery O'Connor, in his short story, 'Good Country People', describes this 'obvious' presentation of facial expression as follows:

> *Besides the neutral expression that she wore when she was alone, Mrs Freeman had two others, forward and reverse, that she used for all her human dealings. Her forward expression was steady and driving like the advance of a heavy truck. Her eyes never swerved to left or right but turned as the story turned as if they followed a yellow line down the centre of it. She seldom used the other expression because it was not often necessary for her to retract a statement, but when she did, her face came to a complete stop, there was an almost imperceptible movement of her black eyes, during which they seemed to be receding, and then the observer would see that Mrs Freeman, though she might stand there as real as several grain sacks thrown on top of each other, was no longer there in spirit.*

> (O'Connor, 1998)

We should be wary, perhaps, of becoming too *obvious*.

ATTENDING, LISTENING AND THE HEALTH PROFESSIONAL

The attending and listening aspects of counselling are essential skills that can be used in every health professional's job. The skills are clearly not limited only to use within the counselling relationship but can be applied in other interpersonal exchanges. An advantage of paying attention to the development of these particular skills is that becoming an effective listener not only makes for better counselling practice but interpersonal effectiveness and self-awareness are also enhanced. In the following chapters, verbal interventions are explored that will complement the listening and attending described here. Again, such interventions can be used both inside and outside the counselling relationship and can do much to improve every health professional's performance as a carer.

Listening in practice

David is a GP in a busy city centre practice. He gets repeated visits from a young woman, Sarah, whose husband has recently been killed in a road accident. She often makes allusion to the problems of adjusting to her bereavement but presents with fairly minor physical ailments. David gently suggests to her that it may be helpful if they talked about her loss in more detail and offers her an afternoon, booked appointment. At first she is reluctant to accept this but later phones to make such an appointment. During the next few weeks, David meets Sarah on a regular basis and listens to her. During these appointments, he has to make very few verbal interventions: Sarah is able to describe and ventilate her feelings very easily, once she is offered the opportunity. She works through stages of anger, extreme sorrow and meaninglessness and finally to some acceptance. During these stages, David has had to 'do' very little. His supportive attention and ability to listen, without making too many suggestions or offering too much advice has been therapeutic in itself. He realises, however, that he has had to 'learn to listen'. Previously in his career, he tended to be a 'sentence finisher', for other people and has slowly learnt to focus attention on other people and really listen to them.

COUNSELLING SKILLS II: CLIENT-CENTRED SKILLS

8

Counselling skills may be divided into two subgroups: (a) listening and attending and (b) counselling interventions. Listening and attending were considered in the last chapter. This chapter identifies important counselling interventions: the things that the counsellor says in the counselling relationship.

The term 'client-centred', first used by Carl Rogers (1951) refers to the notion that it is the client, himself, who is best able to decide how to find the solutions to his problems in living. 'Client-centred' in this sense may be contrasted with the idea of 'counsellor-centred' or 'professional-centred', both of which may suggest that someone other than the client is the 'expert'. Whilst this may be true when applied to certain concrete 'factual' problems: housing, surgery, legal problems and so forth, it is difficult to see how it can apply to personal life issues. In such cases, it is the client who identifies the problem and the client who, given time and space, can find his way through the problem to the solution.

Murgatroyd (1986) summarises the client-centred position as follows:

- a person in need has come to you for help;
- in order to be helped clients need to know that you have understood how they think and feel;
- they also need to know that, whatever your own feelings about who or what they are or about what they have or have not done, you accept them as they are – you accept their right to decide their own lives for themselves;
- in the light of this knowledge about your acceptance and understanding of them they will begin to open themselves to the possibility of change and development;
- but if they feel that their association with you is conditional upon them changing, they may feel pressurised and reject your help.

The first issues identified by Murgatroyd, the fact of the client coming for help and needing to be understood and accepted, have been discussed in previous chapters. What we need to consider now are ways of helping people to express themselves, to open themselves and thus to begin to change. It is worth noting, too, the almost paradoxical nature of Murgatroyd's last point: that if clients feel that their association with you is conditional upon them changing, they may reject your help. Thus we enter into the counselling relationship without even being desirous of the other person changing!

In a sense, this is an impossible state of affairs. If we did not hope for change, we presumably would not enter into the task of counselling in the first place! On another level, however, the point is a very important one. People change at their own rate and in their own time. The process cannot be rushed and we cannot will other people to change. Nor can we expect them to change to become more the sort of person that we would like them to be. We must meet them on their own terms and observe change as they wish and will it to be (or not, as the case may be). This sort of counselling, then, is a very altruistic sort. It demands of us that we make no demands of others.

Client-centred counselling is a process rather than a particular set of skills. It evolves through the relationship that the counsellor has with the client and vice versa. In a sense, it is a period of growth for both parties, for each learns from the other. It also involves the exercise of restraint. The counsellor must restrain herself from offering advice and from the temptation to 'put the client's life right' for him. The outcome of such counselling cannot be predicted nor can concrete goals be set (unless they are devised by the client, at his request). In essence, client-centred counselling involves an act of faith: a belief in the other person's ability to find solutions through the process of therapeutic conversation and through the act of being engaged in a close relationship with another human being.

Certain, basic client-centred skills may be identified, although as we have noted, it is the total relationship that is important. Skills exercised in isolation amount to little: the warmth, genuineness and positive regard must also be present. On the other hand, if basic skills are not considered, then the counselling process will probably be shapeless or it will degenerate into the counsellor becoming prescriptive. The skill of standing back and allowing the client to find his own way is a difficult one to learn. The following skills may help in the process:

- questions;
- reflection;
- selective reflection;
- empathy building;
- checking for understanding.

Each of these skills will now be considered in turn, and in the last chapter a wide range of exercises is offered for the development of the skills. Each skill can be learned. In order for that to happen, each must be tried and practised. There is a temptation to say, 'I do that anyway!' when reading a description of some of these skills. The point is to notice the doing of them and to practise doing them better! Whilst counselling often shares the characteristics of everyday conversation, if it is to progress beyond that it is important that some, if not all, of the following skills are used effectively, tactfully and skilfully.

QUESTIONS

Two main sorts of questions may be identified in the client-centred approach: closed and open questions.

Closed questions

A closed question is one that elicits a 'yes', 'no' or similar one-word answer. Or it is one where the counsellor can anticipate an approximation of the answer, as she asks it. Examples of closed questions are as follows:

- What is your name?
- How many children do you have?
- Are you happier now?
- Are you still depressed?

Too many closed questions can make the counselling relationship seem like an interrogation! They also inhibit the development of the client's telling of his story and place the locus of responsibility in the relationship firmly with the client. Consider, for instance, the following exchange between marriage guidance counsellor and client:

Counsellor: Are you happier now ... at home?
Client: Yes, I think I am ...
Counsellor: Is that because you can talk more easily with your wife?
Client: I think so ... we seem to get on better, generally.
Counsellor: And has your wife noticed the difference?
Client: Yes, she has.

In this conversation, made up only of closed questions, the counsellor clearly 'leads' the conversation. She also tends to try to influence the client towards accepting the idea that he is 'happier now' and that his wife has 'noticed the difference'. One of the problems with this sort of questioning is that it gives little opportunity for the client to disagree profoundly with the counsellor. In this exchange, for example, could the client easily have disagreed with the counsellor? It would seem not.

On the other hand, the closed question is useful in clarifying certain specific issues. For example, one may be used as follows:

Client: It's not always easy at home ... the children always seem to be so noisy ... and my wife finds it difficult to cope with them ...
Counsellor: How many children have you?
Client: Three. They're all under ten and they're at the sort of age when they use up a lot of energy and make a lot of noise ...

Here, the closed question is fairly unobtrusive and serves to clarify the conversation. Notice, too, that once the question has been asked, the counsellor allows the client to continue to talk about his family, without further interruption.

Open questions

Open questions are those that do not elicit a particular answer: the counsellor cannot easily anticipate what an answer will 'look like'. Examples of open questions include:

- What did you do then?
- How did you feel when that happened?
- How are you feeling right now?
- What do you think will happen?

Open questions are ones that encourage the client to say more, to expand on his story or to go deeper. An example of their use is as follows:

Counsellor: What is happening at home at the moment?
Client: Things are going quite well. Everyone's much more settled now and my son's found himself a job. He's been out of work for a long time ...
Counsellor: How have you felt about that?
Client: It's upset me a lot ... It seemed wrong that I was working and he wasn't ... he had to struggle for a long time ... he wasn't happy at all ...
Counsellor: And how are you feeling right now?
Client: Upset ... I'm still upset ... I still feel that I didn't help him enough ...

In this conversation, the counsellor uses only open questions, and the client expands on what he thinks and feels. More importantly, perhaps, this example illustrates the counsellor 'following' the client and noting his paralinguistic and non-verbal cues. In this way, she is able to help the client to focus more on what is happening in the present. This is an example of the 'concreteness' and 'immediacy' referred to in Chapter 5.

Open questions are generally preferable, in counselling, to closed ones. They encourage longer, more expansive answers and are rather more free of value judgements and interpretation than are closed questions. All the same, the counsellor has to monitor the 'slope' of intervention when using open questions. It is easy, for example, to become intrusive by asking too piercing questions, too quickly. As with all counselling interventions, the timing of the use of questions is vital.

When to use questions

Questions can be used in the counselling relationships for a variety of purposes. The main ones include:

- Exploration: 'What else happened ... ?', 'How did you feel then?'
- For further information: 'How many children have you got?', 'What sort of work were you doing before you retired?'
- To clarify: 'I'm sorry, did you say you are going to move or did you say you're not sure?', 'What did you say then ... ?'
- Encouraging client to talk: 'Can you say more about that?', 'What are your feelings about that?'

Other sorts of questions

There are other ways of classifying questions and some to be avoided! Examples of other sorts of questions include:

Leading questions

These are questions that contain an assumption which places the client in an untenable position. The classic example of a leading question is, 'Have you stopped beating your wife?'! Clearly, however the question is answered, the client is in the wrong! Other examples of leading questions are:

> Is your depression the thing that's making your work so difficult? Are your family upset by your behaviour? Do you think that you may be hiding something … even from yourself?

The later, pseudo-analytical questions are particularly awkward. What could the answer possibly be?

Value-laden questions

A question such as 'Does your homosexuality make you feel guilty?' not only poses a moral question but guarantees that the client feels difficult answering it!

'Why' questions

These have been discussed in Chapter 5, and the problems caused by them in the counselling relationship suggest that they should be used very sparingly, if at all.

Confronting questions

Examples of these may include, 'Can you give me an example of when that happened?' and 'Do you still love your wife?' Confrontation in counselling is quite appropriate once the relationship has fully developed but needs to be used skilfully and appropriately. It is easy for apparent 'confrontation' to degenerate into moralising. Heron (1986) and Schulman (1982) offer useful approaches to effective confrontation in counselling.

Funnelling

Funnelling (Kahn and Cannell, 1957) refers to the use of questions to guide the conversation from the general to the specific. Thus, the conversation starts with broad, opening questions and, slowly, more specific questions are used to focus the discussion. An example of the use of funnelling is as follows:

> *Counsellor:* You seem upset at the moment, what's happening?
> *Client:* It's home … things aren't working out …
> *Counsellor:* What's happening at home?
> *Client:* I'm always falling out with Jane and the children …
> *Counsellor:* What does Jane feel about what's happening?
> *Client:* She's angry with me …
> *Counsellor:* About something in particular?
> *Client:* Yes, about the way I talk to Andrew, my son …
> *Counsellor:* What is the problem with Andrew?

In this way, the conversation becomes directed and focused and this may pose a problem. If the counsellor does use funnelling in this way, it is arguable that the counselling conversation is no longer client-centred but counsellor-directed. Perhaps, in many situations – particularly where shortage of time is an issue – a combination of following and leading may be appropriate. Following refers to the counsellor taking the lead from the client and exploring the avenues that he wants to explore. Leading refers to the counsellor taking a more active role and pursuing certain issues that she feels are important. If in doubt, however, the 'following' approach is probably preferable, as it keeps the locus of control in the counselling relationship firmly with the client.

Funnelling in Practice

Andy is a volunteer telephone counsellor on a local AIDS 'Helpline'. A young man of 18 rings in to ask about the symptoms of AIDS and for general information about the condition. Andy, in return, asks some open questions of the young man in order to establish a 'phone relationship'. As the conversation progresses, Andy gradually asks more specific questions and helps the young man to express more particular, personal anxieties about his own sexuality and his fear that he may be homosexual. Andy, through using the 'funnelling' approach to the use of questions, is able to help the person through a difficult personal crisis that continues to be worked through in subsequent counselling sessions.

REFLECTION

Reflection (sometimes called 'echoing') is the process of reflecting back the last few words, or a paraphrase of the last few words, that the client has used, in order to encourage him to say more. It is as though the counsellor is echoing the client's thoughts and as though that echo serves as a prompt. It is important that the reflection does not turn into a question, and this is best achieved by the counsellor making the repetition in much the same tone of voice as the client used. An example of the use of reflection is as follows:

> *Client:* We had lived in the South for a number of years. Then we moved and I supposed that's when things started to go wrong ...
> *Counsellor:* Things started to go wrong ...
> *Client:* Well, we never really settled down. My wife missed her friends and I suppose I did really ... though neither of us said anything ...
> *Counsellor:* Neither of you said that you missed your friends ...
> *Client:* We both tried to protect each other, really. I suppose if either of us had said anything, we would have felt that we were letting the other one down ...

In this example, the reflections are unobtrusive and unnoticed by the client. They serve to help the client to say more, to develop his story. Used skilfully and with good timing, reflection can be an important method of helping the client. On the other hand, if it is overused or used clumsily, it can appear stilted and is very noticeable. Unfortunately, it is an intervention that takes some practice and one that many people anticipate learning on counselling courses. As a result, when people return from counselling courses, their friends and relatives are often waiting for them to use the technique and may comment on the fact! This should not be a deterrent, as the method remains a useful and therapeutic one.

SELECTIVE REFLECTION

Selective reflection refers to the method of repeating back to the client a part of something he said that was emphasised in some way or which seemed to be emotionally charged. Thus selective reflection draws from the middle of the client's utterance and not from the end. An example of the use of selective reflection is as follows:

Client: We had just got married. I was very young and I thought things would work out OK. We started buying our own house. My wife hated the place! It was important, though ... we had to start somewhere ...

Counsellor: Your wife hated the house ...

Client: She thought it was the worst place she'd lived in! She reckoned that she would only live there for a year at the most and we ended up being there for five years!

The use of selective reflection allowed the client in this example to develop further an almost throwaway remark. Often, these 'asides' are the substance of very important feelings, and the counsellor can often help in the release of some of these feelings by using selective reflection to focus on them. Clearly concentration is important, in order to note the points on which to selectively reflect. Also, the counselling relationship is a flowing, evolving conversation which tends to be 'seamless'. Thus, it is little use the counsellor storing up a point which she feels would be useful to selectively reflect! By the time a break comes in the conversation, the item will probably be irrelevant! This points up, again, the need to develop 'free-floating attention': the ability to allow the ebb and flow of the conversation to go where the counsellor takes it and for the counsellor to trust her own ability to choose an appropriate intervention when a break occurs.

EMPATHY BUILDING

This refers to the counsellor making statements to the client that indicate that she has understood the feeling that the client is experiencing. A certain intuitive ability is needed here, for often empathy-building statements refer more to what is implied than what is overtly said. An example of the use of empathy-building statements is as follows:

Client: People at work are the same. They're all tied up with their own friends and families ... they don't have a lot of time for me ... though they're friendly enough ...
Counsellor: You sound angry with them ...
Client: I suppose I am! Why don't they take a bit of time to ask me how I'm getting on? It wouldn't take much! ...
Counsellor: It sounds as though you are saying that people haven't had time for you for a long time ...
Client: They haven't. My family didn't bother much ... I mean, they looked as though they did ... but they didn't really ...

The empathy-building statements, used here, are ones that read between the lines. Now, sometimes such reading between the lines can be completely wrong and the empathy-building statement is rejected by the client. It is important, when this happens, for the counsellor to drop the approach altogether and to pay more attention to listening. Inaccurate empathy-building statements often indicate an overwillingness on the part of the counsellor to become 'involved' with the client's perceptual world – at the expense of accurate empathy! Used skilfully, however, they help the client to disclose further and indicate to the client that they are understood.

CHECKING FOR UNDERSTANDING

Checking for understanding involves either (a) asking the client if you have understood them correctly or (b) occasionally summarising the conversation in order to clarify what has been said. The first type of checking is useful when the client quickly covers a lot of topics and seems to be 'thinking aloud'. It can be used to further focus the conversation or as a means of ensuring that the counsellor really stays with what the client is saying. The second type of checking should be used sparingly or the counselling conversation can get to seem rather mechanical and studied. The following two examples illustrate the two uses of checking for understanding:

Example 1
Client: I feel all over the place at the moment ... things aren't quite right at work ... money is still a problem and I don't seem to be talking to anyone ... I'm not sure about work ... sometimes I feel like packing it in ... at other times I think I'm doing OK ...
Counsellor: Let me just clarify ... you're saying things are generally a problem at the moment and you've thought about leaving work?
Client: Yes ... I don't think I will stop work but, if I can get to talk it over with my boss, I think I will feel easier about it.

Example 2

Counsellor: Let me see if I can just sum up what we've talked about this afternoon. We talked about the financial problems and the question of talking to the bank manager. You suggested that you may ask him for a loan. Then you went on to say how you felt you could organise your finances better in the future ... ?

Client: Yes, I think that covers most things ...

Some counsellors prefer to use the second type of checking at the end of each counselling session and this may help to clarify things before the client leaves. On the other hand, there is much to be said for not 'tidying up' the end of the session in this way. If the loose ends are left, the client continues to think about all the issues that have been discussed, as he walks away from the session. If everything is summarised too neatly, the client may feel that the problems can be 'closed down' for a while or even worse, that they have been 'solved'! Personal problems are rarely simple enough to be summarised in a few words, and checking at the end of a session should be used sparingly.

These, then, are particular skills that encourage self-direction on the part of the client and can be learned and used by the counsellor. They form the basis of all good counselling and can always be returned to as a primary way of working with the client in the counselling relationship.

IS THE CLIENT-CENTRED APPROACH ENOUGH?

The 1990s have seen many changes in health provision. They have also seen dramatic changes in people's financial, work and life situations. These changes have contributed to a considerable debate about the appropriateness of the client-centred approach to counselling as an *exclusive* approach. Writing of the development of humanistic psychology in counselling, Dryden *et al*. have this to say:

> The object of person-centred counselling ... is to help the client 'to become what he/she is capable of becoming' (Rogers, 1951), or, to employ an even more well-worn phrase associated with Maslow, to achieve self-actualization (Maslow, 1962). These terms have a slightly hollow ring about them in the enterprise economy of the late 1980s in Britain, in which the division between the 'haves' and the 'have nots' is sharply apparent. Striving for self-actualization is easier if one is well-off, well-housed, has a rewarding and secure job and lives in a pleasant environment than if one is unemployed, poor, ill-housed, and lives in a run-down neighbourhood. Terms like self-actualization simply do not feature in and do not derive from the culture of the 1980s.
>
> (Dryden *et al*., 1989)

A similar point was made rather more directly when, discussing the changing needs of clients who seek counselling, Howard suggested about counsellors that:

It is time we shed our naivety and the 'syrupy' illusions of Carl Rogers and his many cohorts.

(Howard, 1990)

These writers raise important questions that relate to issues in this study. There have been considerable changes in life in the UK since the 1960s. The political climate has changed, employment patterns and patterns of health and sickness have also changed, some would say irreversibly (Bowen, 1990). Ashton and Seymour (1988) sum up some of these changes as follows:

Fundamental changes are taking place both in the way we view ill-health and the way individuals, families and governments respond to it. In the United Kingdom ministerial reputations and careers are being made and lost out of the health-related issues of AIDS, drugs, heart disease and the environmental conditions of the inner cities. The once sacred National Health Service is under attack for failing to deliver the goods and the long assumed immunity to accountability of physicians is falling away week by week. In Liverpool, 26 per cent of adult men are unemployed and nationally the infant mortality rate has just risen for the first time in 16 years.

(Ashton and Seymour, 1988)

Ashton and Seymour begin to raise the question of whether or not the client-centred approach is appropriate in AIDS counselling. In Chapter 10, it is noted that education and advice both have their part to play in effective AIDS counselling. It is also noted that the concept of AIDS counselling involves a wide and diverse range of counselling. Thus it seems likely that a more *prescriptive* approach to counselling may well be appropriate in the AIDS field. On the other hand, Rogers was not only advocating a particular set of skills or counselling interventions, he was also suggesting a particular *attitude* towards counselling which involved respect for the client, appreciation of his or her range of choices and the fact that it was the client who, in the end, made his or her decision for him- or herself. This aspect of the Rogerian approach may still be appropriate in all types of counselling.

Murgatroyd and Woolfe (1982) note that approaches to counselling and caring for people with different problems of living are also changing. They suggest that there has been a move away from the client-centred approach of Rogers towards an interest in short-term, crisis-oriented counselling for which more directive, action-oriented procedures are usually advocated.

A number of commentators and researchers have also moved away from the client-centred approach to counselling towards a more *challenging* one and see confrontation and challenge as an essential part of the counselling process (Dorn, 1986; Ellis, 1987; Ellis and Dryden, 1987). Farrelly and Brandsma propose four 'challenge related hypotheses' for consideration within the counselling movement:

- Clients can change if they choose.
- Clients have more resources for managing problems in living and developing opportunities than they or most helpers assume.
- The psychological fragility of clients is overrated both by themselves and others.
- Maladaptive and antisocial attitudes and behaviours of clients can be significantly altered no matter what the degree of severity or chronicity (Farelly and Brandsma, 1974).

In a similar vein, Howard *et al.* suggest that action and challenge are an essential part of human make-up and that people have a 'bias towards action' which requires them, directly or indirectly, to:

- change from a passive to a more active state;
- change from a state of dependency on others to relative independence;
- change from behaving in a few ways to acting in many ways;
- change in interests – with erratic, shallow and casual interests giving way to mature, strong and enduring interests;
- change from a present-oriented time perspective to a perspective encompassing past, present and future;
- change from solely subordinate relationships with others to relationship as equals or superiors;
- change from lack of a clear sense of self to a clearer sense of self and control of self (Howard *et al.* 1987).

As with most things, there needs to be a middle path. Sometimes, the client-centred approach will suffice. At other times, a more confronting approach may be appropriate. Also, there are situations in which the giving of clear information is important. In Chapter 10, some of these situations are explored in greater detail. The most obvious, current situation is that of people who, for whatever reason, find themselves in the HIV/AIDS field.

Despite criticisms and limitations, the client-centred approach continues to be useful and practical in a variety of health care settings. As Davis and Fallowfield suggest:

Rogers presented his theories as a basis for development, and not as complete and absolute frameworks. He was at pains to express his ideas tentatively and clearly, pointing out what was unknown or less than certain.

(Davis and Fallowfield, 1991)

However, we are likely to see changes. The client-centred approach may be time consuming and it is difficult to evaluate for effectiveness. As we have noted, elsewhere, health care profession in the UK and in other countries is changing. The push towards *evidenced-based practice* is everywhere and counsellors, like all other practitioners, are going to have to be able to demonstrate how well or otherwise their practice 'works'.

Finally, Tyrrell offers the follow critique of the client-centred approach to counselling:

Client centred therapy can certainly make people feel better by meeting their need for attention from a well-meaning outsider. However, there has never been any evidence that client centred approaches are effective.

Depressed people for example need to learn skills and approaches to life and there is a high percentage of client dissatisfaction and frustration with the therapists' passive stance and refusal to give opinions or make suggestions.

[It is] impossible to be non-influential ... towards the end of his life Carl Rogers expressed regret at promoting the idea that it was possible to avoid influencing a client. His students sat him down and showed him a video of him working with a client, pointing out how he would lean forward and appear interested when the client talked of something that got his attention, obviously influencing the client. Recent research by Howard Friedman of Stanford University indicates that it is impossible not to influence another person if you are in the same room as them.

Again client centred therapy or counselling does poorly as far as efficacy research is concerned and is also contra-indicated for the treatment of depression. Of course it is essential to feel safe in a non-judgemental setting but there has to be more offered than just this for most people in urgent need of help. Going over what hurts can make it worse. 'Psychological archaeology' – ruminating over past hurts – is what depressives do already, so encouraging more of the same as a therapy model is dubious to say the least.

(Tyrrell, 2004)

The client-centred approach in practice

Mary, a health visitor, is asked by one of her young single-parent clients about her young daughter's inability to sleep. Mary uses client-centred interventions and draws out the details surrounding the family situation. In allowing the young mother to talk through her financial and emotional worries she allows some of the pressure on the mother to be dispelled. She follows this up with some practical suggestions about how to help the daughter to sleep, including the suggestions of a regular bedtime, a planned routine during the evening and a 'winding down' period before going to bed. The combination of allowing the mother to talk out her own anxieties and offering practical suggestions enables both mother and daughter to live more comfortably.

CLIENT-CENTRED SKILLS AND THE HEALTH PROFESSIONAL

Whilst the discussion, in this chapter, has focused on the use of client-centred interventions in the counselling relationship, the range of skills involved is clearly useful in a wide range of health contexts. Workers in the primary health care team may use them as part of their assessment programme whilst professionals in longer-term care can use them as supportive measures and as a means of evaluating the effectiveness of care. In nursing, they may be used to draw up care plans and to implement, effectively, the use of nursing models – particularly self-care models. In the next chapter, consideration will be made of how to combine these client-centred interventions with those that help clients to express and handle emotions and feelings.

9 COUNSELLING SKILLS III: HELPING WITH FEELINGS

A considerable part of the process of helping people in counselling is concerned with the emotional or 'feelings' side of the person. In UK and US cultures, a great premium is placed on the individual being able to 'control' feelings, and thus overt expression of emotion is often frowned upon. As a result, we learn to bottle up feelings, sometimes from a very early age. Dorothy Rowe has summed up the situation well:

> *Just as we were born with the ability to breathe so we were born with the ability to express our emotions fully and to be aware of other people's emotions. We can keep our capacity to experience the full range and totality of our feelings and our capacity to empathise with other people. We can use these capacities to know ourselves, to know other people and let them be themselves. We can do this. But we rarely do. Society, the group we belong to, will not let us.*
>
> (Rowe, 1987)

In this chapter, we will consider the effects of such suppression of feelings and identify some practical ways of helping people to identify and explore their feelings. The skills involved in managing feelings can be seen to augment the skills discussed in the previous chapter – the basic client-centred counselling skills.

THE CULTURAL CONTEXT

It should always be borne in mind that the expression of emotion is a cultural issue. Whereas in Europe and the US it is seen as normal and reasonable to express strong feelings, this is certainly not the case in most south-east Asian countries. In Thailand, for example, a person loses a very considerable amount of 'face' if he or she openly expresses anger. More usually, the Thai person will simply wait for strong feelings to fade away. It is *not* considered helpful or therapeutic to a person for someone to 'help' him express his feelings. Mostly, in Thailand, friends and family will help to distract a person who is upset and encourage him to return to a more balanced and calm frame of mind.

It is always easy for us to be both blind to other cultures and also to believe that our own culture is somehow 'right'. The wise counsellor does well to study those people from cultures different from his or her own. Certainly, anyone who engages in cross-cultural counselling needs to have such an understanding. Also, the studying (and, if possible, the *experiencing*) of other cultures can do much to help us understand the range and 'difference' of the human condition. If we tend to think, 'We are all the same under the skin', then we are probably wrong. There is probably no one 'human nature' that is churning away in each of us. Instead, each of us has been programmed or socialised by the cultures in which we grow up. There is nothing unusual for the Thai person to avoid getting angry and it does not worry him or her. Similarly, there is everything wrong in the Thai person seeing someone from another culture publicly displaying anger. In the Thai person's eyes, the angry foreigner has lost considerable face. The Thai person, then, has had a different cultural and social conditioning from the 'Western' person, and deals with emotions, and with life, differently. If we are going to be competent counsellors and able to help a range of people, we must understand this diversity. It is with these caveats and variations in mind that the rest of this chapter should be read.

TYPES OF EMOTION

Heron (1977a) distinguishes between at least four types of emotion that are commonly suppressed or bottled up: anger, fear, grief and embarrassment. He notes a relationship between these feelings and certain overt expressions of them. Thus, in counselling, anger may be expressed as loud sound, fear as trembling, grief through tears, and embarrassment by laughter. He notes, also, a relationship between those feelings and certain basic human needs. Heron argues that we all have the need to understand and know what is happening to us. If that knowledge is not forthcoming, we may experience fear. We need, also, to make choices in our lives, and if that choice is restricted in certain ways, we may feel anger. Thirdly, we need to experience the expression of love and of being loved. If that love is denied us or taken away from us, we may experience grief. To Heron's basic human needs may be added the need for self-respect and dignity. If such dignity is denied us, we may feel self-conscious and embarrassed. Practical examples of how these relationships 'work' in everyday life and in the counselling relationship may be illustrated as follows:

- A twenty-year-old girl is attempting to live in a flat on her own. Her parents, however, insist on visiting her regularly and making suggestions as to how she should decorate the flat. They also regularly buy her articles for it and gradually she senses that she is feeling very uncomfortable and distanced from her parents. In the counselling relationship she discovers that she is very angry: her desire to make choices for herself is continually being eroded by her parents' benevolence.
- A forty-five-year-old man hears that his mother is seriously ill and, subsequently, she dies. He feels no emotions except that of feeling 'frozen' and unemotional. During a counselling session he suddenly discovers the need to cry profoundly. As he does so, he realises that, many years ago, he had decided that crying was not a masculine thing to do. As a result, he blocked off his grief and felt numb, until, within the safety of the counselling relationship, he was able to discover his grief and express it.
- An eighteen-year-old boy, discussing his college work during a

counselling session, begins to laugh almost uncontrollably. As he does so, he begins to feel the laughter turning to tears. Through his mixed laughter and tears he acknowledges that 'No one ever took me seriously ... not at school, at home ... or anywhere'. His laughter may be an expression of his lack of self-esteem, and his tears, the grief he experiences at that lack.

In the last example it may be noted how emotions that are suppressed are rarely only of one sort. Very often, bottled-up emotion is a mixture of anger, fear, embarrassment and grief. Often, too, the causes of such blocked emotion are unclear and lost in the history of the person. What is perhaps more important is that the expression of pent-up emotion is often helpful in that it seems to allow the person to be clearer in his thinking once he has expressed it. It is as though the blocked emotion 'gets in the way' and its release acts as a means of helping the person to clarify his thoughts and feelings. It is notable that the suppression of feelings can lead to certain problems in living that may be clearly identified.

THE EFFECTS OF BOTTLING UP EMOTION

Physical discomfort and muscular pain

Wilhelm Reich, a psychoanalyst with a particular interest in the relationship between emotions and the musculature noted that blocked emotions could become trapped in the body's muscle clusters (Reich, 1949). Thus he noted that anger was frequently 'trapped' in the muscles of the shoulders, grief in muscles surrounding the stomach and fear in the leg muscles. Often, these trapped emotions lead to chronic postural problems. Sometimes, the thorough release of the blocked emotion can lead to a freeing up of the muscles and an improved physical appearance. Reich believed in working directly on the muscle clusters in order to bring about emotional release and subsequent freedom from suppression and out of his work was developed a particular type of mind–body therapy, known as 'bioenergetics' (Lowen, 1967; Lowen and Lowen, 1977).

In terms of everyday counselling, trapped emotion is sometimes 'visible' in the way that the client holds himself, and the skilled counsellor can learn to notice tension in the musculature and changes in breathing patterns that may suggest muscular tension. We have noted throughout this book how difficult it is to interpret another person's behaviour. What is important, here, is that such bodily manifestations be used only as a clue to what may be happening in the person. We cannot assume that a person, who looks tense, is tense, until he has said that he is.

Health professionals will be very familiar with the link between body posture, the musculature and the emotional state of the person. Frequently, if patients and clients can be helped to relax, then their medical and psychological condition may improve more quickly. Those health professionals who deal most directly with the muscle clusters (remedial gymnasts and physiotherapists, for example) will tend to notice physical tension more readily but all carers can train themselves to observe these important indicators of the emotional status of the person in their care.

Difficulty in decision-making

This is a frequent side effect of bottled-up emotion. It is as though the emotion makes the person uneasy and that uneasiness leads to lack of confidence. As a result, that person finds it difficult to rely on his own resources and may find decision-making difficult. When we are under stress of any sort it is often the case that we feel the need to check decisions with other people. Once some of this stress is removed by talking through problems or by releasing pent-up emotions, the decision-making process often becomes easier.

Faulty self-image

When we bottle up feelings, those feelings often have an unpleasant habit of turning against us. Thus, instead of expressing anger towards others, we turn it against ourselves and feel depressed as a result. Or, if we have hung on to unexpressed grief, we turn that grief in on ourselves and experience ourselves as less than we are. Often, in counselling, as old resentments or dissatisfactions are expressed, so the person begins to feel better about himself.

Setting unrealistic goals

Tension can lead to further tension. This tension can lead us to set ourselves unreachable targets. It is almost as though we set ourselves up to fail! Sometimes, too, failing is a way of punishing ourselves or it is 'safer' than achieving. Release of tension, through the expression of emotion, can sometimes help in a person's taking a more realistic view of himself and his goal setting.

The development of long-term faulty beliefs

Sometimes, emotion that has been bottled up for a long time can lead to a person's view of the world being coloured in a particular way. He learns that 'People can't be trusted' or 'People always let you down in the end'. It is as though old, painful feelings lead to distortions that become part of that person's world-view. Such long-term distorted beliefs about the world do not change easily but may be modified as the person comes to release feelings and learns to handle his emotions more effectively.

The 'last straw' syndrome

Sometimes, if emotion is bottled up for a considerable amount of time, a valve blows and the person hits out either literally or verbally. We have all experienced the problem of storing up anger and taking it out on someone else: a process that is sometimes called 'displacement'. The original object of our anger is now replaced by something or someone else. Again, the talking through of difficulties or the release of pent-up emotion can often help to ensure that the person does not feel the need to explode in this way.

Clearly, no two people react to the bottling up of emotion in the same way. Some people, too, choose not to deal with life events emotionally. It would be curious to argue that there is a 'norm' where emotions are concerned. On the other hand, many people complain of being unable to cope with emotions, and if the client perceives there to be a problem in the emotional domain, then that perception may be expressed as a desire to explore his emotional status. It is important, however, that the counsellor does not force her particular set of beliefs about feelings and emotions on the client, but waits to be asked to help. Often the request for such help is a tacit request: the client talks about difficulty in dealing with emotion and that, in itself, may safely be taken as a request for help. A variety of methods is available to the counsellor to help in the exploration of the domain of feelings, and those methods will be described. Sometimes, these methods produce catharsis – the expression of strong emotion: tears, anger, fear, laughter. Drawing on the literature on the subject, the following statements may be made about the handling of such emotional release:

- Emotional release is usually self-limiting. If the person is allowed to cry or get angry, that emotion will be expressed and then gradually subside. The supportive counsellor will allow it to happen and not become unduly distressed by it.
- Physical support can sometimes be helpful in the form of holding the person's hand or putting an arm round him. Care should be taken, however, that such actions are unambiguous and that the holding of the client is not too 'tight'. A very tight embrace is likely to inhibit the release of emotion. It is worth remembering, also, that not everyone likes or wants physical contact. It is important the counsellor's support is not seen as intrusive by the client.
- Once the person has had a cathartic release he will need time to piece together the insights that he gains from such release. Often all that is needed is that the counsellor sits quietly with the client while he occasionally verbalises what he is thinking. The postcathartic period can be a very important stage in the counselling process.
- There seems to be a link between the amount we can 'allow' another person to express emotion and the degree to which we can handle our own emotion. This is another reason why the counsellor needs self-awareness. To help others explore their feelings we need, first, to explore our own. Many colleges and university departments offer workshops on cathartic work and self-awareness development that can help in both training the counsellor to help others and in gaining self-insight.
- Frequent 'cathartic counselling' can be exhausting for the counsellor,

and, if she is to avoid 'burnout', she needs to set up a network of support from other colleagues or via a peer-support group. We cannot hope to constantly handle other people's emotional release without its taking a toll on us.

METHODS OF HELPING THE CLIENT TO EXPLORE FEELINGS

These are practical methods that can be used in the counselling relationship to help the client to identify, examine and, if required, release emotion. Most of them will be more effective if the counsellor has first tried them on herself. This can be done simply by reading through the description of them and then trying them out, in one's mind. Alternatively, they can be tried out with a colleague or friend. Another way of exploring their effectiveness is to use them in a peer-support context. The setting up and running of such a group is described in Chapter 12 of this book; Chapter 13 contains various exercises that can be used to improve counselling skills. All of the following activities should be used gently and thoughtfully and timed to fit in with the client's requirements. There should never be any sense of pushing the client to explore feelings because of a misplaced belief that 'A good cry will do him good!'

Giving permission

Sometimes in counselling, the client tries desperately to hang on to strong feelings and not to express them. As we have seen, this may be due to the cultural norm which suggests that holding on is often better than letting go. Thus a primary method for helping someone to explore his emotions is for the counsellor to 'give permission' for the expression of feeling. This can be done simply through acknowledging that 'It's all right with me if you feel you are going to cry ... '. In this way the counsellor has reassured the client that expression of feelings is acceptable within the relationship. Clearly, a degree of tact is required here. It is important that the client does not feel pushed into expressing feelings that he would rather not express. The 'permission giving' should never be coercive nor should there be an implicit suggestion that 'You must express your feelings!'

Literal description

This refers to inviting the client to go back in his memory to a place that he is, until now, only alluding to, and describing that place in some detail. An example of this use of literal description is as follows:

Client: I used to get like this at home ... I used to get very upset ...
Counsellor: Just go back home for a moment ... describe one of the rooms in the house ...
Client: The front room faces directly out onto the street ... there is an armchair by the window ... the TV in the corner ... our dog is laying on the rug ... it's very quiet ...

Counsellor: What are you feeling right now?
Client: Like I was then ... angry ... upset ...

The going back to and describing in literal terms a place that was the scene of an emotional experience can often bring that emotion back. When the counsellor has invited the client to literally describe a particular place, she asks him, then, to identify the feeling that emerges from that description. It is important that the description has an 'I am there' quality about it and does not slip into a detached description, such as, 'We lived in a big house which wasn't particularly modern but then my parents didn't like modern houses much ... '.

Locating and developing a feeling in terms of the body

As we have previously noted, very often feelings are accompanied by a physical sensation. It is often helpful to identify that physical experience and to invite the client to exaggerate it, to allow the feeling to 'expand' in order to explore it further. Thus, an example of this approach is as follows:

Counsellor: How are you feeling at the moment?
Client: Slightly anxious.
Counsellor: Where, in terms of your body, do you feel the anxiety?
Client: (rubs stomach) Here.
Counsellor: Can you increase that feeling in your stomach?
Client: Yes, it's spreading up to my chest.
Counsellor: And what's happening now?
Client: It reminds me of a long time ago ... when I first started work ...
Counsellor: What happened there ... ?

Again, the original suggestion by the counsellor is followed through by a question to elicit how the client is feeling following the suggestion. This gives the client a chance to identify the thoughts that go with the feeling and to explore them further.

Empty chair

Another method of exploring feelings is to invite the client to imagine the feeling that he is experiencing as 'sitting' in a chair, next to him and then have him address the feeling. This can be used in a variety of ways and the next examples show its applications:

Example 1
Client: I feel very confused at the moment, I can't seem to sort things out ...
Counsellor: Can you imagine your confusion sitting in that chair over there ... what does it look like?
Client: It looks like a great big ball of wool ... how odd!
Counsellor: If you could speak to your confusion, what would you say to it?
Client: I wish I could sort you out!

Counsellor: And what's your confusion saying back to you?

Client: I'm glad you don't sort me out – I stop you from having to make any decisions!

Counsellor: And what do you make of that?

Client: I suppose that could be true ... the longer I stay confused, the less I have to make decisions about my family ...

Example 2

Counsellor: How are you feeling about the people you work with ... you said you found it quite difficult to get on with them ... ?

Client: Yes, it's still difficult, especially my boss.

Counsellor: Imagine your boss is sitting in that chair over there ... how does that feel?

Client: Uncomfortable! He's angry with me!

Counsellor: What would you like to say to him?

Client: Why do I always feel scared of you ... why do you make me feel uncomfortable?

Counsellor: And what does he say?

Client: I don't! It's you that feels uncomfortable, not me ... You make yourself uncomfortable ... (to the counsellor). He's right! I do make myself uncomfortable but I use him as an excuse ...

The 'empty chair' can be used in a variety of ways to set up a dialogue between either the client and his feelings or between the client and a person that the client talks 'about'. It offers a very direct way of exploring relationships and feelings, and deals directly with the issue of 'projection': the tendency we have to see qualities in others that are, in fact, our own. Using the empty chair technique can bring to light those projections and allow the client to see them for what they are. Other applications of this method are described in detail by Perls (1969).

Contradiction

It is sometimes helpful if the client is asked to contradict a statement that he makes, especially when that statement contains some ambiguity. An example of this approach is as follows:

Client: (looking at the floor) I've sorted everything out now: everything's OK.

Counsellor: Try contradicting what you've just said ...

Client: Everything's not OK ... Everything isn't sorted out ... (laughs) ... that's true, of course ... there's a lot more to sort out yet ...

Mobilisation of body energy

As we saw previously, there is the idea that emotions can be trapped within the body's musculature; it is sometimes helpful for the counsellor to suggest to the client that he stretches, or takes some very deep breaths. In the process, the client may become aware of tensions that are trapped in his body and begin to recognise and identify those tensions. This, in turn, can lead to the client talking about and expressing some of those tensions. This is particularly helpful if, during the counselling conversation, the client becomes less and less 'mobile' and adopts a particularly hunched or curled-up position in his chair. The invitation to stretch serves almost as a contradiction to the body position being adopted by the client at that time.

Exploring fantasy

We often set fairly arbitrary limits on what we think we can and cannot do. When a client seems to be doing this, it is sometimes helpful to explore what may happen if this limit was broken. An example of this is as follows:

> *Client:* I'd like to be able to go abroad for a change, I never seem to go very far on holiday.
> *Counsellor:* What stops you?
> *Client:* Flying, I suppose . . .
> *Counsellor:* What's the worst thing about flying?
> *Client:* I get very anxious.
> *Counsellor:* And what happens if you get very anxious?
> *Client:* Nothing really! I just get anxious!
> *Counsellor:* So nothing terrible can happen if you allow yourself to get anxious?
> *Client:* No, not really . . . I hadn't thought about it like that before . . .

Rehearsal

Sometimes the anticipation of a coming event or situation is anxiety provoking. The counsellor can usefully help the client to explore a range of feelings by rehearsing with him a future event. Thus the client who is anticipating a forthcoming interview may be helped by having the counsellor act the role of an interviewer, with a subsequent discussion afterwards. The client who wants to develop the assertive behaviour to enable him to challenge his boss might benefit from role-playing the situation in the counselling session. In each case, it is important that both client and counsellor 'get into role' and that the session does not just become a discussion of what may or may not happen. The actual playing through and rehearsal of a situation is nearly always more powerful than a discussion of it. Alberti and Emmons (1982) offer some useful suggestions about how to set up role-plays and exercises for developing assertive behaviour and Wilkinson and Canter (1982) describe some useful approaches to developing socially skilled behaviour. Often, if the client can practise effective behaviour, then the appropriate thoughts and feelings can accompany that behaviour. The novelist, Kurt Vonnegut, wryly commented that 'We are what we pretend to be – so take care what you pretend to be' (Vonnegut, 1968). Sometimes, the first stage in changing is trying out a new pattern of behaviour or a new way of thinking and feeling. Practice, therefore, is invaluable.

This approach develops from the idea that what we think influences what we feel and do. If our thinking is restrictive, we may begin to feel that we can or cannot do certain things. Sometimes, having these barriers to feeling and doing challenged can free a person to think, feel and act differently.

These methods of exploring feelings can be used alongside the client-centred interventions described in the previous chapter. They need to be practised in order that the counsellor feels confident in using them, and the means to developing the skills involved are identified in later chapters of this book. The domain of feelings is one that is frequently addressed in counselling.

Counselling people who want to explore feelings takes time and cannot be rushed. Also, the development and use of the various skills described here is not the whole of the issue. Health professionals working with emotions need, also, to have developed the personal qualities that have been described elsewhere: warmth, genuineness, empathic understanding and unconditional positive regard. Emotional counselling can never be a mechanical process but is one that touches the lives of both client and counsellor.

Helping with feelings in practice: I

Jane is a student nurse on a busy medical ward. She develops a close relationship with Arthur Davis, an elderly man who has been treated for heart failure. Suddenly and unexpectedly, Mr Davis dies. Jane finds herself unable to come to terms with this and seeks the help of an older tutor in the school of nursing. The tutor helps her to talk through her feelings and she cries a great deal. Through the process of talking and crying she comes to realise that Arthur Davis reminded her of her own father, who had also died suddenly and for whom she had been unable to grieve. In grieving for Mr Davis, she was enabled to work through some of her grief for her own father.

Helping with feelings in practice: II

Andrew is a radiographer in a large casualty department. He has recently had difficulties in his marriage which he feels affect his work in the department. He is able to talk this through with his superintendent, who has had training as a counsellor. During the course of the conversation, Andrew feels close to tears. His superintendent says, 'What would happen if you allowed yourself to cry?' Andrew smiles wryly and says, 'Nothing.' With that, he bursts into tears and is 'allowed' to cry. Afterwards, he finds it much easier to talk through his problems in a rational and systematic way and feels able to make more sense of what is happening at home. The superintendent's skilful and well-timed intervention allows Andrew the prompt that he needed to enable him to express bottled-up feelings.

HELPING WITH FEELINGS AND THE HEALTH PROFESSIONAL

As with other counselling interventions, the ones that deal with the expression of feelings have a wider application than just the counselling relationship. There are many occasions in the health care world in which the professional is called upon to help and support the person who is in emotional distress. Sometimes, such situations arise suddenly and without warning. The professional who has considered the skills involved in helping with the expression of emotion is likely to be better equipped to deal with these emergencies when they arise.

INFORMATION GIVING AND COUNSELLING IN SPECIFIC HEALTH CARE CONTEXTS

10

The climate of health care and the way in which people organise and live their lives are changing. As we have seen, there have been criticisms of the client-centred approach to counselling. There are also situations in which giving clear and unequivocal advice is likely to be appropriate in counselling. In this chapter, three things are considered: information giving, counselling people in the HIV/AIDS field and talking to children. All three are contemporary and important aspects of the counselling field in the health care professions.

INFORMATION GIVING

First, an important distinction needs to be made between *information giving* and *advice giving*. Information giving involves sharing with others facts, theories, statistics and other information gleaned from a variety of sources. Advice giving, on the other hand, suggests opinion: the *counsellor's* opinion. Whilst I have no intention of getting into the thorny debate about whether or not information can ever be 'objective' nor whether or not it can be proved to be 'true', there seems little doubt that information giving rarely involves a *moral* or *ethical* judgement that information giving implies.

So far, this book has focused mostly on the client being 'drawn out' by the counsellor and on that client finding his or her way through problems, to solutions. There are occasions, however, when those in a counselling role will be asked for specific information. This is true in all types of counselling but particularly true in health care settings where the counsellor in question may have valuable and useful information to be shared with the client. Examples of situations in which information is required are not difficult to think of, and a short list of some of them would include:

- the person who needs information about contraception;
- the person who is a newly diagnosed diabetic;
- the person who has recently been discharged from psychiatric hospital after many years in that institution;
- the person who is considering a career change but is unaware of options.

In all of these situations, the counsellor is called upon to give information. If he or she does not *have* that information then there is little point in bluffing or in trying to help the client to find it. In most cases it is more economical and safer to refer the person to another agency.

Certain guidelines can be offered about information giving. Information given in counselling should be:

- accurate;
- up to date;
- appropriate to the context;
- worded in such a way that the client will understand it;
- sufficient to satisfy the client's needs at the time.

Many health care professionals use jargon as a form of shorthand and as a means of quickly communicating with other colleagues. It is not difficult for such professionals to *forget* that they have learned this jargon and to assume that it is common currency amongst other people. It is vital that any health professional giving information does so using words that are straightforward, unambiguous and clear. This never means 'talking down' to the client but it does mean that the counsellor should check with the client that he or she has understood the information that has been given. It is not uncommon for people to 'hear what they want to hear' – particularly when they are frightened or want to hear good news. Others are bemused by professionals and are uncertain how to seek clarification. The good counsellor will make him or herself approachable enough to be questioned – at length, if necessary – by the client. Many of these points have been summarised in the context of medicine, by Myerscough:

> *In addition to availability of information, a further element contributes greatly to the success of the exposition. This is the doctor's skill in choosing vocabulary suitable to the patient. The form of words and choice of terms will differ from one patient to another; it will be influenced by their education, cultural and occupational background and other factors. Terms the doctor may regard as 'innocent' and reassuring may readily create serious anxiety. For example, when a woman with a cervical erosion is told that she has 'just a small ulcer on the neck of the womb', she may infer the presence of serious disease, imminently or actually malignant, and be too alarmed to try to clarify what the doctor's words really mean.*

(Mysercough, 1989)

HIV/AIDS COUNSELLING: SOME CONSIDERATIONS

This section considers some of the issues involved in the health professional as AIDS counsellor. It is important to state from the outset that just as not all health care professionals will need to develop counselling skills in general, nor will all health care professionals need to develop AIDS counselling skills. It is also important to note that most other health professionals will also need to develop basic counselling skills in this field.

It is possible to argue that the skills involved in counselling the person with AIDS are not fundamentally different from counselling anyone. On the other hand, the evidence suggests that people with AIDS often have particular problems that can best be helped by someone who has specific skills and knowledge (Andersen and MacElveen-Hoen, 1988; MacCaffrey, 1987; Sketchley, 1989).

It is notable, too, that health care professionals are becoming increasingly interested in the issue of counselling as part of the nursing role (Hopper *et al.*, 1991; Tschudin, 1991). Also, it is clear from the developing literature on the topic that AIDS and AIDS counselling are issues of growing concern to health care professionals and educators in the UK (see, for example, Dennis, 1991; Howe, 1989; Hurtig and Fandrick, 1990; McGough, 1990).

Client groups

People who need AIDS counselling are not a homogenous group. A list of the people who are likely to require counselling in this field is offered by Bor:

- clients who have concerns or queries about AIDS, regardless of their clinical status;
- clients who are referred for the human immunodeficiency virus (HIV) antibody test;
- clients who are HIV antibody negative but who continue to present with AIDS-related worries;
- clients who are HIV antibody positive and symptomless;
- clients who are HIV antibody positive and who are becoming unwell;
- clients who have developed AIDS;
- clients who are being offered, or who are being considered for, antiviral treatments;
- the sexual contacts, loved ones, or family of any of those already listed, if the client has given his or her permission;
- the close contacts of a deceased client, who may also later require bereavement counselling;
- staff with concerns about AIDS or those who are occupationally exposed to HIV (in conjunction with the occupational health department) (Bor, 1991).

It seems clear that different sorts of counselling skills and approaches are likely to be needed in AIDS counselling and that 'AIDS counselling' is not one particular entity. Bor, Miller, Perry *et al.*, (1989) conclude that 'There are many different counselling approaches and no evidence yet that one is better than another'.

For people who are substance abusers, Cook *et al.* suggest risk reduction counselling, which includes:

1 assisting the client to acknowledge the personal risks of HIV infection;
2 explaining the range of changes that will reduce infection and transmission risks, addressing attitudinal and environmental obstacles (for example, feelings of having no control, resistance from partners) and rehearsing behaviours as needed;

3 reinforcing changes in a way that helps the client to assume increasing control over health behaviours so that early accomplishments can be sustained and built upon (Cook *et al.*, 1988).

Faltz offers the following guidelines for working with substance-abusing clients. Some of these may well be appropriate for other client groups:

- Be willing to listen and encourage constructive expression of feelings.
- Express caring and concern for the individual.
- Hold the individual responsible for his or her actions.
- Ensure consistent consequences for negative behaviours.
- Talk to the individual about specific actions that are disruptive or disturbing.
- Do not compromise your own values or expectations.
- Communicate your plan of action to other staff members or professionals working with the client.
- Monitor your own reactions to the client (Faltz, 1989).

A wide range of other sorts of clients has been discussed in the AIDS counselling literature including 'the worried well' – discussed in a little more detail later (Bor, Miller, Perry *et al.*, 1989), those who want or need to keep their diagnosis secret (Bor, Miller and Salt, 1989), the counselling of antenatal women (Miller and Bor, 1990), children (Miller, Goldman, Bor *et al.*, 1989), those with haemophilia (DiMarzo, 1989) and ethnic minorities (Fullilove, 1989). Another group that might ask for counselling are bisexual people. The Off Pink Collective (1988), having noted the paucity of research into bisexuality, writes as follows:

> *Up until now the fact that maybe over a third of the population has strong attractions to or sexual activities with both sexes has generally been ignored. Sexual self-identities have been seen as either heterosexual, or gay or lesbian. But in reality people are not in distinct groups. As far as disease transmission is concerned, it is actual behaviour rather than self-identity that counts and many self-identified heterosexuals and gay men and lesbians behave bisexually. Contrary to a frequent association of bisexuality with promiscuity, it is our experience that many self-identified bisexuals are recurrently celibate, and increasingly so as part of a safer sex life.*

(Off Pink Collective, 1988)

Reviewing the literature on AIDS, AIDS counselling and sexuality tends to confirm the view that whilst bisexual people are noted to be at risk, they are less widely written about than are gay or heterosexual people.

There are specific issues in counselling for the counsellor who faces a person who is unsure about whether or not to be tested. McCreaner identifies the aims of pre-test counselling as follows:

- To ensure that any decision to take the test is fully informed and based on an understanding of the personal, medical, legal and social implications of a positive result. At one level, this is a mere practical application of the traditional medical ethic of informed consent to a procedure.

- To provide the necessary preparation for those who will have to face the trauma of a positive result. Such preparation is vital in that patients who have been prepared for a positive result are able to face that result much more equably.
- To provide the individual, whether he eventually elects not to be tested, or elects to be tested and is found positive or found to be negative, with necessary risk-reduction information on the basis of which he can reduce the risk of either acquiring HIV infection or passing it on to others (McCreaner, 1989).

For the person who has AIDS, Sketchley (1989) suggests that there are frequently four stages to be worked through in the counselling relationship:

1 Crisis: a stage in which the predominant emotions are shock, fear and denial,
2 Adjustment to the news: in which social disruption and withdrawal are common as the person struggles to accept the diagnosis,
3 Acceptance: a stage in which the person adopts a new sense of self within the limitations imposed by the illness,
4 Preparation for death: a stage in which the issues of fear of dependence, pain, being abandoned, isolation and death, itself, may predominate.

These stages are not at all dissimilar to the stages worked through by any person who has to face the prospect of dying (Stedeford, 1989). The counsellor who seeks to help the person with AIDS may also have to work on his or her feelings about his or her *own* death.

AIDS counselling is carried out by many people. At one level, various telephone counselling services exist for people who are worried that they may have AIDS and for those who need support. At another level, there are people who are identified specifically as AIDS counsellors (Leukefeld, 1988). They are often attached to hospitals, hospices and national AIDS organisations and offer help to people with AIDS, their friends and families (Dilley *et al.*, 1989).

It is notable that different cities have organised their counselling and support systems in different ways. In 1987, the Canadian Federal Centre for AIDS observed that the AIDS programme in San Francisco was much more community oriented (with correspondingly more counselling agencies) than was the programme in New York (where many more people were being cared for in hospital).

Increasingly, health care professionals will find themselves fulfilling the role of AIDS counsellor, for as Bor (1991) points out, they are at the forefront of professional care-giving to patients and families affected with or affected by AIDS. If AIDS continues to increase in incidence (and there is every evidence that it will), then health care professionals will find themselves caring for more and more people who have developed a range of infections suffered by people with AIDS. At least two things follow from this. All health care professionals will have to have a considerable knowledge about the nature of AIDS. They will also have to explore their own values and attitudes to the problem and to develop counselling strategies and skills.

On the first issue, the question of health care professionals developing their knowledge base, the problem is a difficult one. Just as the AIDS virus itself seems to be changing (Connor and Kingman, 1989), so does the research and knowledge base. No worker in the field can expect to stay completely up to date. On the other hand, certain issues stay the same. The mode of transmission of the virus is well documented and everyone should have a clear idea about what constitutes safe sex and what to do to avoid becoming a person with AIDS (Miller, 1987; Miller, 1990).

In summary of the issues involved in HIV/AIDS counselling, Sketchley (1989) suggests that counselling people with AIDS involves three domains:

- educational issues;
- advice;
- psychosocial issues.

The worried well

This is not a particularly comfortable expression but it has been used to describe people who do not suffer from a particular disease or disorder but who are, nevertheless, worried about themselves. Green and Davey (1992) suggest that, in the early days of AIDS counselling, many of the people that sought advice fell into the category of the worried well.

The worried well are not a homogenous group. They can range from people who are edging towards what some psychiatrists might want to call 'neurosis', to people who simply want to know what they should do about aspects of their lives. Traditionally, the worried well have sometimes been given little sympathy from medical and health care professionals, who sometimes would prefer to deal with frank illness or tangible problems. It is important, however, not to 'pathologise' further the person who is both worried and well. The label should not become a diagnosis.

Perhaps the main point is that the worried well should be taken seriously. They are as entitled as anyone else to be listened to and given appropriate help. Trivialisation or glib reassurance that 'Everything will work out OK' or that 'There is nothing to worry about' fall well short of the sort of help that people are seeking. Once again, the keyword seems to be *listening*. If we can listen to the worried and well person, we are likely to help to alleviate some of the worry and help to ensure that he or she remains well. Sickness or disability are not prerequisites for seeking counselling.

AIDS counselling in adolescence and childhood

The prevention of the spread of HIV/AIDS may depend, in the West, on the appropriate education and counselling of children and adolescents. Hein has suggested that there are important differences between adolescents and adults in sexual behaviour and AIDS epidemiology that should be considered in planning appropriate responses to the AIDS epidemic. The differences are:

- A higher percentage of adolescent cases is acquired by heterosexual transmission.
- A higher percentage of infected adolescents is asymptomatic.
- A higher percentage of infected adolescents are from minorities.
- Special ethical and legal considerations pertain to minors.
- Adolescents differ from adults in sociocognitive reasoning.
- There are special economic and medical implications for infected adolescents who are pregnant.
- Unified community support systems for infected adolescents are not available.
- Adolescents as a population include a higher percentage of 'sexual adventurers', who have many sexual contacts and rarely use contraceptives.
- Convenient and appropriate health services are relatively unavailable for adolescents (Hein, 1989).

It would seem, too, that health professionals who counsel young people in this field are likely to find some differences between what adolescents *know* about HIV/AIDS and what they *do*:

> Surveys of sexual activity among high school students and among college students conducted since the AIDS epidemic indicate that a higher percentage of youths engage in unsafe sexual activity in spite of having a high level of knowledge about AIDS and about the value of condoms in protecting against HIV infections.
>
> (Henggeler *et al.*, 1992)

Added to all this is the controversy that has surrounded the teaching of young people who have been identified as HIV positive. Often, it would seem, the counsellor of young people in this field is likely to need to consider the attitudes of parents, teachers and other people who come into contact with children and adolescents. Gostin summarises some of emotive attitudes that have been observed in this area:

> From the earliest times of the HIV epidemic, exclusion of school children infected with HIV from their classrooms was an issue debated with great emotion. Parents of children infected with HIV sued school boards for denying children state education, giving homebound instruction, or making the child wait for inordinate periods while the board developed a policy. In other cases, HIV-infected children were permitted to attend school, but they were

clearly singled out as different by being placed alone in a separate 'modular' classroom, by being required to use a separate bathroom and to be accompanied by an adult on all field trips, or even being isolated inside a glass booth.

(Gostin, 1990)

Clearly, the whole area of counselling children and adolescents in the area of HIV/AIDS is a complicated one. The health professional as counsellor needs to know, not only about the syndrome, modes of infection and means of prevention, but about children, adolescents and their ways of viewing and operating in the world. Counselling in this area calls for all of the skills described so far in this book and, further, for particular and accurate knowledge.

Training in AIDS counselling for health care professionals

Many courses in AIDS counselling are already available to both health care professionals and other carers. The question remains, however, to what degree *all* health care professionals should undergo some basic training in the field. At the moment, perhaps, it is for individual health care professionals to identify their own needs and wants. It is questionable how long this state of affairs can be allowed to continue. If, as is suspected, the incidence of AIDS continues to grow, the AIDS issue is going to be everyone's business. In the meantime, more research needs to be undertaken to establish exactly how best to train health care professionals in helping those with AIDS.

From a review of the literature, three elements of training appear to be important:

- information about AIDS;
- values clarification;
- counselling skills.

It would appear that any training programme for health care professionals would need to include these elements. First, health care professionals need up-to-date and accurate information about the prevention, incidence, nature and characteristics of AIDS and HIV. They also need information about the psychosocial issues involved in being a person with AIDS.

Values clarification is an approach to helping people to explore their beliefs, values and attitudes. Again, it would seem vital that these are examined with health care professionals prior to those health care professionals working in the capacity of AIDS counsellors.

Finally, given that the focus of the role is counselling, a grounding in basic counselling skills is essential to any programme of this sort. The skills of questioning, reflecting, empathy building and checking for understanding can be augmented by skills in confrontation and effective information giving (Heron, 1986; Nelson-Jones, 1995). Whilst, as we have noted, the counselling approach in AIDS counselling may not always be of the client-centred type, client-centred skills can serve as the basis of a broader range of effective counselling skills.

This section has discussed some of the issues involved in considering the training of health care professionals as AIDS counsellors as part of their nursing role. It has been identified that not all health care professionals will want or need to take part in such work but that those who do will need to explore their own attitudes, develop a broad and accurate knowledge base and develop a range of effective interpersonal and helping skills.

Emotions and AIDS

Given that individuals vary in their response to life-threatening situations, it is difficult to generalise about the ways in which people react to the knowledge that they are HIV positive or have AIDS. George, however, identifies the following emotions that he suggests are frequently associated with the experience of having AIDS:

- shock;
- relief;
- anger;
- guilt;
- decreased self-esteem;
- loss of identity;
- loss of a sense of security;
- loss of personal control;
- fear of what may happen in the future;
- sadness and depressed mood;
- obsessions and compulsions;
- positive adjustment (George, 1989).

Presumably, too, this list could be easily added to. It is notable that only one of George's items is positive and he suggests that positive adjustment to the realisation of having AIDS may occur with little intervention from professionals. This suggests that the AIDS counsellor may well have to face a wide range of negative emotions.

COUNSELLING CHILDREN

'Counselling', in this context, may be too strong a term. I prefer to use the expression 'talking with children'. Many people, for a variety of reasons, find that quite difficult. For some, children seem to be 'different' from adults: they are smaller, they talk a different language and it seems a long time since the adult listener was their age. However, children need to be able to talk and need, very much, someone they can trust and have listen to them.

It is possible to draw principles from the world of counselling to shed light on how we might begin to think about helping children.[1] 'Adult'

[1] I am indebted to my friend and colleague, Jim Richardson, for his help and advice on talking to children.

counselling usually involves two people: the counsellor and the client. The counsellor is usually the person who asks questions, reflects back feelings and thoughts and checks that he or she has understood what the client has said. In the client-centred tradition of counselling, it is taken as given that it is the client who will find his or her *own* solutions to his or her problems. There seems no immediate reason why such an approach cannot be used in communicating with children. It seems that the main point of helping children should be to allow those children to express their thoughts and feelings and to identify strategies for dealing with difficulties – whatever those 'difficulties' might be.

There are numerous occasions on which children may need to talk through difficulties and problems. Examples include, prior to surgical or medical intervention; in coming to terms with acute or chronic illness or disability; following the death of a parent, relative or close friend; after another family crisis has occurred or in coming to terms with new, anxiety-provoking ideas and realisations revealed to the child during his or her developmental progress. Whether or not all of these situations would be deemed 'counselling' situations is not the point: the basic skills of counselling apply to them all. The person who listens and helps children is already functioning in the role of a counsellor.

The literature often identifies *listening* as the most important skill in communicating effectively with other people (Calnan, 1983; Egan, 1990; Tschudin, 1991). The ability to sit and listen to a child as she or he talks through what is happening to her or him is the starting point of any therapeutic relationship. In many situations, the mere fact of being heard is all that is required. In other situations, help and advice will be appropriate. Whilst the *client-centred* approach to counselling has been widely advocated as appropriate to helping adults, it is possible that, if information giving is necessary as part of this process for children, they may need more direction and prescription. In the end, though, like adults, children have to come to terms with their problems in their own individual ways. Like adults, no one can make a decision about a problem *for* a child: they, like adults, have to make their own decisions in their own time. However, there are certain issues that can help in the process of offering counselling to children. An understanding of the processes and peculiarities of development in childhood can help in the evolution of empathy and in the skill of listening.

Issues in communicating with children

Children's communication abilities vary with their age and experience (Prosser, 1985). The health care professional will have to be sensitive not only to subtle non-verbal communicative means but also to sometimes idiosyncratic use of language. In particular, children may have unusual ways of describing situations or feelings for which they do not, yet, have the language. An example of this is the child who was asked to describe her pain and referred to it as 'like a sausage' (Jerrett and Evans, 1986). It is important to try to get 'inside' children's frames of reference and to try to understand what *they* mean by the words they use. This calls for considerable empathy: a quality that Rogers (1957) identified as a necessary and sufficient condition for therapeutic change. Empathising with children may be more difficult than is the case with adults: it is certainly just as essential. Children's interpersonal responses are influenced by their interpretation of the context and situation. This may, in the light of adult logic, be quite unexpectedly different from an adult's interpretation.

Children's dependence on their parents/carers may mean that, particularly in the situation in which they feel frightened or vulnerable, they might prefer to communicate with a stranger obliquely, e.g. via a parent. A fine distinction is drawn between treating the child as an individual on the one hand and as an enmeshed member of a supportive family on the other (Jackson and Vessey, 1992). None of us exists in isolation. We are all closely bound up with the lives of the people with whom we live and work. For the child, the ego boundary – the difference between 'me here' and 'you out there' – may be even less pronounced than is the case with adults.

Children have a tendency towards literal, concrete communication. Witticisms, sarcasms and word games may be lost on the child, clouding communication. Again, Carl Rogers saw the ability to be concrete in dealing with others as an essential feature of the counselling process.

Most family members use a 'shorthand' when talking to each other. Family names, for example, may not be 'proper' names. Often, too, families develop secret or private languages (Crystal, 1987) through which to communicate with each other. There may, for example, be family words for certain meals, for drinks or for certain events. The genesis of these names may be lost in family history. More importantly, the child may not *know* that this is a 'family' word and may think that *everyone* uses language in this way. It is important for the person who talks to a child to clarify any unusual use of language in order to have a more complete understanding of any given situation.

Indirect communication, perhaps using a doll or a soft toy, may be successful with the shy or wary child, as this diffuses the focus from the child and introduces an element of play and therefore normality. A child at a stage of development characterised by animistic or magical thinking will find this form of communication natural.

Paralinguistic devices such as variations in the speed, rhythm, tone and volume of speech as well as extra 'padding' words such as 'um', 'ah' and 'well' which have little direct meaning are extensively used by adults and may be misinterpreted by children. When children do begin to use these communication styles they may do so inexpertly and this in turn may be awkward for adults to understand.

To make communication between adults and children as effective as possible it is important that the adult firmly establishes what the child's understanding is of the issue in question. This is particularly important when the discussion centres on an abstraction about which the child may have no experience. An example of this is the topic of death: if the child has an inaccurate perception of what death is he may find it extremely difficult to understand an adult-level conversation on this topic (Lansdown, 1992). Effective talking with the child can only occur when the adult is clear about the terms which are understandable to the child on the basis of his experience and stage of cognitive development.

Avoid rushing the child – allow him a little time to get to know you. Let him dictate the pace. The flustered child is unlikely to be able to – or want to – talk with the adult who is pressurising him. Watch the child for signs of tiredness and withdrawal – in these circumstances communication is less likely to succeed.

It was acknowledged in Chapter 1 that many adults want some form of *spiritual* counselling and that this may or may not take on a religious connotation. What is less commonly recognised is *children's* need for talking about spiritual matters. There are some examples of the situations in which health care and other professionals might come into contact with children's spiritual needs:

- the nurse on the night shift who is embarrassed when a little boy asks if she will listen to his prayers;
- the medical student who is told by a girl that she is worried because she is dying but does not believe in God;
- the parent whose child asks her mother if God does not like her and that is the reason she is dying;
- the doctor who has no experience of talking to children who are concerned that they are having an anaesthetic and might die;
- the social worker who wants to know the right words to comfort a suffering child but does not know how to talk to him;
- the occupational therapist who is working with children but does not know how to answer their questions about 'God';
- the student health care practitioner who is uncertain whether or not to share her own religious beliefs with children who ask questions;
- the student nurse who is an atheist but is asked 'religious' questions by children for whom she cares.

Practical guidelines for talking to children

From the issues already discussed and from the considerable literature on counselling and talking with children, the following guidelines may be identified:

- Listen to the child – although his or her message may not be immediately clear he or she has much to say (Coles, 1992).
- Find out what the child likes to be called. Do not assume that he or she will like you to call him by a nickname or a name used in the family. Give the child your own name – introduce yourself!
- Be aware of levels and stages of child development. This can help you to pitch your questions and responses at the correct level. Observe the child's response for signs of success in this.
- Respond to the individual child as an individual. Do not assume that 'All children are much the same'. Children are complete human

beings in their own right. When meeting a child for the first time the only thing that you can assume is that you are about to meet a *new* person.

- Talk to children 'normally': neither talk down to them nor patronise them and be aware of any overuse of endearments such as 'dear' or 'love'. Try to keep speech clear, avoid very erudite words and expressions. Keep sentences short. Repeat/rephrase as necessary, based on response.
- Respect the child. Remember that he or she is a human being just like you, only a little younger.
- Think about the environment in which you talk to the child. If you are working in a hospital or clinical setting, find a quiet room in which to talk: children's wards and out-patients, departments are often excruciatingly noisy places. Alternatively, talk as you play with the child.
- Use play to communicate with smaller children.
- Do not try to copy children's slang or adapt their mannerism. I recall a conversation with my adolescent son in which I tried to use some of the slang that he used with his friends. His suggestion was, 'You shouldn't even try, because even when you get the words right, it doesn't sound right.' 'Why?' 'Because you're too old.'
- Believe children. Trust must be the basis of any relationship and it is particularly important with children.
- Remember that most children are taught not to talk to strangers. Therefore, some children will prefer talking to you only in the company of one of their parents. Do not assume that children will *want* to talk to you. Also, as Shapiro suggests:

> *Children are used to being talked about by people who care for them; it happens all the time with their parents, and they can accept this as a part of life. They do not necessarily distrust the therapist who also talks to their parents, as long as the therapist's intentions are made clear from the beginning of the treatment.*
>
> (Shapiro, 1984)

- Allow the child to determine the issue of proximity. Do not stand or sit too close or automatically put your arm around him or her. Allow the child to decide on these issues. Be aware of what might, for the child, constitute a threat. Sometimes, it is necessary to be creative and to find out where the *child* would like to sit and talk. In her excellent book *Children and Counselling*, Margaret Crompton writes as follows about the issue of *where* to counsel children:

> *... Yet somewhere can always be found. During my work with children in 1989–90, I carried materials in a large shopping bag. Since it was not possible to work with Mark in his foster home and there was no office within miles, I met him once a week from school and asked: 'Where shall we go today?' The answer was*

*always the same, despite the possibility of an interesting castle
and an inviting river: 'To the café'.*

(Crompton, 1992)

Crompton's book is essential reading for anyone who is considering
either a career in working with children or who needs further information about counselling and talking with children.

Talking to children is an activity which many adults will undertake
without hesitation. With a little attention to some ground rules, the
likelihood of successful communication can be maximised, and the
potential for this activity to offer benefit, comfort and pleasure to both
the child and to the adult can be safeguarded. The key to success lies in
the adult's appreciation of the various facets of the child as a dynamic,
developing human being with sometimes imperfect, unpractised psychological, social and communication skills. Everyday communication with
children merges subtly with counselling – communication with a therapeutic purpose (Macleod Clark *et al.*, 1991). With practice in the basic
skills of talking to children, the person should come to recognise when
basic skills are no longer sufficient and specialist counselling assistance
is required. This will signal the need for referral. Thus, familiarity with
the ground rules of communicating with children may help you to
recognise your own limitations in this field.

Street, in discussing the question of *family counselling*, suggests that
the following four questions need to be asked of families that present
themselves for counselling. The questions impinge, directly, on the
process of talking to children in therapeutic settings:

- Does the family have information on which to base an appropriate
  view of the task?
- Is the communication in the family clear and open or does it need to
  be clarified?
- Is it possible to specify the needs of everyone in the family?
- What negotiations for adaptions to change need to be made? (Street,
  1989).

OTHER CONTEXTS

This chapter has only hinted at the variety of arenas in which
counselling may take place. Many others exist. There has been debate,
for instance, about *race*. Lago and Thompson suggest that the following
may be the major themes in this field:

- In order to understand the relationships between black and white
  people today, a knowledge of the history between differing racial
  groups is required.
- Counsellors will also require an understanding of how contemporary
  society works in relation to race, the exercise of power, the effects of
  discrimination, stereotyping, how ideologies sabotage policies, and so
  on.

- Counsellors require a personal awareness of where they stand in relation to these issues (Lago and Thompson, 1989).

Other writers have discussed the issues of sexual orientation (Beane, 1981; Lourea, 1985), sexual dysfunction (Bancroft, 1983; Fairburn *et al.*, 1983). Yet others have described the particular issues involved in counselling the unemployed and those who need career guidance (Ball, 1984; Hopson, 1985). The literature on sexuality counselling is considerable and those who need further information about job-related counselling are referred to the various journals on the topic, which include the *British Journal of Guidance and Counselling* and *Employee Counselling Today*. Other contexts, which may involve the giving of clear information are identified in Dryden *et al.* (1989) and include the following:

- pastoral counselling;
- counselling in death and bereavement;
- counselling people with disabilities and chronic illnesses;
- counselling people with alcohol and drug problems.

The range of counselling situations remains vast. Indeed, it may be argued that the term 'counselling' is also an umbrella term for a wide range of varied activities carried out by a number of different sorts of professionals. Within that spectrum, the full range of counselling approaches from the client-centred to the confronting may be found.

11 PROBLEMS AND SUPPORT IN COUNSELLING

Counselling takes time and energy on the part of the counsellor. The fact of being intimately involved in someone else's world means that both counsellor and client form a close and, sometimes, painful relationship. If counselling is to be successful, it will involve change on the part of the client. It may also involve change on the part of the counsellor. Now most of us resist change – we prefer to stay as we are. In counselling it often seems as though the client wants problem-resolution without having to change himself! Clearly, life-problems cannot change without the person who experiences them changing too. The nature of the counselling relationship, then, is one that develops, regresses, modulates and is finally outgrown. Along that dimension, various difficulties can arise and in this chapter a number of such problems are identified and explored.

CONFIDENTIALITY

Should what is said in a counselling situation remain confidential? On the face of it, the answer seems fairly straightforward: that, in usual circumstances, what the client tells the counsellor should remain only with those two people. On the other hand, there are numerous situations in which the client may disclose things that the counsellor feels *must* be disclosed to another person. Some examples of such situations might include the following:

- the person who says that she is going to kill herself;
- the client who tells the counsellor that he is abusing one of his children;
- the person who seems, in the counsellor's opinion, to be showing signs of mental illness.

These situations and many others call for considerable soul-searching on the part of the counsellor. Various possible equations can be worked out for anticipating and coping with the question of confidentiality in counselling:

- The counsellor may offer total confidentiality to the client. In this case, the counsellor must be prepared to stick to his or her word, and *everything* that is said must remain confidential. One of the considerable strengths of the *Samaritan* movement is that it offers this level of confidentiality. On the other hand, the health professional is often in a different situation from a Samaritan and is accountable to the health care organisation in which he or she works. It may be debatable whether or not such total confidentiality can be offered by a health care professional.

- The counsellor may tell the client at the beginning of the relationship that the relationship will *not* be a confidential one and that certain people may have to know about the content of counselling conversations. This is the reverse side of the previous option. Whilst some clients may feel that this lack of confidentiality is inhibiting, then at least the contract between the two people is clear. Also, the client can be reassured that people will only be given information on a 'need to know' basis.

- The counsellor may avoid discussing the question of confidentiality as an issue in its own right but consult the client, during the relationship, as to the degree to which that person is comfortable about information being shared with other professional colleagues.

Sometimes, of course, the nature of the content of a counselling relationship is not of the 'confidential' sort. Some conversations do not contain very much 'personal' information but many do. All health professionals working as counsellors need to address and face the issue of confidentiality in counselling. Munro *et al.* offer these other useful guidelines:

- The client should know where she stands in relation to confidentiality. For example, if case discussion is routine within an agency, the client should be told this.

- Where referral to another agency or consultation with another family member seems appropriate, the client's prior permission should be sought.

- When a client specifically requests confidentiality regarding a particular disclosure, this must be respected.

- Where confidentiality has to be broken because of the law or because of danger to the client's life, she should be informed as soon as possible.

- Records of interviews should be minimal, noting only what is essential within the particular agency setting. Records should be locked up, shared only with authorised recipients who would also be bound by confidentiality, and destroyed when the counselling relationship is terminated.

- An atmosphere of confidentiality is even more important than any verbal reassurance of it. If, for example, during the interview notetaking is considered essential, the counsellor could offer to let the client see what is being written or even write it herself.

- Confidentiality, when part of a professional code of ethics, should be upheld (Munro *et al.*, 1989).

What must be borne in mind is that *carrying* someone else's confidential thoughts and feelings can be painful and distracting. When someone shares an important, personal and even dangerous thought or feeling, part of the responsibility that goes with that thought or feeling is transferred to the person who receives it. If, for example, I tell you that I am planning to kill myself, the fact that you now *know* this means that you have to decide whether or not you (as another human being) are responsible for doing something about it. Also, you have to consider whether or not you *can* do anything about it. A person who sets him or herself up as a counsellor must be prepared to shoulder other people's problems. It is not simply a question of sitting and listening, noting what the other person says and moving on. When we hear intimate thoughts and feelings, they stay with us. If the relationship is not a confidential one, we can sometimes share that burden with other colleagues. If we remain in a *totally* confidential relationship, then we must be prepared to live with whatever we hear.

TRANSFERENCE AND COUNTER-TRANSFERENCE

As the client discloses himself to the counsellor, so an element of dependence creeps into the relationship. Because the counsellor is accepting of what the client has to say, the client may begin to cast the counsellor in the role of a person from the past who has also adopted this accepting, allowing position: a trusted parent. Transference refers to the client's coming to view the counsellor as if she were the all-forgiving, positive parent. The net result of this perception is that the client may come to view the counsellor as having exceptionally positive qualities: the client may temporarily come to view the counsellor as one of the most important people in his life.

Counter-transference, on the other hand, refers to the feelings that the counsellor develops for the client. Usually, too, these are positive in nature and fed by the positive feelings that the client expressed for the counsellor. A problem arises, however, if the counsellor does not notice that she is being cast in the 'good parent' role and begins unawares to play 'mother' (or 'father') to the client's 'son' (or 'daughter'). What happens, then, is that old child–parent relationships are played out by the client with the counsellor and little progression is achieved. The counsellor unconsciously colludes with the role that the client has cast her in, and the relationship staggers on until the client finds little reward in it or discovers that the counsellor is 'only human' after all, or the counsellor finds the whole relationship too claustrophobic and releases herself from the relationship.

Two practical approaches may be taken to the question of transference and counter-transference. One is that the counsellor learns to notice what happens as the relationship develops and looks out for growing dependence on the part of the client. As the dependence develops, the counsellor can encourage the client, also, to become aware of it and make the counselling relationship itself the subject of discussion. Thus a joint focus is maintained in the counselling sessions: the client's life-problems and the counsellor–client relationship. Much can be learned from the latter that will help with the former, for the quality of the client–counsellor relationship can do much to inform both parties about other relationships the client may have. It is as though the client–counsellor relationship represents one, intense example of how the client relates to other people in everyday life.

The second approach to dealing with transference and counter-transference is for the counsellor to consider having an experienced colleague act as supervisor during the counselling relationship. The supervisor serves as a person with whom the counselling relationship can be discussed confidentially and who may offer suggestions as to how she sees the counselling developing. Thus another, arguably objective, point of view is offered which may enable the counsellor to gain a little more objectivity herself. Three types of 'contract' may usefully be used in the counsellor–supervisor relationship:

1 The supervisor agrees only to listen to the counsellor, talking through her difficulties in the counselling relationship.
2 The supervisor agrees to make occasional comments as the counsellor talks.
3 The supervisor agrees to make intensive interventions during the conversation and may act in a 'devil's advocate' capacity to explore, in detail, the relationship that the counsellor has built up with the client.

These three contracts, agreed at the beginning of the counsellor–client relationship can serve to determine the degree of involvement that the supervisor has. Obviously and at any time, the contract can be changed to meet the altering needs of the counsellor.

Through regular meetings with a supervisor, the counsellor can work through the sometimes painful period of the counsellor–client relationship in which transference is at its most acute.

Another basis for counsellor–supervisor meetings is for the counsellor to write out the counsellor–client dialogue, after the counselling session, as she remembers it. This then serves as a basis for counsellor–supervisor discussions and can also help in identifying the counsellor's growing skill in using counselling interventions effectively.

The supervisor's role in the relationship is not as 'counselling expert' but as one who listens and perhaps offers her perception of what is going on between counsellor and client. No counsellor gets to the point where she does not 'need' a supervisor. The support offered by such a person is useful to the health practitioner who is just beginning a counselling role and also to the expert who has had many years of experience.

Transference in practice

Geoff is an occupational therapist in a unit aiming to rehabilitate those with long-term psychiatric illnesses, in a large psychiatric hospital. He is trying to encourage the development of effective social skills with a small group of five patients and organises role modelling, practice and reinforcement of socially acceptable behaviour. He finds one, younger, patient very difficult to cope with and begins to feel that he does not like that patient. He allows the situation to continue for some time but finds himself becoming increasingly hostile towards the young man. Finally, Geoff is able to talk through his feelings with the Head OT, with whom he has a good relationship. The Head OT, who has had counselling training, is able to explore with Geoff what it is that makes the young patient so unacceptable to Geoff. During the course of their conversations, it becomes apparent that the young man reminds Geoff partly of himself as a younger person and partly of his younger brother, with whom he had never got on. The identification of this 'transference' relationship allows Geoff to explore ways in which the young patient is different from both Geoff and his brother. In this way, Geoff becomes able to 'disidentify' with the associations he had made and to see the patient more clearly for his own strengths and weaknesses. Geoff is able to return to the social skills group and work with the young man in more constructive ways.

DEALING WITH 'BLOCKS' IN COUNSELLING

Periodically, in many counselling relationships, a point may be reached where the client appears to be making little progress and the relationship seems to be 'stuck'. At least two practical approaches may be taken to this problem. First, the counsellor can acknowledge to the client that she perceives the relationship to be 'stuck' and thus verbalises and makes explicit what has previously only been hinted at. This, in itself, can serve to push the relationship on and open up discussion on other things that are not being talked about. Sometimes the block is caused, unknowingly, by the counsellor herself. If the client is discussing a problem that is also a problem for the counsellor, then the counsellor may unawares skirt round the issue rather than face it. Few of us like our own, unresolved, problems brought out into the open, particularly by someone else! This highlights, further, the need for the prospective counsellor to develop self-awareness and to explore some of her own life-problems before helping others to tackle theirs.

A second approach to dealing with blocks in the counselling relationship is to allow or even encourage the block to remain unresolved. This paradoxical way of working can sometimes be particularly effective. It is as though, if we allow the problem to exist, then problem resolution is encouraged. On the other hand, the more we fight blocks, the more they continue to be a problem. The facing up to, accepting and 'staying with' the block can be a productive means of allowing the relationship to develop. Sometimes, the longer we can stay confused about where the relationship is going, the more successful the outcome.

COPING WITH SILENCE

There are many occasions on which the counselling relationship falls into silence. So too are there different sorts of silences, from the meditative, thoughtful silence through to the hostile, angry silence. One thing is important, here: that the counsellor learns to differentiate between the sort of silence in which a counsellor intervention is called for and the sort of silence in which the client is quietly thinking things through. Normally, when the client is 'asking' for the counsellor to say something, he will make eye contact with her and look towards her. When he is thinking about things his eyes will usually be defocused or, sometimes, looking upwards (Bandler and Grinder, 1982). It is important that, because of anxiety about the silence, the counsellor does not 'overtalk'. It is tempting to imagine that every silence needs filling, and if the client isn't talking, then the counsellor should! Thoughtful silences are often some of the most productive aspects of counselling. Occasionally, too, however, it is helpful for the counsellor to ask, 'What are you thinking?' or 'What's the thought?'. These are particularly useful when the client suddenly falls silent, or stops his train of conversation and glances to one side. Often these are indicators of sudden insight which may (or may not) be usefully verbalised.

CONFRONTATION IN COUNSELLING

There are times when the counselling relationship cannot be purely client-centred. There are occasions on which the counsellor needs to draw attention to particular behaviours or beliefs that are negatively affecting the client's life. There are times, too, when we have to confront the client with bad news: news of a sudden death, for example. At other times, still, we need to be able to tell the client of the effect they are having on us.

The prospect of confrontation often causes anxiety. Two classic ways of reacting to that anxiety in the counsellor are outlined by Heron (1986) (Figure 11.1). He describes two extremes: the 'pussyfooting' approach, where the counsellor skirts gently all round the topic but never comes to the point, and the 'sledgehammer' approach, where the counsellor allows her anxiety about confrontation to build up to the point where it is all blurted out in one go and the situation may degenerate to the point where a verbal attack is made on the client. This, perhaps, is a version of the 'last straw' syndrome, described previously. Neither approach is very effective. A more constructive approach is the assertive, confronting approach in which the counsellor clearly and quietly states what it is she wants to confront the client on and remains ready, if necessary, to repeat the confrontation. Such repetition may be necessary because there can be no guarantee how the client will react to clear, assertive confrontation. Some people respond by becoming submissive and quiet. The temptation, here, may be to 'back off' and to withdraw the confrontation. On the other hand, some people respond by becoming angry and again (though for different reasons) the counsellor may feel tempted to withdraw. The most effective approach, however, would seem to be to stay with the confrontation and to ensure that it is heard. A note of caution needs to be sounded, however, in that it is easy for the counsellor to 'overtalk' in these situations and to overstate the confrontation because of the anxiety generated by the task. Effective confrontation usually involves the confrontation being made and then time allowed for it to sink in.

Another approach to confrontation is the 'sandwich' approach. Three stages are involved in this method. In the first stage (or the 'top slice of the sandwich'), warning of the confrontation is given by the counsellor to the client. This is immediately followed up by the confrontation itself (the 'filling of the sandwich'). The third stage involves the counsellor offering the client support, without withdrawing the confrontation in any way (the 'bottom layer of the sandwich'). An example of this in action is as follows, where the counsellor has to give the client news of a relative's death:

> *Counsellor:* I have some very bad news for you. I'm sorry to tell you that your mother died earlier this afternoon. I know it will be a great shock to you and I want you to know that I will stay with you.

What are the principles behind the sandwich approach? First, the 'warning' that comes before the confrontation allows the client to anticipate the coming confrontation. It is important, however, that the confronting statement follows almost immediately, so that the client does not have to imagine, for too long, what form the confrontation will take. The final layer of the sandwich offers the client some means of support after experiencing the confrontation. Notice that in this offering of very bad news, the language used is completely unambiguous. It is vital, when breaking bad news, that there can be no doubt as to the meaning of the confrontation. Thus all euphemisms should be avoided for the sake of clarity.

The sandwich approach in practice

Joe is a social worker with a caseload that covers a large housing estate. He is asked by his Director to follow up a report that has been sent in by a local school teacher that suggests that one of the children in her class may have received non-accidental injuries in the home. Joe visits the child's house and meets his parents. His first task is to develop rapport with the parents and he does this by introducing himself and by discussing his role and by then discreetly asking the parents about themselves. He follows this, directly, by suggesting that he has some difficult issues to talk about and moves straight into outlining what those issues are. He then offers the parents the chance to talk things through in detail, to establish their reactions to the accusations. He then 'backs off' and allows the parents to react to the report, having used the 'sandwich' method of breaking difficult and upsetting news to the parents.

This approach can be used in a variety of confronting contexts. Examples of the sorts of situations in which the counsellor may be required to confront the client may be enumerated as follows:

- when the counsellor has to give the client difficult or shocking information (e.g. death of a relative, notice of a diagnosis, challenging in suspected cases of child abuse);
- when the client is using compulsive, negative self-statements (e.g. 'I'll never be able to walk again ... I've never been any good at anything ... ');
- when the client is using 'games' in the relationship and manipulating the counsellor (e.g the 'Yes, but' game, where the client answers every suggestion the counsellor makes with the phrase, 'Yes, I would, but ... '. For further details of this sort of game playing, see Berne, 1964; Harris, 1969 and James and Jongeward, 1971);
- when contractual issues need to be clarified (e.g. previously agreed times of meeting and of finishing the counselling sessions);
- when 'excuses' need to be challenged. Wheeler and Janis (1980) identify the following sorts of excuses that a client may use:
  - complacency: the 'it won't happen to me' attitude,
  - rationalisation: the 'it's not as bad as it looks' approach,
  - procrastination: the 'nothing needs to be done at the moment' argument,
  - passing the buck: the 'I'm not the one who needs to do something' idea.

Arguably, all of these excuses may have to be confronted at various stages in certain counselling relationships. Care needs to be taken, however, that counselling of this sort does not degenerate into heavy-handed patronage of the client by the counsellor.

Of all the aspects of counselling, perhaps effective confrontation is the most difficult and needs the most practice. It is worth reflecting on how you handle confrontation!

Confrontation in practice

Julia is a speech therapist working with a young child, Clare, who has hearing problems. During one of their appointments, Clare's mother begins to tell Julia of Clare's difficult behaviour at home and is very critical of the child. She does this with the child sitting in front of both Julia and her mother. Julia reaches out and gently holds the mother's arm and says, 'I would appreciate it if we could talk about this in a few minutes when Clare goes in to see the doctor'. The mother, however, continues to talk negatively about her daughter. Julia repeats, 'I want to stop you and suggest that we talk in a few minutes'. After a third repetition of the request by Julia, Clare's mother stops talking but is encouraged to talk more freely when her daughter is not present. At a later appointment,

Julia, Clare and her mother are more easily able to talk freely between themselves. Clare's mother has been able to 'offload' to Julia, without hurting her daughter's feelings. In the instance described here, Julia has confronted the mother and used the 'broken record' method to ensure that what she wanted to say got through. 'Broken record' refers to the technique of repeating, calmly, the confronting statement, until it is 'heard'.

Figure 11.1

Confrontation and its variants.

'Pussyfooting' approach:	the counsellor is vague, unclear and has a tendency to go 'round the houses'.
'Sledgehammer' approach:	the counsellor becomes aggressive and interventions become an attack on the person.
'Confronting' approach:	the counsellor stays calm, keeps to the point and is prepared to repeat her confronting statement.

THE LIMITS OF COUNSELLING

Much of the counselling that health professionals will be involved in will concern what may be called the 'worried well': people who have particular life-problems but who are essentially mentally well. Whilst the question of where 'wellness' ends and mental illness begins is by no means clear cut, the health professional should always bear in mind her limitations. It is tempting, once we have established a close relationship with another person, to believe that we alone can help them. Sometimes it is with extreme reluctance that we call in other advice or help. It is, however, important that we only take on relationships that we can handle and in which we can be therapeutic. Clients who may present problems that the health professional working as counsellor may not be able to deal adequately with, include:

- the person who is clinically depressed and talking of suicide;
- the person who is hallucinated or deluded;
- the person who has an organic mental illness;
- the person whose behaviour is potentially dangerous to himself or others.

Making judgements about when to counsel and when to refer to another agency is always difficult and it is helpful if the practitioner can talk through, in confidence, the problems of the person whom she feels may benefit from further referral. Referrals for psychiatric help are normally made through the person's general practitioner or sometimes through occupational health agencies.

What is perhaps more difficult is persuading clients that you are not the best person to help them. Suggesting referral to other agencies may be seen either as a rebuff or as a sign that you view them as being seriously mentally ill. Bearing in mind the previous discussion regarding confrontation, the person who cannot be helped through counselling must be approached about the possibility of referral: to do otherwise is to limit the possibilities that person has of regaining his health.

BURNOUT IN COUNSELLING

The process of counselling and of coping with others can take its toll on the counsellor and health professional. The word 'burnout' (derived from the idea that once a rocket has burnt up its fuel it is then of no use but it continues to circulate in space) has been used to denote the overall feeling that a person can experience when exhausted by being intimately involved in human relationships. Gerard Corey (cited by Murgatroyd, 1986) has suggested that there are a number of causes of burnout which the counsellor and health professional needs to bear in mind if she is to avoid it:

- doing the same type of helping over and over again with little variation;
- giving a great deal of one's own emotional and personal energy to others whilst getting very little back;
- being under a constant pressure to produce results in a certain time-scale when the time-scale and the pressure are unrealistic;
- working with a difficult group: for example, those who are highly resistant to change, those who have been 'sent' for help but who do not wish to be helped, or those for whom the chances of change are small because of the nature of their difficulties (for example, the terminally ill);
- the absence of support from immediate colleagues and an abundance of criticism – what might be called 'the atmosphere of certain doubt';
- lack of trust between those who engage in helping and those who manage the organisational resources that make helping possible – a feature sometimes present in voluntary organisations;
- not having the opportunity to take new directions, to develop one's own approach or to experiment with new models of working – being unnecessarily constrained;
- having few opportunities for training, continuing education, super-vision or support;
- unresolved personal conflicts beyond the helping and counselling work, which interfere with the helper's ability to be effective, for example marital problems, health problems.

Burnout in practice

Ann is a district nurse working mainly with elderly patients. Recently, her case load has increased and she has also taken on an Open University course. Her eldest child, who is 11, is having difficulty in settling at his new secondary school. Ann slowly finds that she is losing interest in the elderly people that she is visiting. She also finds that she is avoiding working on her Open University assignments and she begins to wonder how she had ever been interested in the course at all. Her general disenchantment is brought to a head when she visits a younger patient who begins to tell her about her marital problems. Ann realises that she has no interest at all in what the woman has to say and just wants to leave the house. Later, Ann discontinues her Open University course and begins to consider whether or not she should remain a district nurse. She is suffering from 'burnout'. It is only after she has had a number of long talks with her husband that she realises the degree of emotional exhaustion that she has been experiencing. It is only then that her husband also begins to realise how difficult life has become for her. Together, they map out a plan to reorganise family life a little, so that Ann has some 'time for herself'. Her husband agrees to take over more of the household chores and both Ann and her husband find time to sit down and listen to their son talk about his problems at school. She does not go back to the Open University course but enrols, instead, at a local evening class. Slowly, her interest in her work returns and she feels less afraid to talk about the negative feelings she sometimes has.

It is unreasonable to suppose that we can continue to work with and for others without paying attention, also, to our own needs. The person who wants to avoid burnout needs to consider at least the following preventative measures:

- Vary your work as much as is possible.
- Consider your education and training needs and plan ahead.
- Take care of your physical health.
- Consider new ways of developing counselling skills and try them out.
- Develop an effective supervision or peer-support system.
- Nurture your friendships and relationships with others.
- Develop a range of interests away from work.
- Attend 'refresher' workshops, occasionally – as a means of 'updating' and also as a means of experiencing new ideas and methods.
- Initiate your own projects, without relying on others to approve them.
- Seek positive and reliable feedback on your performance from other people.

PEER SUPPORT: CO-COUNSELLING

If we are to avoid burnout and subsequent disillusionment with the task of counselling, it is vital that we have an adequate peer-support system. Co-counselling offers one such means of ensuring that two people regularly review their life situation and their counselling practice.

Co-counselling was originally devised by Harvey Jackins in the US

(Jackins, 1965, 1970) and further developed by John Heron in the UK (Heron, 1978). Basically, it involves two people who have trained as co-counsellors, meeting on a regular basis for two hours. For the first hour, one of the partners is 'counsellor' or helper and the other is 'client' or talker. In the second hour, roles are reversed and the 'counsellor' becomes the 'client' and vice versa. The 'counselling' role in co-counselling, however, is not the traditional role of counsellor: the role demands more that the person listens and gives attention to her partner than would usually be the case. In this respect, co-counselling offers a bonus to the practising counsellor in that it is an excellent way of developing and enhancing listening skills. In its most basic form, the hour spent in the role of 'counsellor' is one of listening only, while the client verbally reviews any aspect of her life that she chooses: her emotional status, life-problems, recent difficulties, future plans and so forth. An important aspect of co-counselling is that what is talked about during the co-counselling sessions remains confidential to those sessions. Nothing that is talked about is discussed away from the session. For this reason, it is helpful if the two people meet only for co-counselling. To this end, co-counselling 'networks' have been set up which enable those trained to contact others.

Having the sustained and supportive attention of another person can be very liberating. It can create the circumstances in which a person is truly able to work things out for herself. Whilst the co-counselling format allows for certain verbal interventions on the part of the 'counsellor', those interventions never extend to giving advice, making suggestions or comparing experiences. In this sense, co-counselling is truly self-directed and client-centred. Courses in co-counselling training are usually of 40 hours in length, run either as a one-week course or as a series of evening classes. Such courses are offered by a variety of colleges and extra-mural departments of universities.

These are some of the practical problems that can occur in counselling, and some methods of facing those problems and getting personal support. Sometimes it can be useful to consider some practical questions before setting out to counsel. A list of useful questions is as follows:

- Why has this person come to me?
- Can I help them?
- Have I the necessary knowledge and skills to help?
- What are my beliefs about the nature of the counselling process?
- Why do I want to help this person?
- Do they remind me of anyone I know? This is particularly useful when it comes to the possible development of transference and counter-transference. It is important to keep in mind the fact that this person only looks like someone else you know: he is, of course, a separate person!

PROBLEMS AND SUPPORT IN COUNSELLING AND THE HEALTH PROFESSIONAL

All of the issues discussed in this chapter apply to a wide range of situations in which health professionals may find themselves apart from the counselling situation. In other words, the issues of transference and counter-transference apply to most relationships in which professional and client develop a close relationship. The question of therapeutic distance applies equally to both counselling and all other professional relationships, and so does the issue of burnout. In all aspects of health provision, the need for self and peer support is a particularly pertinent one. The building of a network of support throughout the professional's career is a necessity if she is to function effectively and caringly. In order to care effectively for others, we must learn to care for ourselves. In the next chapter, the methods of developing specific counselling skills are described in detail.

LEARNING COUNSELLING SKILLS

12

Three routes are open to the practitioner who wishes to develop a range of counselling skills: working on her own, working as a pair with a colleague or friend or learning in a small group. Each of these routes will be considered in turn and linked to the practical exercises for skills development offered in this book. Given that this book is all about counselling skills, it might be reasonable to question exactly what we might mean by *skill*. Barnett (1994) has suggested four criteria for the application of the term 'skill' that are relevant to counselling. Skills involve:

- a situation of some complexity;
- a performance that addresses the situation, is deliberate and is not just a matter of chance;
- an assessment that the performance has met the demands of the situation;
- a sense that the performance was commendable.

THE INDIVIDUAL WORKING ON HER OWN

The first consideration, here, needs to be, what knowledge do I need in order to function as an effective counsellor? This may be answered by reference back to the three domains of knowledge referred to in Chapter 3: propositional, practical and experiential knowledge. Figure 12.1 identifies some of the types of knowledge in each of the three domains that the health professional needs to consider.

The person working on her own has a variety of options. She can, for instance, enrol on a counselling skills course. A variety of these are offered by colleges and university departments, ranging from one-year certificate courses, through two-year diploma courses to Master's degree courses in counselling psychology.

Such courses usually offer a wide curriculum covering both the theory and the practice of counselling.

An alternative method is for the person to 'train herself'. This may involve attendance at a number of short counselling workshops in order to identify skilled counselling examples from effective rolemodels, backed up by reading on the topic, reinforced by practice with real clients. Such a solo programme can be helped if the individual can rely on a friend or colleague who is prepared to discuss progress and/or difficult clients. It is also helpful if the person working on her own keeps a journal in which she notes down her progress as a counsellor.

Essential to this method of training is the development of 'conscious use of self' described in Chapter 3. It is important if progress is to be

Figure 12.1

Aspects of knowledge required for counselling.

Propositional knowledge

- Types of counselling
- Maps of the counselling process
- Psychological approaches to counselling
- Psychology, sociology, philosophy, politics, theology

Practical knowledge

- Listening and attending skills
- Counselling interventions, including:
  - being prescriptive
  - being informative
  - being confronting
  - being cathartic
  - being client-centred
  - being supportive
  - starting and finishing the session
  - coping with transference and counter-transference
  - coping with silence
  - avoiding burnout

Experiential knowledge

- Experience of a wide range of different types of people
- Experience of a wide range of human problems
- Self-awareness
- Life experience

made, that the health professional works at using herself intentionally and notices what she does, both in the counselling relationship and also away from it. Such noticing can bring to attention behaviours and language that are effective and those that are not. It is not until we notice what we do that we can begin to modify or change our behaviour.

The problems associated with learning to be a counsellor should not be underestimated. Truell reports a small-scale study of students' experiences of learning counselling and notes the following:

- Counselling training can cause significant disruption in the trainee's relationship with friends and family.
- Counselling trainees report significant negative feelings during their training.
- A sizeable number of trainees developed unrealistic beliefs and non-useful ways of coping.
- Counsellor trainers are not addressing these issues effectively.
- When trainees experience class discussions on the unrealistic beliefs associated with counselling, some will benefit positively.
- Trainees need a variety of supports to help reduce the negative effects of learning counselling, specifically, classroom discussion and one-to-one contact with a non-marking staff member.
- Trainees also considered personal counselling and focused supervision to be useful methods for harm reduction (Truell, 2001).

However, Truell does not indicate how the term 'significant' is being used in the first two items just listed.

Quotes on training

Any training that does not include the emotions, mind and body is incomplete; knowledge fades without feeling.

Anonymous

Just because you're trained for something doesn't mean you're prepared for it.

Anonymous

Training is useless unless you have a purpose, it's knowing for what purpose to train for that can break men's fulfilment.

Anonymous

There is nothing training cannot do. Nothing is above its reach. It can turn bad morals to good; it can destroy bad principles and recreate good ones; it can lift men to angelship.

Mark Twain

WHAT CONSTITUTES AN *EFFECTIVE COUNSELLOR?*

The whole notion of training in counselling raises the question of what we might consider to be an effective counsellor. McLeod (1993) suggested the following fairly exhaustive list of areas that might be considered when attempting to assess counselling competence:

- *Interpersonal skills*. Competent counsellors are able to demonstrate appropriate listening, communicating, empathy, presence, awareness of non-verbal communication, sensitivity of voice quality, responsiveness to expressions of emotion, turn-taking, structuring of time, use of language.
- *Personal beliefs and attitudes*. Capacity to accept others, belief in the potential for change, awareness of ethical and moral choices. Sensitivity to values helped by client and self.
- *Conceptual ability*. Ability to understand and assess the client's problems, to anticipate future consequences of actions, to make sense of immediate process in terms of a wider conceptual scheme, to remember information about the client. Cognitive flexibility. Skill in problem-solving.
- *Personal 'soundness'*. Absence of personal needs or irrational beliefs which are destructive to counselling relationships, self-confidence, capacity to tolerate strong or uncomfortable feelings in relation to clients, secure personal boundaries, ability to be a client. Absence of social prejudice, ethnocentrism and authoritarianism.

- *Mastery of technique.* Knowledge of when and how to carry out specific interventions, ability to access effectiveness of interventions, understanding of rationale behind techniques, possession of a sufficiently wide repertoire of interventions.
- *Ability to understand and work within social systems.* Including awareness of the family and work relationship of the client, the impact of the agency on the client, the capacity to use support networks and supervision. Sensitivity to the social worlds of clients who may be from different gender, ethnic background, sexual orientation or age group.

WORKING IN PAIRS

Perhaps a more amicable (and less lonely!) way of developing counselling skills is through working with another person. That person can be a member of the family, a friend or a colleague. It is useful if a 'contract' is set up between the two people so that they meet at a regular time each week during which they devote that time to practising counselling skills. In the section in this book on pairs exercises, a whole range of activities is offered which can be worked through by two people. The time spent together can be divided in two and thus one person spends, say, one hour in the role of client and one hour in the role of counsellor. This style of working is not 'role play', as role play suggests acting as a person other than yourself. In the pairs work suggested here, it is recommended that both 'client' and 'counsellor' work on real-life issues during their spell as 'client'. In this way, the self-awareness argued for in previous chapters can be enhanced whilst counselling skills are being developed. Clearly, the subject matter discussed during these sessions must be confidential to the sessions. For this reason, it is often useful if a pair can meet solely for the purpose of practising counselling skills, though this may be difficult to arrange.

At the end of each training session, it is helpful if both parties go through a self- and peer-evaluation procedure. This involves one person verbalising her current strengths, weaknesses and things she has learned during the session, to her partner. Then the partner offers that person both negative and positive feedback on that person's performance during the training session. When both self and peer aspects of the evaluation process have been worked through, the two people swap roles and the other person talks through her strengths, weaknesses and things she has learned and then invites feedback from the other person. During the self-evaluation aspects of the process, all that is required of the other person is that she listens. No comments are necessary whilst the other person is evaluating herself – that comes afterwards in the peer aspect of the process.

Regular meetings between the two partners can be further supplemented by attendance at short training workshops and by further reading on the subject of counselling, counselling psychology and psychotherapy.

WORKING IN A GROUP

The most effective way of training as a counsellor, outside of attendance at a formal course of training, is through the setting up of a small training group. This can be made up from colleagues who are interested in developing counselling skills and may be usefully started by the implementation of a one-day workshop to develop basic skills. Such a workshop can be run at a weekend or, if a one-day slot cannot be found to suit all members of the group, the 'workshop' can be spread over a number of meetings of the group.

An alternative to the self-help or 'do-it-yourself' group is the more formal educational group, set up by the educational body responsible for training staff in the health organisation. Both groups can use the outline programme described in Figure 12.2 for running a counselling skills workshop.

- Setting the learning climate
- Identifying the needs/wants of the group
- Programme planning
- Working through the programme
- Evaluating learning

Figure 12.2

Stages in a counselling skills workshop.

Figure 12.2 offers a sample programme outline for such a workshop on counselling skills. It may be given to workshop participants before the workshop or it may be allowed to 'unfold' as the workshop develops. The advantage of giving it out prior to the workshop is that it offers minimal but essential structure. Many people attending workshops seem to prefer and expect structure, and this programme can satisfy that need. On the other hand, the advantage of allowing the programme to 'unfold' is that it ensures that the workshop is a dynamic and organic process that responds to the needs and wants of the participants as those needs and wants arise. In the end, it may be a question of the personal preference of the person setting up the workshop and, perhaps, of his or her previous experience in running groups of this sort.

Setting the learning climate

This is the first stage of the counselling skills workshop. It involves at least the following activities:

- introductions;
- expectations;
- rationale for the workshop.

The 'introductions' aspect involves helping group members to get to know each other and to remember each other's names. A variety of 'icebreakers' is described in the literature, which some people prefer to use as a means of starting the workshop (Brandes and Phillips, 1984; Burnard, 1985; Heron, 1973). Three examples of such icebreakers are as follows:

Icebreaker one

Group members stand up and move around the room. At a signal from the group leader, they stop and pair off with their nearest colleague. The pairs then spend a few minutes sharing their thoughts on one of the following:

- childhood memories;
- interests away from work;
- personal interests in counselling.

After a few minutes, the leader suggests that the group moves on and pairs up with other people. They then spend a few minutes in those pairs discussing similar issues.

Icebreaker two

Group members, in turn, recall three positive and formative experiences from their lives and share those experiences with the rest of the group.

Icebreaker three

The group leader asks each person in turn to imagine that she were one of the following objects: a book, a piece of music or a film. The group member is then asked to describe herself as though she was that object. Thus, the leader asks one of the following questions:

- If you were a book, what book would you be? Describe yourself as that book.
- If you were a piece of music, what piece would you be? Describe yourself as that piece of music.
- If you were a film, what film would you be? Describe yourself as that film.

Again, the use of such icebreakers may be a question of personal preference. Some group leaders (and workshop participants) may find them difficult to use or to take part in. They seem to suit the more extroverted (and possibly younger) participants. They do, however, serve to allow people to unwind a little and thus prepare for some of the pairs and group activities described later.

A quieter method of introducing a counselling skills workshop is to invite members in turn to identify the following things about themselves:

- their name;
- their present job;
- their background;
- their interests away from work.

After group members have disclosed themselves to the group in this way, each member is invited to repeat his or her name slowly and in turn. This slow name-round is often usefully repeated two or three times until all members are sure of each other's names.

Following these introductory activities, group members may be invited to pair off and to discuss their expectations about the coming workshop and about future group meetings. Such expectations may include both negative and positive things. The point, here, is that all members should be given the opportunity to explore how they feel about the coming time together and are able to share fantasies, hopes and anxieties. Following this ten-minute exercise, the group may be invited to re-form, and those expectations are discussed. It is usually helpful to discuss negative expectations first, followed by the positive.

Once expectations have been fully explored (a process that may take between 30 minutes and one hour), the group leader may offer a rationale for the workshop. That rationale will include the leader's explanation of her reasons for organising the workshop in this manner. It will also include details of what the workshop is intended to be about. It may also include the negotiation, with the group, of basic ground rules for the workshop. These may include such things as:

- rules about smoking;
- issues relating to coffee, tea and meal breaks;
- a 'proposal' clause;
- a 'voluntary' clause.

A proposal clause raises the idea that any member of the group may feel free to propose changes to the format or structure of the group at any time. It may also be used to promote the idea of group members taking responsibility for ensuring that they get what they want from the workshop. If they are not, then they should feel free to propose a change of activity.

A voluntary clause stresses the idea that each member of the group should feel free to take part or not to take part in any aspect of the workshop or the group meetings. As all counselling workshops are organised for adults, its seems reasonable to assume that they will decide, as individuals, what does and what does not enhance their learning. It seems reasonable, too, that no part of the workshop should be compulsory.

Identifying the needs/wants of the group

This next process is one that naturally leads into programme planning. The group is invited to form into small groups of three and four. Each group 'brainstorms' onto a large sheet of paper the things that they require from the workshop. Such requirements may be particular skills, various sorts of knowledge or some sort of personal development. It is useful, too, at this stage to identify any particular resources in the group. Thus some group members may have particular counselling exercises that they feel others may benefit from. Others may have

Figure 12.3

Layout for a brainstorming exercise.

NEEDS/WANTS	OFFERS
Identify here anything that you need to gain from this counselling workshop. You can list theories, skills – anything.	Identify here anything you are prepared to share with the group (skills, knowledge, activities, etc.).

particular knowledge about counselling theory. Figure 12.3 identifies a layout of the sheet for use in the small group.

When the small groups have had sufficient time to complete the brainstorming exercise, they may be invited to prioritise their list of needs and wants. Once this is completed, a feedback session will ensure that group priorities are identified, and offers made by individuals are recognised.

Out of the previous activity develops the programme for the counselling workshop. This stage involves negotiating the timing of activities required by the group. It also involves fitting in those activities with any pre-planned activities that the leader has brought to the workshop. It is useful, at this stage, to offer group members a skeleton programme plan which contains various 'blanks' into which go the activities identified in the exercise in Figure 12.3. An example of a 'typical' programme is offered in Figure 12.4. The 'sessions' referred to in the outline programme are times when the exercises that follow in this book may be used to develop specific counselling skills. Alternatively, those sessions can be made up of exercises offered by other group members.

Working through the programme

Once the programme has been negotiated, all that remains is for the sessions to be undertaken as planned. Given that the workshop and subsequent group meetings are about counselling, it is useful if the experiential learning cycle is observed though each session (Burnard, 1985; Kolb, 1984). Experiential learning is learning through doing, through immediate, personal experience. A modification of the cycle is identified in Figure 12.5.

First, a brief theory input is offered to the group. This may be on a particular aspect of counselling or a description of a counselling skill. It is helpful, too, if the group can see some examples of 'excellent practice' in counselling in order for them to be able to base their own counselling skills on these exemplars. Such examples of good practice may be shown on video or film, or skilled practitioners may be invited to demonstrate counselling practice 'live', in front of the groups. This use of exemplars is particularly useful in the early stages of counselling skills workshops and counselling skills development. Once group members have established a basic range of their own skills, the exemplars can be dropped.

Then an activity is undertaken by the group, either as a whole or with the group split into pairs, in order to practise a particular counselling skill. When the activity has finished (and details of how to set up and run those activities are offered with each exercise in the pages that follow), group members are invited to reflect on the experience and draw new learning from it. That learning is then applied, and implications for future behaviour are discussed. It is vital that all new learning is carried over from the workshop situation to the 'real' situation with clients; new counselling skills have to be practised as soon as possible away from the workshop to maximise the efficacy of the activity.

Evaluating learning

At the end of the workshop, the group needs to evaluate its learning. This can be done formally, through the use of a written evaluative questionnaire (Clift and Imrie, 1981; Patton, 1982) prepared prior to the workshop. Alternatively it can be carried out through the process of self- and peer evaluation.

9.00–10.00	Introductions
10.00–10.30	Coffee
10.30–12.00	Identification of needs/wants and programme planning
12.00–1.00	First skills training session
1.00–2.00	Lunch
2.00–3.00	Second skills training session
3.00–3.15	Tea
3.15–4.15	Third skills training session
4.15–5.00	Evaluation

Figure 12.4

Example of a 'skeleton' counselling skills workshop programme.

Brief theory input
Application of new learning: counselling skills exercise
Development of new learning out of that reflection
Reflection on the exercise, in the group

Figure 12.5

The experiential learning cycle applied to counselling skills development.

Such self- and peer evaluation involves the following stages:

- identification of criteria for evaluation;
- group members silently evaluating themselves using those criteria;
- group members, in turn, verbalising their evaluation to the group;
- group members, in turn, inviting feedback from the group on their own performance during the workshop.

This process may be followed by a closing 'round' of (a) what each group member, in turn, liked least about the workshop, followed by a round of (b) what each member liked most about the workshop. This serves to round off the proceedings and to reinforce themes and learnings gained within the workshop.

This format for running a one-day workshop can be adapted for use at subsequent meetings of the counselling skills learning group. At each meeting, a short period can be used to 'warm up' the group, using icebreakers or similar activities. Then the group members can decide on what they want to achieve during the meeting. A series of counselling skills exercises can be used, drawn from this book or from others (see, for example, Egan, 1990; Heron, 1973; Lewis and Streitfield, 1971; Pfeiffer and Jones, 1974 and ongoing; Wilkinson and Canter, 1982). After each exercise a reflective period can be instituted to allow consideration of how the new skill may be implemented in the 'real' situation. Finally, the meeting can close with an evaluation activity.

These, then, are three approaches to counselling skills training that can be used separately or in combination. All three emphasise the need for practice and for practical experience. All three need to be combined with constant reflection on the qualities of the effective counsellor. Counselling without certain skills can be fruitless. Skills without human qualities will be mechanical. All health professionals who practise counselling as an aspect of their job need to consider a balance between counselling skills, up-to-date knowledge and the development of a human and caring approach to people.

Clearly, any courses of training should be evaluated thoroughly in order to continue to enhance and improve that course. Dryden *et al.* (1995) have suggested what might be reviewed during an internal audit of a counselling course. They recommend that the following information might be sought:

- number of applications received, applicants interviewed, places offered and places accepted;
- number of students in each cohort or year group, drop outs and reasons for leaving;
- number of students passing the course;
- information on employment changes of students as a result of taking the course;
- student feedback and evaluation including summary of comments;
- external examiner's report or evaluation;
- staff response to critical feedback from students or external examiner;
- changes or solutions to problems during the year;
- proposed developments or improvements for future courses;
- staff professional and academic development activities;
- extraordinary achievements of the course or students;
- organisational problems beyond the responsibility of the staff team.

LEARNING COUNSELLING SKILLS AND THE HEALTH PROFESSIONAL

As we have noted throughout this book, the skills described as 'counselling skills', also have wider application outside of the counselling relationship and can be used to enhance professional practice in any branches of the caring and health professions. The format for organising the learning of counselling skills, described in this chapter, can also be adapted to be used for learning or developing a whole range of interpersonal skills related to health care, including interviewing, stress management, self-awareness, assertiveness, assessment and evaluation.

13 Counselling skills exercises

In the previous chapter, details were given as to how to develop counselling skills, working alone, in pairs or in a small group. This chapter offers a range of counselling skills exercises and activities. The first group is for the individual working on her own, the second group is pairs activities and the third is group activities. The second and third group may be used in combination by a group of colleagues working together to enhance their counselling skills. Each exercise should be worked through slowly and plenty of time allowed for 'processing' or discussing the activity afterwards.

As we noted in the last chapter, a useful format for a counselling skills training session is as follows:

- identification of how the group wants to spend the time;
- a theory input and some examples of good counselling practice, either 'live' or shown on video or film;
- using a variety of exercises to develop counselling skills;
- evaluation activities.

The following exercises will serve as the 'exercises to develop counselling skills'. Built into each of the pairs and group exercises is the means to evaluate learning at the end of each activity. It is recommended that the evaluation procedure is followed fairly closely so that the maximum amount of learning may be gained from each exercise. No claims are made that the list of exercises is exhaustive of all possible exercises, and many more may be gleaned from the literature. Many exercises may also be developed by group members themselves.

The 'pairs' format is particularly useful. In this, the group breaks into pairs, each member of which spends some time in the role of 'counsellor' and of 'client'. After a period of practising specific counselling skills, the partners swap roles. This format can be used on a regular basis for practising counselling and may be combined with receiving feedback on skills development from the partner.

All of the work done individually, in pairs or in a group must be followed up quickly by real-life experience. Thus the counsellor must learn to develop the 'conscious use of self' referred to throughout this book. In this way, the health professional can make full use of any learning gained by putting it into practice, in real counselling situations. Like all skills, counselling skills must be reinforced if they are to become a regular part of the person's repertoire of behaviour.

ACTIVITIES   **EXERCISES FOR THE PERSON WORKING ON HER OWN**

Exercise No. 1

Aim of the Exercise
To clarify beliefs and values, prior to undertaking counselling.

Process of the Exercise
Write out in a free style a paper which expresses your current set of values and beliefs about human beings, counselling and about yourself. Do not try to make the paper 'academic' in any way and do not worry about style or presentation. Once you have written the paper, consider whether or not it highlights any ambiguities or contradictions in your construing of the world. If so, consider whether or not you will attempt to resolve those contradictions. Consider, also, ways in which your beliefs and values affect your work and your attitude towards counselling. You may or may not choose to show the paper to someone else and have her comment on it.

Exercise No. 2

Aim of the Exercise
To consider aspects of yourself and your work that will help or hinder your counselling.

Process of the Exercise
'Brainstorm' onto a sheet of paper all those aspects of yourself and your work that you bring to your counselling work. Include in your list those aspects of yourself and your work that you anticipate will cause difficulties. Allow yourself to think and write quickly. Once the list has become fairly lengthy, organise it into 'pluses' and 'minuses'. Consider, then, the degree to which one list is longer than the other and the implications of that. Consider, also, what you intend to do about the 'minuses'.

Exercise No. 3

Aim of the Exercise
To enable a continuous means of personal evaluation to be maintained.

Process of the Exercise
Keep a journal from the point of taking up counselling. Use the following headings to order the journal:

- recent skills developed;
- recent problems encountered and problem-solving methods used;
- new references to books and journals noted;
- aspects of personal growth.

Journals may usefully be kept by all members of a group working together on developing counselling skills. At each meeting of the group, time can be set aside to discuss journal entries.

Exercise No. 4

Aim of the Exercise
To develop 'conscious use of self'.

Process of the Exercise
Set aside a time each day when you notice what it is you do and how you do it. Notice patterns of behaviour, speech, proximity to others, use of touch, hand and arm gestures, social skills and so on. Try out new behaviour and new counselling skills as they develop. Allow this time to develop and lengthen until you become more aware of how you react and interact.

Exercise No. 5

Aim of the Exercise
To develop the ability to 'notice'.

Process of the Exercise
Noticing (sometimes called 'staying awake' or 'conscious awareness') involves setting aside time each day to notice everything that is going on around you. Notice sounds, smells, colours, activity, objects and so on. Allow this period of noticing to develop and lengthen. Use the activity, particularly, when you are with other people.

Exercise No. 6

Aim of the Exercise
To develop observational skills, 'conscious use of self' and the ability to 'notice'.

Process of the Exercise
Spend 20 minutes each evening, sitting in the same place and at the same time. Allow your attention to focus only on those things that you see, hear, smell or feel, outside of yourself. Do not attempt to evaluate what comes in through your senses, but only notice them. Regular use of this activity (akin to certain types of meditation) will improve your ability to keep your attention 'out' and will improve your observational skills.

Exercise No. 7

Aim of the Exercise
To experience physical changes in the body, to become more aware of the body and to relax physically.

Process of the Exercise

Find a place that is quiet and warm in which you can lay down for about half an hour, undisturbed. Once you have lain down take three deep breaths. Then allow your attention to focus on the muscles in your face. Let them relax. Then focus your attention on the muscles in your shoulders and upper arms. Let them relax. Focus your attention on the muscles in your lower arms and hands. Stretch out your fingers. Then let your arms relax. Then put your attention on the muscles in your chest and stomach. Let those muscles relax. Then focus on the muscles in your legs and stretch your feet forward. Then let all the muscles in your legs relax. Then notice how all the muscles in your body are relaxed. Allow yourself to notice what it feels like to be relaxed. Notice, too, parts of the body that you find difficult to relax. After about 10 minutes, stretch gently, allow yourself to sit up and then slowly, stand up. Notice the difference in the way you feel before and after the activity.

This exercise may also be used as a stress reduction activity with clients who find it difficult to relax. It can also be dictated onto a tape for use as a means of deep relaxation.

Exercise No. 8

Aim of the Exercise
To identify personal strengths and weaknesses in terms of counselling interventions.

Process of the Exercise
Consider Heron's (1986) 'Six category intervention analysis':

- prescriptive interventions: giving advice, offering suggestions;
- informative interventions: offering information;
- confronting interventions: challenging;
- cathartic interventions: helping the client to express emotion;
- catalytic interventions: 'drawing out' the client;
- supportive interventions: encouraging, validating the client.

Identify the two categories that you feel you are least skilled in using at the moment. Then consider the two categories that you are most skilled in using at the moment. Consider the implications of your assessment and anticipate ways that you can enhance your deficiencies.

Exercise No. 9

Aim of the Exercise
To plan future objectives.

Process of the Exercise
Write down a list of the counselling skills or aspects of counselling that you need to improve upon. Make each of them a specific, behavioural objective and ones that are attainable. Then determine how you will meet those objectives.

ACTIVITIES   **EXERCISES FOR PEOPLE WORKING IN PAIRS**

Exercise No. 10

Aim of the Exercise
To experience problems associated with listening.

Equipment Required/Environmental Considerations
The pair should sit facing each other in chairs of equal height. It is helpful if the room is comfortably warm and free from distractions and interruptions.

The Process of the Exercise
The pair divides themselves into A and B. A talks to B on any subject for four minutes and B does not listen! After the four minutes, roles are reversed and B talks to A, who does not listen! After the second round, the pair discuss the activity.

Evaluation Procedure
At the end of the exercise each person should report to the other what she disliked and what she liked about the activity. They may also comment on what they will be able to carry over from it into the 'real' counselling situation.

Exercise No. 11

Aim of the Exercise
To experience problems with the non-verbal aspects of listening.

Equipment Required/Environmental Considerations
The pair should sit facing each other in chairs of equal height. It is helpful if the room is comfortably warm and free from distractions and interruptions.

The Process of the Exercise
The pair divides themselves into A and B. A talks to B for four minutes about any topic and B listens but contradicts the first four aspects of the SOLER behaviours identified by Egan (1990). Thus B does not sit squarely in relation to A. She folds her arms and her legs. She leans away from her partner and makes no eye contact with her. After four minutes, roles are reversed and B talks to A, while A listens but offers contradictory behaviours. After the second four minutes, the pair discuss the exercise.

Evaluation Procedure
At the end of the exercise each person should report to the other what she disliked and what she liked about the activity. They may also comment on what they will be able to carry over from it into the 'real' counselling situation.

Exercise No. 12

Aim of the Exercise
To experience effective listening and to enhance listening skills.

Equipment Required/Environmental Considerations
The pair should sit facing each other in chairs of equal height. It is helpful if the room is comfortably warm and free from distractions and interruptions.

The Process of the Exercise
The pair divides themselves into A and B. A talks to B for four minutes about any topic and B listens, observing the SOLER behaviours. Thus she sits squarely in an open position. She leans slightly towards her partner and maintains good eye contact. She also relaxes and does nothing but listen. It is important that this is not a conversation but a listening exercise! After four minutes, roles are reversed and B talks to A, who listens appropriately. After the second four minutes the pair discuss the exercise and compare it with the previous two.

Evaluation Procedure
At the end of the exercise each person should report to the other what she disliked and what she liked about the activity. They may also comment on what they will be able to carry over from it into the 'real' counselling situation.

Exercise No. 13

Aim of the Exercise
To practise effective listening and to evaluate the effectiveness of the listening.

Equipment Required/Environmental Considerations
The pair should sit facing each other in chairs of equal height. It is helpful if the room is comfortably warm and free from distractions and interruptions.

The Process of the Exercise
The pair divides themselves into A and B. A talks to B for four minutes on any topic. B listens and periodically 'recaps' what A has said, to A's satisfaction. After four minutes, roles are reversed and B talks to A, who listens and periodically recaps. After a further four minutes, the pair discuss the exercise.

Evaluation Procedure
At the end of the exercise each person should report to the other what she disliked and what she liked about the activity. They may also comment on what they will be able to carry over from it into the 'real' counselling situation.

Exercise No. 14

Aim of the Exercise
To discriminate between open and closed questions.

Equipment Required/Environmental Considerations
The pair should sit facing each other in chairs of equal height. It is helpful if the room is comfortably warm and free from distractions and interruptions. A pencil and paper are needed for this activity.

The Process of the Exercise
Both partners jot down the following sequence: O,O,C,C,O,C,O,C. Then the pair divides themselves into A and B. A then asks questions of B on any of the following topics:

- current issues at work;
- recent holidays;
- the current political situation.

The questions are asked in the sequence noted (i.e. 'open question, open question, closed question, closed question' and so on) until they have all been asked. Then the pair swap roles and B asks questions of A, in that sequence and on one of those topics.

Evaluation Procedure
At the end of the exercise each person should report to the other what she disliked and what she liked about the activity. They may also comment on what they will be able to carry over from it into the 'real' counselling situation.

Exercise No. 15

Aim of the Exercise
To practise 'funnelling' in questioning.

Equipment Required/Environmental Considerations
The pair should sit facing each other in chairs of equal height. It is helpful if the room is comfortably warm and free from distractions and interruptions.

The Process of the Exercise
The pair divides themselves into A and B. A then asks questions of B on any subject they wish starting with a very broad open question and slowly allowing the questions to become more specific and focused. After four minutes, the pair swap roles and B asks questions of A, moving from the general to the particular.

Evaluation Procedure
At the end of the exercise each person should report to the other what she disliked and what she liked about the activity. They may also comment on what they will be able to carry over from it into the 'real' counselling situation.

Exercise No. 16

Aim of the Exercise
To practise 'reflection' and 'selective reflection'.

Equipment Required/Environmental Considerations

The pair should sit facing each other in chairs of equal height. It is helpful if the room is comfortably warm and free from distractions and interruptions.

The Process of the Exercise

The pair divides themselves into A and B. A talks to B about any subject and A uses only reflection or selective reflection to encourage her to continue. This should be carried on for about six minutes. After six minutes, roles are reversed and B talks to A who uses only reflection or selective reflection as a response. For details of these two techniques, see the chapter on client-centred counselling skills.

Evaluation Procedure

At the end of the exercise each person should report to the other what she disliked and what she liked about the activity. They may also comment on what they will be able to carry over from it into the 'real' counselling situation.

Exercise No. 17

Aim of the Exercise

To practise a range of client-centred counselling skills.

Equipment Required/Environmental Considerations

The pair should sit facing each other in chairs of equal height. It is helpful if the room is comfortably warm and free from distractions and interruptions.

The Process of the Exercise

The pair divides themselves into A and B. A then begins to 'counsel' B but restricts herself only to the following types of interventions:

- open or closed questions;
- reflections or selective reflections;
- checking for understanding;
- empathy-building statements.

The counselling session should continue for at least 10 minutes, then both partners change roles for a further 10 minutes. There should be no sense of play-acting or role-playing about the exercise. Both partners should counsel on 'real' issues and thus develop realistic skills. This exercise, like the previous one, is very difficult because both parties are 'in the know'!

Evaluation Procedure

At the end of the exercise each person should report to the other what she disliked and what she liked about the activity. They may also comment on what they will be able to carry over from it into the 'real' counselling situation.

Exercise No. 18

Aim of the Exercise
To experience being asked a wide range of questions.

Equipment Required/Environmental Considerations
The pair should sit facing each other in chairs of equal height. It is helpful if the room is comfortably warm and free from distractions and interruptions.

The Process of the Exercise
The pair divides themselves into A and B. A then asks a wide range of questions, on any topic at all, for five minutes and B does not respond to them or answer them! After five minutes, roles are reversed and B asks questions of A, who does not respond to them. It is important for both partners to notice how they feel about asking and being asked very personal questions.

Evaluation Procedure
At the end of the exercise each person should report to the other what she disliked and what she liked about the activity. They may also comment on what they will be able to carry over from it into the 'real' counselling situation.

Exercise No. 19

Aim of the Exercise
To notice the difference between being asked questions and making statements.

Equipment Required/Environmental Considerations
The pair should sit facing each other in chairs of equal height. It is helpful if the room is comfortably warm and free from distractions and interruptions.

The Process of the Exercise
The pair divides themselves into A and B. A sits and makes a series of statements, on any topic, to B for five minutes. B listens to the statements but does not respond to them. After five minutes, roles are reversed and B makes a series of statements to A who only listens. Afterwards, the pair discuss the perceived differences between how this exercise felt and how the previous one felt. They discuss, also, the relative merits of questions and statements with regard to counselling.

Evaluation Procedure
At the end of the exercise each person should report to the other what she disliked and what she liked about the activity. They may also comment on what they will be able to carry over from it into the 'real' counselling situation.

Exercise No. 20

Aim of the Exercise
To explore personal history.

Equipment Required/Environmental Considerations
The pair should sit facing each other in chairs of equal height. It is helpful if the room is comfortably warm and free from distractions and interruptions.

The Process of the Exercise
The pair divides themselves into A and B. A talks to B for 10 minutes and reviews her life history to date. Any aspects may be included or left out but some sort of chronological order should be aimed at. After 10 minutes, roles are reversed and B reviews her biography to date, while A listens but does not comment.

Evaluation Procedure
At the end of the exercise each person should report to the other what she disliked and what she liked about the activity. They may also comment on what they will be able to carry over from it into the 'real' counselling situation.

Exercise No. 21

Aim of the Exercise
To explore 'free association'.

Equipment Required/Environmental Considerations
The pair should sit facing each other in chairs of equal height. It is helpful if the room is comfortably warm and free from distractions and interruptions.

The Process of the Exercise
The pair divides themselves A and B. A sits and verbalises whatever comes into her head, whilst B sits and listens only. Everything possible should be verbalised but A should note the things that she does not verbalise! This process continues for three minutes when the pair swap roles and B attempts 'free association' accompanied by A's attention and listening. Afterwards the pair discuss the implications of the activity for themselves and for their counselling practice.

Evaluation Procedure
At the end of the exercise each person should report to the other what she disliked and what she liked about the activity. They may also comment on what they will be able to carry over from it into the 'real' counselling situation.

Exercise No. 22

Aim of the Exercise
To self-evaluate.

Equipment Required/Environmental Considerations

The pair should sit facing each other in chairs of equal height. It is helpful if the room is comfortably warm and free from distractions and interruptions.

The Process of the Exercise

The pair divides themselves into A and B. A then considers and verbalises all the positive and negative aspects of her counselling practice to date. Negative considerations should be made first. When A has finished, B goes through the same process. Afterwards, the pair consider the implications of their evaluations for their counselling practice.

Evaluation Procedure

At the end of the exercise each person should report to the other what she disliked and what she liked about the activity. They may also comment on what they will be able to carry over from it into the 'real' counselling situation.

Exercise No. 23

Aim of the Exercise

To receive feedback on counselling skills.

Equipment Required/Environmental Considerations

The pair should sit facing each other in chairs of equal height. It is helpful if the room is comfortably warm and free from distractions and interruptions.

The Process of the Exercise

The pair divides themselves into A and B. A then offers B both positive and negative feedback as to how she perceives the other's counselling skills. Negative comments should be made first. Then B offers A feedback on her counselling skills. Afterwards both partners consider the implications of this feedback for their counselling practice and compare it with their own, self-evaluation.

Evaluation Procedure

At the end of the exercise each person should report to the other what she disliked and what she liked about the activity. They may also comment on what they will be able to carry over from it into the 'real' counselling situation.

ACTIVITIES   EXERCISES FOR PEOPLE WORKING IN GROUPS

Exercise No. 24

Aim of Exercise
To increase the listening and attending skills of group members.

Number of Participants
Any number between 5 and 20.

Time Required
Between 1 and 1½ hours.

Equipment Required/Environmental Considerations
The group should sit in chairs of equal height and in a circle. It is helpful if the room is comfortably warm and does not contain too many distractions.

The Process of the Exercise
The group holds a discussion on any topic. One ground rule applies throughout the exercise: once the first person has spoken, before anyone else contributes to the discussion, she must first summarise what the person before her has said, to that person's satisfaction! After half an hour, the group discusses the activity.

Evaluation Procedure
Learning from the exercise is evaluated by two 'rounds'. First, each person in turn says what she did not like about the exercise. Then, each person in turn says what she did like about the activity. A third round can be used to establish how each person will use the learning gained, in the future.

Variations on the Exercise
1 The facilitator chooses a topic for discussion, e.g.

   * qualities of the effective counsellor;
   * how we can become better counsellors;
   * how this group is developing?

2 The larger group can break into small groups of four or five to carry out the exercise and then have a plenary session back in the larger group.

Exercise No. 25

Aim of Exercise
To practise asking questions in a group and to experience being asked questions.

Number of Participants
Any number between 5 and 20.

Time Required

Between 1 and 1½ hours.

Equipment Required/Environmental Considerations

The group should sit in chairs of equal height and in a circle. It is helpful if the room is comfortably warm and does not contain too many distractions.

The Process of the Exercise

Each person, in turn, spends five minutes in the 'hotseat'. When occupying the hotseat, she may be asked questions, on any subject, by any member of the group. If she wishes not to answer a particular question, she may say 'pass'. At the end of the person's five minutes in the hotseat, she nominates the next person to occupy it, until all members of the group have had a five-minute turn.

Procedure

Learning from the exercise is evaluated by two 'rounds'. First, each person in turn says what she did not like about the exercise. Then, each person in turn says what she did like about the activity. A third round can be used to establish how each person will use the learning gained, in the future.

Variations on the Exercise

1   The time in the 'hotseat' may be varied from 2 to 10 minutes depending upon the size of the group and the time available.
2   A large group may be split up into smaller groups.
3   With a group in which members know each other very well, the 'pass' facilitity may be abandoned!

Exercise No. 26

Aim of Exercise

To experience clear communication within the group.

Number of Participants

Any number between 5 and 20.

Time Required

Between 1 and 1½ hours.

Equipment Required/Environmental Considerations

The group should sit in chairs of equal height and in a circle. It is helpful if the room is comfortably warm and does not contain too many distractions.

The Process of the Exercise

The group holds a discussion, on any topic, and observes the following ground rules:

- Speak directly, using 'I' rather that 'you', 'we' or 'one'.
- Speak directly to others, using the first person.

- Stay in the present.
- Avoid theorising about what is going on in the group.

Either the facilitator acts as guardian of the ground rules or the group monitors itself.

Evaluation Procedure

Learning from the exercise is evaluated by two 'rounds'. First, each person in turn says what she did not like about the exercise. Then, each person in turn says what she did like about the activity. A third round can be used to establish how each person will use the learning gained, in the future.

Variations on the Exercise

No topic is chosen by or for the group: the material for discussion evolves out of what is happening in the 'here and now'.

Exercise No. 27

Aim of Exercise

To experience participation in a 'leaderless' group and to consider the dynamics of such an activity.

Number of Participants

Any number between 5 and 20.

Time Required

Between 1 and 1½ hours.

Equipment Required/Environmental Considerations

The group should sit in chairs of equal height and in a circle. It is helpful if the room is comfortably warm and does not contain too many distractions. An object to use as a 'conch' is required.

The Process of the Exercise

The group has a discussion, on any topic. In order to speak, however, members must be in possession of the 'conch': an object which signifies that, at that moment, the person holding it is leading the group. Other people who wish to speak must non-verbally negotiate for possession of the conch. After about half an hour, the group drops the 'conch' rule and freely discusses the activity.

Evaluation Procedure

Learning from the exercise is evaluated by two 'rounds'. First, each person in turn says what she did not like about the exercise. Then, each person in turn says what she did like about the activity. A third round can be used to establish how each person will use the learning gained, in the future.

Variations on the Exercise

1   The facilitator chooses a topic for the group to discuss.

2 A rule may be introduced whereby each person may only make one statement when in possession of the 'conch'.

Exercise No. 28

Aim of Exercise
To practise using client-centred counselling interventions in a group.

Number of Participants
Any number between 5 and 20.

Time Required
Between 1 and 1½ hours.

Equipment Required/Environmental Considerations
The group should sit in chairs of equal height and in a circle. It is helpful if the room is comfortably warm and does not contain too many distractions.

The Process of the Exercise
The group members are only allowed to:

- ask questions of each other;
- practise reflections;
- offer empathy-building statements;
- check for understanding of each other.

After half an hour, the group discusses the exercise, having dropped the rule about types of interventions.

Evaluation Procedure
Learning from the exercise is evaluated by two 'rounds'. First, each person in turn says what she did not like about the exercise. Then, each person in turn says what she did like about the activity. A third round can be used to establish how each person will use the learning gained, in the future.

Variations on the Exercise
1 One group member is invited to facilitate a general discussion with the group, using only: (a) questions, (b) reflections, (c) empathy-building statements or (d) checking for understanding. Afterwards, the group offers that person feedback on her performance.
2 Group members, in turn, facilitate a discussion using only the aforementioned types of interventions, for periods of 10 minutes each.

Exercise No. 29

Aim of Exercise
To explore silence in a group context.

Number of Participants
Any number between 5 and 20.

Time Required
Between 1 and 1½ hours.

Equipment Required/Environmental Considerations
The group should sit in chairs of equal height and in a circle. It is helpful if the room is comfortably warm and does not contain too many distractions.

The Process of the Exercise
The group facilitator suggests to the group that they sit in total silence for a period of five minutes. When the five minutes is over, the group discusses the experience.

Evaluation Procedure
Learning from the exercise is evaluated by two 'rounds'. First, each person in turn says what she did not like about the exercise. Then, each person in turn says what she did like about the activity. A third round can be used to establish how each person will use the learning gained, in the future.

Variations on the Exercise
The group may sit in silence with their eyes closed.

Exercise No. 30

Aim of Exercise
To explore a variety of facets of counselling.

Number of Participants
Any number between 5 and 20.

Time Required
Between 1 and 1½ hours.

Equipment Required/Environmental Considerations
The group should sit in chairs of equal height and in a circle. It is helpful if the room is comfortably warm and does not contain too many distractions. A large sheet of paper or a black- or whiteboard is required for this activity.

The Process of the Exercise
The group carries out a 'brainstorming' activity. One member of the group acts as 'scribe' and jots down on a large sheet of paper or a black/whiteboard all comments from the group on one of the following topics. No contributions are discarded and group members are to be encouraged to call out any associations they make with the topic:

- qualities of an effective counsellor;

- problems/difficulties of this group;
- activities for improving counselling skills;
- qualities of the ineffective counsellor;
- skills required for effective counselling;
- problems that health professionals are likely to encounter in counselling.

Evaluation Procedure

Learning from the exercise is evaluated by two 'rounds'. First, each person in turn says what she did not like about the exercise. Then, each person in turn says what she did like about the activity. A third round can be used to establish how each person will use the learning gained, in the future.

Exercise No. 31

Aim of Exercise

To receive feedback from other group members.

Number of Participants

Any number between 5 and 20.

Time Required

Between 1 and 1½ hours.

Equipment Required/Environmental Considerations

The group should sit in chairs of equal height and in a circle. It is helpful if the room is comfortably warm and does not contain too many distractions.

The Process of the Exercise

Each member of the group, in turn, listens to other members of the group offering them positive feedback, i.e. things they like about that person. The feedback is given in the form of a 'round', with each person in turn offering feedback until every group member has spoken. The group member receiving feedback is not allowed to 'respond' to the comments but must listen in silence!

Evaluation Procedure

Learning from the exercise is evaluated by two 'rounds'. First, each person in turn says what she did not like about the exercise. Then, each person in turn says what she did like about the activity. A third round can be used to establish how each person will use the learning gained, in the future.

Variations on the Exercise

With a group where members know each other very well, a round of negative feedback may be offered to each group member, if she requires it. This activity should be handled with care!

Exercise No. 32

Aim of Exercise
To carry out a peer and group evaluation.

Number of Participants
Any number between 5 and 20.

Time Required
Between 1 and 1½ hours.

Equipment Required/Environmental Considerations
The group should sit in chairs of equal height and in a circle. It is helpful if the room is comfortably warm and does not contain too many distractions.

The Process of the Exercise
The group identifies six criteria for evaluating members of the group, e.g.

- contribution to activities;
- self-disclosure;
- contribution of new ideas to the group, etc.

Then each group member silently jots down her own evaluation of herself under these six headings. When all members have finished, each reads out her notes to the rest of the group and invites feedback from other group members on those six criteria. The process is repeated until all group members have both verbalised their evaluation and received feedback from other group members.

Evaluation Procedure
Learning from the exercise is evaluated by two 'rounds'. First, each person in turn says what she did not like about the exercise. Then, each person in turn says what she did like about the activity. A third round can be used to establish how each person will use the learning gained, in the future.

Variations on the Exercise
The feedback from the group may be offered systematically: each group member, in turn, working round the group, offers the individual feedback on her performance.

Exercise No. 33

Aim of Exercise
To explore a spontaneous and leaderless group activity: the 'Quaker' group.

Number of Participants
Any number between 5 and 20.

Time Required
Between 1 and 1½ hours.

Equipment Required/Environmental Considerations
The group should sit in chairs of equal height and in a circle. It is helpful if the room is comfortably warm and does not contain too many distractions.

The Process of the Exercise
The group has no topic for discussion and no leader. Group members are encouraged to verbalise what they are feeling and what they are thinking as those thoughts and feelings occur but there is no obligation for anyone else to respond to the statements offered. The group may fall into silence at times and at others be very noisy! The group exercise should be allowed to run for at least three-quarters of an hour. After that period, group members can freely discuss how it felt to take part in the activity.

Evaluation Procedure
Learning from the exercise is evaluated by two 'rounds'. First, each person in turn says what she did not like about the exercise. Then, each person in turn says what she did like about the activity. A third round can be used to establish how each person will use the learning gained, in the future.

Variations on the Exercise
A topic may be chosen for the group to consider, but no direction is offered by the group facilitator, and group members make statements about the topic as and when they choose.

COUNSELLING SKILLS AND THE HEALTH PROFESSIONAL

These are a range of counselling skills exercises that have been used by the writer in a variety of contexts to help in the development of counselling and interpersonal skills. They can be modified and adapted to suit the specific needs of particular groups of health professionals. Often, too, as we have noted, the best exercises are those that you devise yourself: the group that learns to identify its particular needs and then develops exercises to explore a particular skill can quickly become an autonomous learning group.

Learning to practise as a counsellor can be an exciting and challenging process. It is hoped that this book has offered some signposts towards directions in which counselling expertise may be gained by the health professional. The rest is up to the individual or the group.

EXTRACT FROM A COUNSELLING CONVERSATION

14

This annotated extract of counsellor–client discussion is offered as an example of *one* way in which counselling may be conducted. It is not claimed to be *typical* of counselling (although many of the interventions used by the counsellor are used by *many* counsellors). It is offered as an illustration of some counselling interventions and as the focus of possible discussion about the hows and whys of counselling. Most of the interventions illustrated in this sample are discussed in chapters of the book.

The conversation described here is free-ranging and exploratory in nature. Conversations that took place later might be more focused. The early stages of counselling are often 'ground-clearing' in nature: they allow the client to open up and to begin to explore a range of issues. Often the 'real' issues don't emerge until the client has been allowed to 'wander' a little through a number of issues.

Counsellor: Hello, how can I help?[1]

Client: Well, I don't know really. I just need to talk some things through. I don't really know where to start.[2]

Counsellor: Tell me a little bit about yourself.[3]

Client: I'm 32, married with two small children. I work as a nursing assistant in a small cottage hospital. We've been married for ten years and ... things ... aren't working out ...[4]

Counsellor: Things aren't working out ...[5]

Client: Well, not properly. Me and my wife are unhappy with the way things are at the moment.

Counsellor: What's your wife's name?[6]

Client: Jane. She's *says* she's happy enough but I don't really think we communicate very well.

Counsellor: Jane says she's happy enough ...[7]

Client: She hasn't actually *said* that but I always get the impression that things are alright for her. On the other hand, we don't talk very much to each other. We sort of live parallel lives, I think.

Counsellor: What do you *need* to talk about?[8]

Client: Almost everything! How we feel about each other and the children. Our relationship ... sex. Everything really.[9]

---

[1]Broad, opening question. Perhaps *too* broad. [2]Client has problems answering it, so ... [3]Counsellor asks a more specific question. The question allows the client to begin to talk about himself. [4]After brief biographical details, the client alludes to problems. [5]Client offers straight *reflection*. [6]Counsellor encourages the client to *personalise* the relationship. [7]Counsellor offers a *selective reflection* and picks up on the tone of voice and emphasis offered by the client. [8]This is a slightly confronting and challenging question. Counsellor tries to get to specifics. [9]Client's response suggests that the intervention may have been *too* direct. His response suggests that *everything* needs to be talked about.

Counsellor: Was there a time when you *did* talk to each other?[10]

Client: Yes. We *always* used to talk ... When we first got married, we talked about everything we did. We had no secrets from each other and we used to go out about twice a week and we couldn't stop talking. Now we can't really *start*!

Counsellor: When did you stop?[11]

Client: We just drifted into it, I suppose ... you know how it is ...

Counsellor: There was nothing, particular, that stopped you ... ?[12]

Client: Well, yes, there was. I ... I had an affair a couple of years ago. I met this girl at work and we got quite serious for a while. I ended up telling Jane and she was, obviously, very upset – so was I – and we talked about it all ... She reckoned she forgave me ... I'm not sure she has ...[13]

Counsellor: You're not sure she forgave you ...[14]

Client: No. I know she hasn't. She brings it up, sometimes, when we have an argument. She sort of throws it in my face. She *hated* Sarah ... I suppose I can't blame her. I suppose I would hate it if *Jane* had an affair ...

Counsellor: Would you?[15]

Client: (Laughs, nervously). I was just wondering about that! It sounds awful, but sometimes I wish she *would* have an affair. That would sort of even things up. It would make things a bit more balanced.

Counsellor: It would make you feel better?[16]

Client: I suppose so. I feel really guilty about what happened with Sarah.[17]

Counsellor: What *did* happen?[18]

Client: Well, we talked about setting up together. At one stage, I was going to leave Jane and move in with Sarah.

Counsellor: Did you discuss that with Jane?

Client: No, not at all. Me and Sarah used to talk about it a lot. Sarah wasn't married or anything – she was only young ... 18 ... and she reckoned we could live together and that it would all work out ...

Counsellor: So what happened?[19]

Client: She gave me an ultimatum. Either I told Jane that I was leaving her or *she* would leave ...

Counsellor: And you chose to stay with Jane?

Client: Yes. I told Sarah that I wasn't going to leave her and the children. I *couldn't* leave ... it would have been the end of things ...

---

[10]As a result, the counsellor 'backs off' a little and asks a more general question about communication. [11]Now, the counsellor returns to a very specific and challenging question. [12]Counsellor, picking up on non-verbal behaviour, persists in trying to focus the conversation. [13]Considerable disclosure on the part of the client and first indication of what may be at the *heart* of some of the problems. [14]Counsellor offers a *reflection* on the issue of forgiveness. [15]A challenge from the counsellor. The client's statement is checked and seems to strike a chord. [16]A slightly judgemental response from the counsellor. [17]Client's response may be in direct response to the counsellor's slightly judgemental tone. Counsellor notes this and moves on. [18]Counsellor invites the client to be specific about the relationship. [19]Again, the counsellor looks for *specifics* and helps the client to focus the discussion.

Counsellor: What's happening now ... ?[20]

Client: I'm feeling upset ... I'm a bit embarrassed ... I think ... (begins to cry).

Counsellor: It's OK if you cry ... you're allowed to have feelings ...[21]

Client: I just ... bottled them up a bit, I suppose ... I just sort of froze after we finished and I went back home ... I just couldn't settle back down with Jane. I felt guilty ...[22]

Counsellor: And how are you feeling now?[23]

Client: Still guilty ... I *wish* I hadn't messed things up at home. It wasn't fair to Jane or the children ...

Counsellor: Or to you?

Client: No, I suppose not. Though I *chose* to go out with Sarah ... no one made me do it![24]

Counsellor: Why did you?

Client: Because I liked her. She had a sense of humour and she liked me. We got on well together and everything. It just sort of happened ...

Counsellor: But you *chose* to go out with her?[25]

Client: Yes, I can remember that. I can remember the day when I made that decision ...[26]

Counsellor: Can you describe it?[27]

Client: I was at work and she came on duty. We talked a bit over coffee and everything and she kept looking at me and smiling. I can remember ... it was 3.30 ... and I said ... (begins to cry again) ... I asked her if she would go out with me ...

Counsellor: That was a tough decision?[28]

Client: It was horrible, looking back! I should never have said it ... I fancied her ... I thought I loved her at the time ...

Counsellor: Did you love her?[29]

Client: Yes! That's the problem ... I did love her ...

Counsellor: What's happening now ... ?[30]

Client: I feel sort of angry ...

Counsellor: Who with?

Client: Sarah ... (goes quiet) ... me ...

Counsellor: You're angry with yourself ...[31]

---

[20]At this point, the client looks at the floor and his tone of voice and facial colour change. The counsellor notes these non-verbal changes and asks the client what is happening. [21]Counsellor 'gives permission' to the client. [22]Client identifies a mixture of feelings. [23]Counsellor brings the client to the 'present time'. It might be possible to return to the feelings 'in the past', later in the counselling session. At this point, though, the counsellor has made a decision to return to the present. [24]Client accepts 'responsibility' for the relationship. [25]Counsellor persists with the 'responsibility' issue, perhaps a little too much. [26]On the other hand, it leads the client to a *specific* remembrance. [27]Counsellor invites client to offer a 'literal description' of the events of the time. Sometimes such invitations lead to further cathartic (emotional) release. [28]Counsellor offers an 'empathy-building' statement. If it is 'right', the client will agree. [29]Challenging and confronting question on the part of the counsellor. [30]Again, the counsellor notes non-verbal changes and invites the client to verbalise what is happening. [31]Counsellor offers a mixture of *reflection* and *empathy building*.

Client: With both of us. We were like adolescents! She *was* adolescent, sort of . . .

Counsellor: And you were older . . .[32]

Client: I suppose I should have known better. I *was* older.

Counsellor: And because you were older, you were supposed to be in control . . . ?

Client: I suppose it doesn't work quite like that, does it? I suppose we were both responsible in some ways for what happened.

Counsellor: What was happening at home, with Jane?[33]

Client: Nothing much. We were getting on OK. The children were quite small and Jane was caught up with them. She gave up work around that time and gave all her time to them.

Counsellor: Leaving you out?[34]

Client: (Grins) That's awful, isn't it? Yes, I suppose I felt left out . . . Sarah was there at the right – the *wrong* time . . . and we just . . .

Counsellor: How do you feel about Sarah now? If you met her again . . . ?[35]

Client: I wouldn't want to. It wouldn't work, now. We wouldn't have much in common any more. I've changed . . .

Counsellor: You *and* Jane have changed?

Client: Yes, I think so.

Counsellor: Does it all date back to when you were going out with Sarah?

Client: Not completely. It goes back further than that.

Counsellor: Let me just check where we've got to so far. You feel that you and Jane aren't communicating and, on the one hand, you feel that this dates back to when you met Sarah. On the other, you feel that it goes back much further . . . ?[36]

Client: Yes, that's it, so far. I guess a lot of it has to do with things that happened way back . . . Those things are going to be more difficult to talk about . . .

Counsellor: Well, we can make a start . . .[37]

Key issues demonstrated in this extract
- the counsellor 'takes the lead' from the client and 'follows' him;
- the counsellor listens, not only to the words that the client uses but also to the non-verbal signals;
- the counsellor clarifies what he or she does not understand or follow;
- the counsellor is prepared to challenge issues raised by the client;
- the counsellor, by his or her approach, indicates that *anything* can be talked about and that *feelings* can be expressed.

---

[32]Counsellor finishes the client's sentence.   [33]Counsellor changes tack and asks about the 'home' situation.   [34]Counsellor seems to respond to an *unspoken* thought and to the client's non-verbal behaviours.   [35]Counsellor checks 'present time' feelings.   [36]The counsellor offers a summary of what has been talked about, so far. In this respect, the counsellor is *checking for understanding.*
[37]The counsellor indicates an openness to listening to 'anything' and quietly gives the client permission to talk further and deeper.

CONCLUSION

15

This book has covered a range of aspects of counselling skills in the health professions. This final chapter offers a summary of the main points. They are offered as a list, perhaps for discussion. Certainly there are few 'laws' of counselling and this list must, necessarily, be provisional and open to revision. In the end, it is my contention that the counsellor is functioning best when he or she 'stays out of the way' of the client and encourages the client to find his or her own way through. In this respect, the counsellor is a fellow-traveller, a supportive friend who, nevertheless, is able to keep a certain detachment and not get drawn, too deeply, into the client's own distress. The *degree* to which such detachment is possible is debatable. If the counsellor 'stands too far back' then he or she will be unable to empathise. If the counsellor is too close to the client, then he or she will be drawn into the client's life-drama and be unable to be of sufficient support, for he or she will become part of that drama. Here is the list of basic issues in counselling in the health care professions:

- There is a useful distinction to be made between *counselling* and *counselling skills*. The person who works as a counsellor may do that as a full- or part-time job. If asked, he or she may say that his or her job is 'a counsellor'. On the other hand, a wide range of people – both within and outside of the health care professions – may find using *counselling skills* very useful in their everyday practice. You don't have to be a *counsellor* to make use of *counselling skills*. Conversely, the *counsellor* will depend on *counselling skills* as part of his or her everyday role. It seems likely that most health professionals will use counselling skills in their work without, necessarily, offering full-scale counselling.
- The key issue in counselling and in the use of counselling skills is *listening*. It is the bedrock of all effective counselling, and all of those who work in the health care professions are likely to benefit from constantly paying attention to the effectiveness of their listening.
- The aim of counselling should be to listen and to understand the client's point of view. It should not be to moralise, to interpret or to offer detailed advice. While it is tempting to develop all sorts of psychological theories about why people are the way they are and why they do the things that they do, in the end, it seems more appropriate, to me, to listen to the other person and to try to discover *her* theory about why and what she does. In the end, few people live their lives according to a particular psychological theory. On the other hand, we all develop a sort of *personal* theory about the world, and it is that theory which guides us. The client's personal theory is the key to understanding what it is that she does in her life.

- Counselling needs a *light touch*. If the atmosphere in a counselling session becomes too heavy and earnest, it is unlikely that much real work will be done. The counsellor who is able to keep the atmosphere relatively 'light' is, almost paradoxically, likely to enable the client to self-disclose and to express emotion far more easily.

- The outcome of counselling should be *action*. Counselling that is only about talking will not suffice. In the end, if we want our lives to be different then we must change. The action and change parts of counselling are often the most difficult, for the client and for the counsellor.

- Counselling skills can be learned. While most people are attracted to counselling because they are interested in other people and, presumably, already have some of the personal qualities that are necessary for being effective, most can also benefit from learning some of the simple skills that have been described in this book. Learning to listen, to ask open questions, to reflect and to offer empathy may seem *too* simple. In the end, though, they are probably more effective than any amount of advice giving and judgement.

- A distinction can be made between *information giving* and *advice giving*. One of the reasons for including a chapter in this book on information giving has been to clarify this point. Information giving involves offering clear information about a certain topic. Thus, to the person who is worried about HIV/AIDS, information about safe sex can be useful. Advice giving, on the other hand, involves the counsellor in making some sort of moral judgement about what is *right* for the client and passing that on to him or her. Most advice is likely to follow the, 'If I were you ... ' pattern. Arguably, it is far less useful, in counselling, than is information giving. It is important to be clear on the two issues.

- Counselling can be tiring. To listen to other people's problems and not to judge can be a draining job. Just being an effective listener takes up a considerable amount of energy. Those who work as counsellors or who regularly use counselling skills should also take care of themselves. If they do regular counselling, they should consider having a *supervisor* who will listen to and support them. Others should make sure that there are parts of their jobs which are entirely different from counselling. Full-time commitment to other people can lead to *burnout* and it is vital that all health care professionals also care for themselves.

- Counselling is learned by *doing*. You cannot learn counselling from a book. Workshops and courses which encourage *experiential learning* – learning through trying things out and then through reflection – are particularly useful. It is also important to monitor continuously your own work as a counsellor. Personal styles of counselling modify and change as the counsellor develops. On the other hand, it is also possible to slip into some bad habits in counselling. For that reason, it is useful every so often to take some sort of refresher course in counselling. It is also important to supplement practical 'hands on' experience with plenty of reading about the topic. While counselling cannot be learned from a book, books obviously have their part to play in informing practice.

- There remains a nagging doubt and a question: does counselling *work*? While all the anecdotal evidence suggests that it does, for some people, there remains a need for further *outcome studies* to be conducted in the field of counselling. We must remain open-minded and humble about the degree to which we *know* that counselling makes a difference. While it seems obvious, to most of us, that talking about problems helps, there is, to date, precious little hard evidence that counselling is the prime means of helping people to come to terms with their psychological, emotional and social problems.

- Linked to the previous point is the danger that we might tend to see *emotional* expression as somehow better than *rationality*. This, in a way, has been a dogma of the past two decades. Ferguson in a wide-sweeping review of the past twenty years makes these comments:

> ... *the change taking place was that the media, keeping pace with the death of argument and alleged 'end of history' had almost wholly stopped asking people, 'What do you think?' and began demanding, instead, 'How do you feel?'. This was a disaster in almost every way.*
>
> *First, it established an orthodoxy of grieving that soon became the centralist norm, and later brought with it a dangerous corollary, what you might call the inviolacy of grief.*
>
> *There grew a tacit understanding that, after a tragedy or disaster, every victim was automatically brave, every perpetrator automatically evil, every reaction one of devastation: and further analysis, further thought, trying to expose a complex issue to a little rigour, would bring automatic opprobrium.*

(Ferguson, 1998)

There might just be an argument that we gain, in life, by suffering, just as much as we do from expressing our feelings; that talking about things does not necessarily and automatically change them. There might also be an argument, sometimes, for coolly and rationally looking at our situation and making life decisions based on such rationality rather than on immediate, emotional reactions as has, in some cases, become the norm. This is not, at all, to deny the place and value of counselling and interpersonal communication but to serve as an astringent to the view that expression of feelings and of almost *everything* is necessarily and always, a good thing. We need, perhaps, to proceed with caution.

APPENDIX: ETHICAL FRAMEWORK FOR GOOD PRACTICE IN COUNSELLING AND PSYCHOTHERAPY

ETHICS FOR COUNSELLING AND PSYCHOTHERAPY

This statement, Ethics for Counselling and Psychotherapy, unifies and replaces all the earlier codes for counsellors, trainers and supervisors and is also applicable to counselling research, the use of counselling skills and the management of these services within organisations. It is intended to inform the practice of each member of the British Association for Counselling and Psychotherapy.

In this statement the term 'practitioner' is used generically to refer to anyone with responsibility for the provision of counselling- or psychotherapy-related services. 'Practitioner' includes anyone under-taking the role(s) of counsellor, psychotherapist, trainer, educator, supervisor, researcher, provider of counselling skills or manager of any of these services. The term 'client' is used as a generic term to refer to the recipient of any of these services. The client may be an individual, couple, family, group, organisation or other specifiable social unit. Alternative names may be substituted for 'practitioner' and 'client' in the practice setting, according to custom and context.

This statement indicates an important development in approach to ethics within the Association. One of the characteristics of contem-porary society is the coexistence of different approaches to ethics. This statement reflects this ethical diversity by considering:

- values;
- principles;
- personal moral qualities.

This selection of ways of expressing ethical commitments does not seek to invalidate other approaches. The presentation of different ways of conceiving ethics alongside each other in this statement is intended to draw attention to the limitations of relying too heavily on any single ethical approach. Ethical principles are well suited to examining the justification for particular decisions and actions. However, reliance on principles alone may detract from the importance of the practitioner's personal qualities and their ethical significance in the counselling or therapeutic relationship. The provision of culturally sensitive and appro-priate services is also a fundamental ethical concern. Cultural factors are often more easily understood and responded to in terms of values. Therefore, professional values are becoming an increasingly significant way of expressing ethical commitment.

Values of counselling and psychotherapy

The fundamental values of counselling and psychotherapy include a commitment to:

- respecting human rights and dignity;
- ensuring the integrity of practitioner-client relationships;
- enhancing the quality of professional knowledge and its application;
- alleviating personal distress and suffering;
- fostering a sense of self that is meaningful to the person(s) concerned;
- increasing personal effectiveness;
- enhancing the quality of relationships between people;
- appreciating the variety of human experience and culture;
- striving for the fair and adequate provision of counselling and psychotherapy services.

Values inform principles. They represent an important way of expressing a general ethical commitment that becomes more precisely defined and action-orientated when expressed as a principle.

Ethical principles of counselling and psychotherapy

Principles direct attention to important ethical responsibilities. Each principle is described below and is followed by examples of good practice that have been developed in response to that principle.

Ethical decisions that are strongly supported by one or more of these principles without any contradiction from others may be regarded as reasonably well founded. However, practitioners will encounter circumstances in which it is impossible to reconcile all the applicable principles, and choosing between principles may be required. A decision or course of action does not necessarily become unethical merely because it is contentious, or other practitioners would have reached different conclusions in similar circumstances. A practitioner's obligation is to consider all the relevant circumstances with as much care as is reasonably possible and to be appropriately accountable for decisions made.

Fidelity: honouring the trust placed in the practitioner

Being trustworthy is regarded as fundamental to understanding and resolving ethical issues. Practitioners who adopt this principle act in accordance with the trust placed in them; regard confidentiality as an obligation arising from the client's trust; restrict any disclosure of confidential information about clients to furthering the purposes for which it was originally disclosed.

Autonomy: respect for the client's right to be self-governing

This principle emphasises the importance of the client's commitment to participating in counselling or psychotherapy, usually on a voluntary basis. Practitioners who respect their clients' autonomy ensure accuracy in any advertising or information given in advance of services offered; seek freely given and adequately informed consent; engage in explicit contracting in advance of any commitment by the client; protect privacy; protect confidentiality; normally make any disclosures of confidential information conditional on the consent of the person concerned; and inform the client in advance of foreseeable conflicts of interest or as soon as possible after such conflicts become apparent. The principle of autonomy opposes the manipulation of clients against their will, even for beneficial social ends.

Beneficence: a commitment to promoting the client's well-being

The principle of beneficence means acting in the best interests of the client based on professional assessment. It directs attention to working strictly within one's limits of competence and providing services on the basis of adequate training or experience. Ensuring that the client's best interests are achieved requires systematic monitoring of practice and outcomes by the best available means. It is considered important that research and systematic reflection inform practice. There is an obligation to use regular and on-going supervision to enhance the quality of the services provided and to commit to updating practice by continuing professional development. An obligation to act in the best interests of a client may become paramount when working with clients whose capacity for autonomy is diminished because of immaturity, lack of understanding, extreme distress, serious disturbance or other significant personal constraints.

Non-maleficence: a commitment to avoiding harm to the client

Non-maleficence involves avoiding sexual, financial, emotional or any other form of client exploitation; avoiding incompetence or malpractice; not providing services when unfit to do so due to illness, personal circumstances or intoxication. The practitioner has an ethical responsibility to strive to mitigate any harm caused to a client even when the harm is unavoidable or unintended. Holding appropriate insurance may assist in restitution. Practitioners have a personal responsibility to challenge, where appropriate, the incompetence or malpractice of others; and to contribute to any investigation and/or adjudication concerning professional practice which falls below that of a reasonably competent practitioner and/or risks bringing discredit upon the profession.

Justice: the fair and impartial treatment of all clients and the provision of adequate services

The principle of justice requires being just and fair to all clients and respecting their human rights and dignity. It directs attention to considering conscientiously any legal requirements and obligations, and remaining alert to potential conflicts between legal and ethical obligations. Justice in the distribution of services requires the ability to determine impartially the provision of services for clients and the allocation of services between clients. A commitment to fairness requires the ability to appreciate differences between people and to be committed to equality of opportunity, and avoiding discrimination against people or groups contrary to their legitimate personal or social characteristics. Practitioners have a duty to strive to ensure a fair provision of counselling and psychotherapy services, accessible and appropriate to the needs of potential clients.

Self-respect: fostering the practitioner's self-knowledge and care for self
The principle of self-respect means that the practitioner appropriately applies all the above principles as entitlements for self. This includes seeking counselling or therapy and other opportunities for personal development as required. There is an ethical responsibility to use supervision for appropriate personal and professional support and development, and to seek training and other opportunities for continuing professional development. Guarding against financial liabilities arising from work undertaken usually requires obtaining appropriate insurance. The principle of self-respect encourages active engagement in life-enhancing activities and relationships that are independent of relationships in counselling or psychotherapy.

Personal moral qualities

The practitioner's personal moral qualities are of the utmost importance to clients. Many of the personal qualities considered important in the provision of services have an ethical or moral component and are therefore considered as virtues or good personal qualities. It is inappropriate to prescribe that all practitioners possess these qualities, since it is fundamental that these personal qualities are deeply rooted in the person concerned and developed out of personal commitment rather than the requirement of an external authority. Personal qualities to which counsellors and psychotherapists are strongly encouraged to aspire include:

Empathy: the ability to communicate understanding of another person's experience from that person's perspective.
Sincerity: a personal commitment to consistency between what is professed and what is done.
Integrity: commitment to being moral in dealings with others, personal straightforwardness, honesty and coherence.
Resilience: the capacity to work with the client's concerns without being personally diminished.
Respect: showing appropriate esteem to others and their understanding of themselves.
Humility: the ability to assess accurately and acknowledge one's own strengths and weaknesses.
Competence: the effective deployment of the skills and knowledge needed to do what is required.
Fairness: the consistent application of appropriate criteria to inform decisions and actions.
Wisdom: possession of sound judgement that informs practice.
Courage: the capacity to act in spite of known fears, risks and uncertainty.

Conclusion

The challenge of working ethically means that practitioners will inevitably encounter situations where there are competing obligations. In such situations it is tempting to retreat from all ethical analysis in order to escape a sense of what may appear to be unresolvable ethical tension. These ethics are intended to be of assistance in such circumstances by directing attention to the variety of ethical factors that may need to be taken into consideration and to alternative ways of approaching ethics that may prove more useful. No statement of ethics can totally alleviate the difficulty of making professional judgements in circumstances that may be constantly changing and full of uncertainties. By accepting this statement of ethics, members of the British Association for Counselling and Psychotherapy are committing themselves to engaging with the challenge of striving to be ethical, even when doing so involves making difficult decisions or acting courageously.

GUIDANCE ON GOOD PRACTICE IN COUNSELLING AND PSYCHOTHERAPY

The British Association for Counselling and Psychotherapy is committed to sustaining and advancing good practice. This guidance on the essential elements of good practice has been written to take into account the changing circumstances in which counselling and psychotherapy are now being delivered, in particular:

- changes in the range of issues and levels of need presented by clients;
- the growth in levels of expertise available from practitioners with the expansion in the availability of training and consultative support/supervision;
- the accumulated experience of this Association over nearly three decades.

The diversity of settings within which counselling and psychotherapy services are delivered has also been carefully considered. These services may be provided by the independent practitioner working alone, one or more practitioners working to provide a service within an agency or large organisation, specialists working in multidisciplinary teams, and by specialist teams of counsellors and psychotherapists. Most work is undertaken face to face but there is also a growing number of telephone and online services. Some practitioners are moving between these different settings and modes of delivery during the course of their work and are therefore required to consider what constitutes good practice in different settings. All practitioners encounter the challenge of responding to the diversity of their clients and finding ways of working effectively with them. This statement therefore responds to the complexity of delivering counselling and psychotherapy services in contemporary society by directing attention to essential issues that practitioners ought to consider and resolve in the specific circumstances of their work.

The term 'practitioner' is used generically to refer to anyone with responsibility for the provision of counselling- or psychotherapy-related services. 'Practitioner' includes anyone undertaking the role(s) of counsellor, psychotherapist, trainer, educator, supervisor, researcher, provider of counselling skills or manager of any of these services. The term 'client' is used as a generic term to refer to the recipient of any of these services. The client may be an individual, couple, family, group, organisation or other specifiable social unit. Alternative names may be substituted for 'practitioner' and 'client' in the practice setting as the terminology varies according to custom and context.

Providing a good standard of practice and care

All clients are entitled to good standards of practice and care from their practitioners in counselling and psychotherapy. Good standards of practice and care require professional competence; good relationships with clients and colleagues; and commitment to and observance of professional ethics.

Good quality of care

1 Good quality of care requires competently delivered services that meet the client's needs by practitioners who are appropriately supported and accountable.

2 Practitioners should give careful consideration to the limitations of their training and experience and work within these limits, taking advantage of available professional support. If work with clients requires the provision of additional services operating in parallel with counselling or psychotherapy, the availability of such services ought to be taken into account, as their absence may constitute a significant limitation.

3 Good practice involves clarifying and agreeing the rights and responsibilities of both the practitioner and client at appropriate points in their working relationship.

4 Dual relationships arise when the practitioner has two or more kinds of relationship concurrently with a client, for example client and trainee, acquaintance and client, colleague and person under supervision. The existence of a dual relationship with a client is seldom neutral and can have a powerful beneficial or detrimental impact that may not always be easily foreseeable. For these reasons practitioners are required to consider the implications of entering into dual relationships with clients, to avoid entering into relationships that are likely to be detrimental to clients, and to be readily accountable to clients and colleagues for any dual relationships that occur.

5 Practitioners are encouraged to keep appropriate records of their work with clients unless there are adequate reasons for not keeping any records. All records should be accurate, respectful of clients and colleagues and protected from unauthorised disclosure. Practitioners should take into account their responsibilities and their clients'

rights under data protection legislation and any other legal requirements.

6   Clients are entitled to competently delivered services that are periodically reviewed by the practitioner. These reviews may be conducted, when appropriate, in consultation with clients, supervisors, managers or other practitioners with relevant expertise.

Maintaining competent practice

7   All counsellors, psychotherapists, trainers and supervisors are required to have regular and on-going formal supervision/consultative support for their work in accordance with professional requirements. Managers, researchers and providers of counselling skills are strongly encouraged to review their need for professional and personal support and to obtain appropriate services for themselves.

8   Regularly monitoring and reviewing one's work is essential to maintaining good practice. It is important to be open to, and conscientious in considering, feedback from colleagues, appraisals and assessments. Responding constructively to feedback helps to advance practice.

9   A commitment to good practice requires practitioners to keep up to date with the latest knowledge and respond to changing circumstances. They should consider carefully their own need for continuing professional development and engage in appropriate educational activities.

10 Practitioners should be aware of and understand any legal requirements concerning their work, consider these conscientiously and be legally accountable for their practice.

Keeping trust

11 The practice of counselling and psychotherapy depends on gaining and honouring the trust of clients. Keeping trust requires:

- attentiveness to the quality of listening and respect offered to clients;
- culturally appropriate ways of communicating that are courteous and clear;
- respect for privacy and dignity;
- careful attention to client consent and confidentiality.

12 Clients should be adequately informed about the nature of the services being offered. Practitioners should obtain adequately informed consent from their clients and respect a client's right to choose whether to continue or withdraw.

13 Practitioners should ensure that services are normally delivered on the basis of the client's explicit consent. Reliance on implicit consent is more vulnerable to misunderstandings and is best avoided unless there are sound reasons for doing so. Overriding a client's known wishes or consent is a serious matter that requires commen-

surate justification. Practitioners should be prepared to be readily accountable to clients, colleagues and the professional body if they override a client's known wishes.

14 Situations in which clients pose a risk of causing serious harm to themselves or others are particularly challenging for the practitioner. These are situations in which the practitioner should be alert to the possibility of conflicting responsibilities between those concerning their client, other people who may be significantly affected, and society generally. Resolving conflicting responsibilities may require due consideration of the context in which the service is being provided. Consultation with a supervisor or experienced practitioner is strongly recommended, whenever this would not cause undue delay. In all cases, the aim should be to ensure for the client a good quality of care that is as respectful of the client's capacity for self-determination and their trust as circumstances permit.

15 Working with young people requires specific ethical awareness and competence. The practitioner is required to consider and assess the balance between young people's dependence on adults and carers and their progressive development towards acting independently. Working with children and young people requires careful consideration of issues concerning their capacity to give consent to receiving any service independently of someone with parental responsibilities and the management of confidences disclosed by clients.

16 Respecting client confidentiality is a fundamental requirement for keeping trust. The professional management of confidentiality concerns the protection of personally identifiable and sensitive information from unauthorised disclosure. Disclosure may be authorised by client consent or the law. Any disclosures should be undertaken in ways that best protect the client's trust. Practitioners should be willing to be accountable to their clients and to their profession for their management of confidentiality in general and particularly for any disclosures made without their client's consent.

17 Practitioners should normally be willing to respond to their client's requests for information about the way that they are working and any assessment that they may have made. This professional requirement does not apply if it is considered that imparting this information would be detrimental to the client or inconsistent with the counselling or psychotherapeutic approach previously agreed with the client. Clients may have legal rights to this information and these need to be taken into account.

18 Practitioners must not abuse their client's trust in order to gain sexual, emotional, financial or any other kind of personal advantage. Sexual relations with clients are prohibited. 'Sexual relations' include intercourse, any other type of sexual activity or sexualised behaviour. Practitioners should think carefully about, and exercise considerable caution before, entering into personal or business relationships with former clients and should expect to be

professionally accountable if the relationship becomes detrimental to the client or the standing of the profession.

19 Practitioners should not allow their professional relationships with clients to be prejudiced by any personal views they may hold about lifestyle, gender, age, disability, race, sexual orientation, beliefs or culture.

20 Practitioners should be clear about any commitment to be available to clients and colleagues and honour these commitments.

Teaching and training

21 All practitioners are encouraged to share their professional knowledge and practice in order to benefit their clients and the public.

22 Practitioners who provide education and training should acquire the skills, attitudes and knowledge required to be competent teachers and facilitators of learning.

23 Practitioners are required to be fair, accurate and honest in their assessments of their students.

24 Prior consent is required from clients if they are to be observed, recorded or if their personally identifiable disclosures are to be used for training purposes.

Supervising and managing

25 Practitioners are responsible for clarifying who holds responsibility for the work with the client.

26 There is a general obligation for all counsellors, psychotherapists, supervisors and trainers to receive supervision/consultative support independently of any managerial relationships.

27 Supervisors and managers have a responsibility to maintain and enhance good practice by practitioners, to protect clients from poor practice and to acquire the attitudes, skills and knowledge required by their role.

Researching

28 The Association is committed to fostering research that will inform and develop practice. All practitioners are encouraged to support research undertaken on behalf of the profession and to participate actively in research work.

29 All research should be undertaken with rigorous attentiveness to the quality and integrity both of the research itself and of the dissemination of the results of the research.

30 The rights of all research participants should be carefully considered and protected. The minimum rights include the right to freely given and informed consent, and the right to withdraw at any point.

31 The research methods used should comply with the standards of good practice in counselling and psychotherapy and must not adversely affect clients.

Fitness to practise

32 Practitioners have a responsibility to monitor and maintain their fitness to practise at a level that enables them to provide an effective service. If their effectiveness becomes impaired for any reason, including health or personal circumstances, they should seek the advice of their supervisor, experienced colleagues or line manager and, if necessary, withdraw from practice until their fitness to practise returns. Suitable arrangements should be made for clients who are adversely affected.

If things go wrong with own clients

33 Practitioners should respond promptly and appropriately to any complaint received from their clients. An appropriate response in agency-based services would take account of any agency policy and procedures.

34 Practitioners should endeavour to remedy any harm they may have caused to their clients and to prevent any further harm. An apology may be the appropriate response.

35 Practitioners should discuss, with their supervisor, manager or other experienced practitioner(s), the circumstances in which they may have harmed a client in order to ensure that the appropriate steps have been taken to mitigate any harm and to prevent any repetition.

36 Practitioners are strongly encouraged to ensure that their work is adequately covered by insurance for professional indemnity and liability.

37 If practitioners consider that they have acted in accordance with good practice but their client is not satisfied that this is the case, they may wish to use independent dispute resolution, for example seeking a second professional opinion, mediation, or conciliation where this is both appropriate and practical.

38 Clients should be informed about the existence of the Professional Conduct Procedure of this Association and any other applicable complaints or disciplinary procedures. If requested to do so, practitioners should inform their clients about how they may obtain further information concerning these procedures.

Responsibilities to all clients

39 Practitioners have a responsibility to protect clients when they have good reason for believing that other practitioners are placing them at risk of harm.

40 They should raise their concerns with the practitioner concerned in the first instance, unless it is inappropriate to do so. If the matter cannot be resolved, they should review the grounds for their concern and the evidence available to them and, when appropriate, raise their concerns with the practitioner's manager, agency or professional body.

41 If they are uncertain what to do, their concerns should be discussed

with an experienced colleague, a supervisor or raised with this Association.

42 All members of this Association share a responsibility to take part in its professional conduct procedures whether as the person complained against or as the provider of relevant information.

Working with colleagues

The increasing availability of counselling and psychotherapy means that most practitioners have other practitioners working in their locality, or may be working closely with colleagues within specialised or multidisciplinary teams. The quality of the interactions between practitioners can enhance or undermine the claim that counselling and psychotherapy enable clients to increase their insight and expertise in personal relationships. This is particularly true for practitioners who work in agencies or teams.

Working in teams

43 Professional relationships should be conducted in a spirit of mutual respect. Practitioners should endeavour to attain good working relationships and systems of communication that enhance services to clients at all times.

44 Practitioners should treat all colleagues fairly and foster equality opportunity.

45 They should not allow their professional relationships with colleagues to be prejudiced by their own personal views about a colleague's lifestyle, gender, age, disability, race, sexual orientation, beliefs or culture. It is unacceptable and unethical to discriminate against colleagues on any of these grounds.

46 Practitioners must not undermine a colleague's relationships with clients by making unjustified or unsustainable comments.

47 All communications between colleagues about clients should be on a professional basis and thus purposeful, respectful and consistent with the management of confidences as declared to clients.

Awareness of context

48 The practitioner is responsible for learning about and taking account of the different protocols, conventions and customs that can pertain to different working contexts and cultures.

Making and receiving referrals

49 All routine referrals to colleagues and other services should be discussed with the client in advance and the client's consent obtained both to making the referral and also to disclosing information to accompany the referral. Reasonable care should be taken to ensure that:

- the recipient of the referral is able to provide the required service;

- any confidential information disclosed during the referral process will be adequately protected;
- the referral will be likely to benefit the client.

50 Prior to accepting a referral the practitioner should give careful consideration to:

- the appropriateness of the referral;
- the likelihood that the referral will be beneficial to the client;
- the adequacy of the client's consent for the referral.

If the referrer is professionally required to retain overall responsibility for the work with the client, it is considered to be professionally appropriate to provide the referrer with brief progress reports. Such reports should be made in consultation with clients and not normally against their explicit wishes.

Probity in professional practice
Ensuring the probity of practice is important both to those who are directly affected but also to the standing of the profession as a whole.

Providing clients with adequate information
51 Practitioners are responsible for clarifying the terms on which their services are being offered in advance of the client incurring any financial obligation or other reasonably foreseeable costs or liabilities.
52 All information about services should be honest, accurate, avoid unjustifiable claims, and be consistent with maintaining the good standing of the profession.
53 Particular care should be taken over the integrity of presenting qualifications, accreditation and professional standing.

Financial arrangements
54 Practitioners are required to be honest, straightforward and accountable in all financial matters concerning their clients and other professional relationships.

Conflicts of interest
55 Conflicts of interest are best avoided, provided they can be reasonably foreseen in the first instance and prevented from arising. In deciding how to respond to conflicts of interest, the protection of the client's interests and maintaining trust in the practitioner should be paramount.

Care of self as a practitioner
Attending to the practitioner's well-being is essential to sustaining good practice.

56 Practitioners have a responsibility to themselves to ensure that their work does not become detrimental to their health or well-being by

ensuring that the way that they undertake their work is as safe as possible and that they seek appropriate professional support and services as the need arises.

57 Practitioners are entitled to be treated with proper consideration and respect that is consistent with this Guidance.

PROFESSIONAL CONDUCT PROCEDURE

It is the responsibility of Members Complained Against and Complainants to ensure that they fully understand the Professional Conduct Procedure and the associated protocols. This procedure forms an essential part of BACP's commitment to the protection of the public. Members are required to inform any client who indicates that they have a complaint or grievance about the existence of this procedure and any other applicable complaints or disciplinary procedures. If requested to do so, practitioners should inform their clients about how they may obtain further information concerning these procedures. Further information may be obtained by contacting BACP directly.

1. Introduction

1.1. Aim

The aim of the Professional Conduct Procedure is to afford protection to the public and to protect the name of BACP and the profession of counselling and psychotherapy as conducted by both individual and organisational members of the Association.

1.2. Bringing a complaint

A complaint can be brought by either:

a) a member of the public seeking or using a service provided by a member of the Association or

b) a member against another member.

1.3. Complaints against non-members

The Association cannot deal with complaints against individuals or organisations who were not members of the Association at the time of the alleged breach of professional conduct.

1.4. Timescale

1.4.1. A complaint must be lodged within three years of the alleged breach.

1.4.2. All records, save for details of the formal complaint, the formal response, the decision of the Professional Conduct Panel, Appeal decision and sanction which are kept for five years, will be kept for a period of two years only.

1.5. Administration

The administration of the Professional Conduct Procedure will follow protocols laid down from time to time by the Association. These will be administered by the Head of Professional Conduct.

1.6. Expenses

The Association is not responsible for travel or any other expenses incurred either by the Complainant or the Member Complained Against (or any support person/representative) in connection with any stage of the complaint. The Association cannot order one party to a complaint to pay another party's costs.

1.7. Dual accountability

The Association may decide to hear a complaint against a member when another organisation is involved in a similar process arising out of the same substantive matters.

1.8. Resolution

Before making the complaint, the Complainant is expected to attempt to resolve the issue with the individual or organisational Member Complained Against. The Complainant must demonstrate that all informal channels or, in the case of organisational members, all internal processes and procedures have been exhausted. If local resolution is impossible or inappropriate, an explanation as to why this is the case will be required.

1.9. Findings

The Association reserves the right to distribute any findings upheld against a member where it considers it right and just to do so in all circumstances and in accordance with the detail in paragraph 4.10 (ii) below.

2. Making a complaint

2.1. The complaint

The complaint must satisfy the following conditions:

a) the allegation is of a breach of a specific clause or clauses of the relevant Code of Ethics & Practice of the Association in force at the time the alleged breach occurred; or gives details of the alleged breach of Professional Conduct that contravenes the minimum standard of good practice outlined in the Ethics for Counselling & Psychotherapy and the Guidance on Good Practice in Counselling & Psychotherapy;

b) it is brought either by a member of the public seeking or using a service provided by a member OR by a current member of the Association;

c) the individual or organisational Member Complained Against is named AND is a current member of the Association AND was a member of the Association at the time the alleged breach occurred;
d) it is in writing, signed and received by the Head of Professional Conduct.

A complaint not satisfying the above conditions will be rejected.

2.2. Notification

The Member Complained Against will be notified that a complaint has been received, given a copy of that complaint and details of the procedure to be followed. The Member Complained Against is not required to respond at this stage, but will be given an opportunity at a later stage if the complaint is accepted under the formal Professional Conduct Procedure (section 3).

2.3. Receipt of a complaint

a) the complaint will be submitted to a Pre-Hearing Assessment Panel;
b) the Pre-Hearing Assessment Panel will decide whether to accept the complaint to be dealt with at a Professional Conduct Hearing, refer it back for further information/clarification, or reject it. The panel has discretion to interview the Complainant and/or Member Complained Against if deemed appropriate;
c) if further information/clarification is requested, upon receipt of same, the complaint will be re-submitted to the Pre-Hearing Assessment Panel which will decide whether to accept it to be dealt with at a Professional Conduct Hearing, or reject it;
d) once the complaint is accepted to be dealt with at a Professional Conduct Hearing, the Head of Professional Conduct will start the formal Professional Conduct Procedure (see section 3);
e) if the complaint is rejected by the Pre-Hearing Assessment Panel, the Complainant and Member Complained Against will be formally notified in writing. The decision of the Pre-Hearing Assessment Panel will be final.

3. The formal Professional Conduct Procedure

3.1. Acceptance of complaint

The Complainant and Member Complained Against will be notified in writing that the complaint will proceed to a Professional Conduct Hearing.

3.2. Responding to a formal complaint

At the time of notification of acceptance of the complaint, a full copy of the formal complaint will be submitted to the Member Complained Against, who will have 28 days to respond to the complaint. Any response to the complaint must be forwarded to the Head of Professional Conduct.

3.3. Evidence

All evidence submitted by either the Complainant or the Member Complained Against shall be available to the parties involved in the complaint. The Head of Professional Conduct will distribute to the parties copies of all submissions made.

3.4. Conduct

It is the duty of the parties taking part in the Professional Conduct Procedure to comply with the protocols laid down by the Association. Such persons shall comply with the implementation of the Professional Conduct Procedure. Any failure to comply may result in the termination of the Professional Conduct Procedure or termination of membership under Article 4.6 of the Memorandum and Articles of Association.

3.5. Suspension of rights of membership

The Chair of the Association may suspend the rights of membership of the Member Complained Against, pending the finalisation of the Professional Conduct Procedure when, having regard to the nature of the complaint, it appears appropriate and just to do so in all the circumstances.

The Head of Professional Conduct will notify the Member Complained Against of the suspension of membership or of any rights of membership.

No liability for any loss suffered, or expenses incurred, will attach to the Association for the suspension of membership or rights of membership even where a complaint is not upheld.

3.6. Lapsed membership

Failure to renew membership by a Member Complained Against during the course of a complaint will not normally terminate the Professional Conduct Procedure.

A member's resignation from membership of the Association will not terminate nor invalidate the hearing of a complaint by the Association.

4. The Professional Conduct Hearing

4.1. Professional Conduct Panel

The Head of Professional Conduct will appoint a panel of not less than three persons to hear the complaint (the Professional Conduct Panel).

4.2. Purpose

The purpose of the Professional Conduct Hearing is to examine the complaint and decide whether the complaint is proved or not. If proved, the panel will decide whether or not any sanction should be imposed.

4.3. Declaration of interest

Members of the Professional Conduct Panel have a duty to declare any interest which may be considered by the Head of Professional Conduct to affect their impartiality, or likely to be thought so to do.

4.4. Venue

Professional Conduct Hearings will be held at or within the vicinity of the Association's headquarters, other than in exceptional circumstances.

4.5. Presence of a representative/support person

When appearing at the Professional Conduct Hearing, the Complainant and Member Complained Against may each be accompanied by a representative who may support and/or speak on behalf of the party concerned.

   The Professional Conduct Hearing will be conducted in accordance with the protocols laid down by the Association.

4.6. Written evidence

Written evidence and/or submissions and witness statements must be submitted in advance by the Complainant and the Member Complained Against. Such papers must be received by the Head of Professional Conduct not less than 28 days prior to the date fixed for the Professional Conduct Hearing. Such papers will be circulated to the Professional Conduct Panel, the Complainant and the Member Complained Against, within a reasonable period prior to the hearing. The Chair of the Professional Conduct Panel may take advice on these papers and/or procedural matters from the Association's solicitor, or the Head of Professional Conduct, or such other relevant person as may be deemed appropriate.

4.7. New evidence

The Chair of the Professional Conduct Panel will determine whether or not new evidence will be accepted on the day of the hearing. The decision will be based on the conditions laid down in the relevant protocol. The Chair of the Professional Conduct Panel may take advice on such matters from the Head of Professional Conduct.

4.8. Attendance by witnesses

The Professional Conduct Panel, Complainant and Member Complained Against may call witnesses to attend the hearing. Parties wishing to call witnesses must notify the Head of Professional Conduct of the names and details of such witnesses not less than 28 days prior to the date fixed for the hearing. Attendance will only be permitted by the Chair of the panel if the witness has supplied a written statement which needs clarification. The panel has discretion to refuse attendance by a witness if it reasonably believes that such attendance is not relevant or will not add any weight to the issue(s) under consideration. Witnesses may be questioned by the panel and either party connected with the case.

4.9. Failure to attend the Professional Conduct hearing

a) Where a Complainant or Member Complained Against fails or refuses, without good reason or notice, to attend a Professional Conduct hearing, the Chair of the Professional Conduct Panel has the power to decide either:

    i) to proceed with the hearing in the absence of one of the parties;

    ii) to adjourn the hearing to a date not less than 28 days in advance;

    iii) to terminate the proceedings or;

    iv) refer the matter for consideration under Article 4.6 of the Memorandum & Articles of Association.

b) What constitutes good reason shall be solely at the discretion of the Chair of the Professional Conduct Panel, who may take advice from the Head of Professional Conduct.

4.10. Notification of findings

i) The decision of the Professional Conduct Panel will be notified in writing to the parties within 28 days of the Professional Conduct hearing.

ii) The decision of the Professional Conduct Panel, together with details of any sanction, will be published in the Association's journal in such detail as deemed appropriate to the findings and at its discretion. (In accordance with paragraph 7.1 such decisions will be based on considerations of public interest and the severity of the findings.)

5. Sanctions

5.1. The Professional Conduct Panel, having regard to the findings, may impose one or more of the sanctions detailed in the relevant protocol.

5.2. Lifting of sanctions

The Member Complained Against may make application to the Head of Professional Conduct for the sanction to be lifted when the conditions laid down in the sanction have been fulfilled.

5.2. (a) The Head of Professional Conduct will appoint not less than three people to consider any evidence of compliance. The Sanctions Panel will decide if the requirements of the sanction have been fulfilled and thus, whether the sanction should be lifted.

5.2. (b) The Member Complained Against will be notified in writing of any decision made (see 5.2.(a)). The lifting of sanction will be published in the Association's journal (if the sanction has been published originally).

5.3. Failure or refusal to comply with sanction

Failure or refusal to comply with the sanction may result in termination of membership. The Chair of the Association will notify any such decision to the Member Complained Against, in writing. This decision will be published in the Association's journal.

6. Formal appeals procedure

6.1. The Member Complained Against may appeal on the grounds detailed in paragraph 6.5. An appeal against the finding of the Professional Conduct Panel must be submitted in writing by the deadline given (see paragraph 6.6), be accompanied by any supporting documentation and served upon the Head of Professional Conduct.

6.2. The grounds for appeal will be considered by an independent person appointed by the Head of Professional Conduct. An appeal can be against the findings of the Professional Conduct Panel and/or sanction imposed.

6.3. If the appeal is accepted under paragraph 6.2, a notice to that effect shall be given to the Head of Professional Conduct and thereupon the appeal procedure set out in paragraph 6.8 hereof shall take effect.

6.4. If there is insufficient evidence to satisfy any of the grounds for appeal (paragraph 6.5), the appellant will be notified in writing by the Head of Professional Conduct. This decision will be final.

6.5. An appeal will be considered on any of the following grounds:

1. That the facts were found against the weight of evidence.
2. That the sanction is disproportionate to the finding of the Professional Conduct Panel and is unjust in all the circumstances.
3. There is evidence to suggest that a procedural impropriety may have had a material effect on the finding and decision of the Professional Conduct Panel.
4. There is new evidence which was not available at the time of the Professional Conduct Hearing (subject to the conditions laid down in the relevant protocol).

6.6. Timescale for appeal

Any appeal must be in writing, specify which grounds it is submitted under and be accompanied by any supporting documentation and served upon the Head of Professional Conduct within 28 days of notification of the decision and/or sanction of the Professional Conduct Panel.

6.7. Professional Conduct Appeal Panel

The Head of Professional Conduct will appoint not less than three people, who were not previously involved in the case, to decide the appeal (The Professional Conduct Appeal Panel). One member of the panel will be a person appointed by the Board of Governors to sit on such panels.

6.8. Format of Appeal Hearing

a) Where there is an appeal as set out in paragraph 6.5 (1), (3) & (4) the appeal will be by way of a re-hearing.

b) Where there is an appeal as set out in paragraph 6.5 (2) only, the Professional Conduct Appeal Panel will meet with the Member Complained Against. The panel will review all the submissions considered by the Professional Conduct Panel, and consider any other mitigating factors submitted by the Member Complained Against.

c) The same rules on representation will apply to the Appeal Hearing as per the original hearing (paragraph 4.5).

6.9. Notification of decision

a) The Chair of the Professional Conduct Appeal Panel will report the panel's decision to the Chair of the Association who will implement its decision. This decision will be final.

b) The decision of the Professional Conduct Appeal Panel will be notified to the respective parties in writing within 14 days of the appeal hearing.

c) Following the hearing of an appeal, where the appeal is rejected, the decision of the Professional Conduct Panel, incorporating any amendment by the Professional Conduct Appeal Panel, may be published in the Association's journal in such detail as deemed appropriate (such decisions will be based on considerations of public interest and severity of the findings).

7. Publication

7.1. The Association reserves the right to publish such details of complaints as it considers appropriate.

7.2. The termination of membership under the Professional Conduct Procedure will be published in the Association's journal.

7.3. Any notification that the Association, under these Procedures, is entitled to publish in its journal may, at its discretion, be published elsewhere by the Association.

8. Effective Date

This Professional Conduct Procedure 2002 will apply to all complaints received by the Association after 1 April 2002.

HEADS OF COMPLAINT

The Professional Conduct Panel is responsible for determining whether the grounds of the complaint are upheld according to the standards of civil law and, if upheld, the head(s) of complaint that have been contravened. It is envisaged that a single act may fall clearly under one head or contravene two or more. The decision about the head must ultimately rest upon consideration of all the circumstances in the case. The information that follows is intended to inform the choice between the three heads of complaint available to the panel. These are:

1. professional misconduct;
2. professional malpractice;
3. bringing the profession into disrepute.

Findings under the first two heads are usually, but not exclusively, concerned with behaviour directly related to someone's professional pursuit. The third head may encompass a wider range of behaviour that extends beyond someone's professional pursuit.

Professional misconduct

A finding of professional misconduct signifies that the practitioner has contravened the ethical and behavioural standards that should reasonably be expected of a member of this profession. 'Misconduct' is defined as acting in contravention of the written and unwritten guidance of the profession.

A finding of 'serious professional misconduct' is appropriate if the misconduct is of sufficient seriousness to merit a period of suspension or permanent exclusion from membership of this Association with a consequential curtailment of opportunities to practise within this profession.

Professional malpractice

A finding of professional malpractice signifies that the service(s) for which the practitioner is responsible has fallen below the standards that would reasonably be expected of a practitioner exercising reasonable care and skill. Examples of 'malpractice' include:

- incompetence;
- negligence;
- recklessness;
- inadequate professional services.

It may be that the seriousness of the malpractice is such that it is considered to amount to misconduct.

This is determined by different, and usually higher, tests than the test of reasonableness in the tort of negligence. The Clerk to the proceedings will advise on the grounds for a finding of 'misconduct'. Care should be taken to avoid any confusion between 'negligence' and 'misconduct'.

A finding of 'serious professional malpractice' is appropriate if the malpractice is of sufficient seriousness to merit a period of suspension or permanent exclusion from membership of this Association with a consequential curtailment of opportunities to practise within this profession.

Bringing the profession into disrepute

A finding of 'bringing the profession into disrepute' signifies that the practitioner has acted in such an infamous or disgraceful way that the public's trust in the profession might reasonably be undermined if they were accurately informed about all the circumstances of the case.

A finding under this head must amount to 'disgraceful conduct in a professional respect'. This involves consideration of three elements:

1 Conduct that is regarded as 'disgraceful' need not amount to moral turpitude or be restricted to acts of serious immorality.
2 The conduct must have had some connection with a professional role in order to be considered as failing 'in a professional respect'. It ought not to be concerned with matters that can reasonably be viewed as solely personal and private.
3 Conduct 'in a professional respect' is not confined to conduct in pursuit of the profession in question.

For example, disgraceful conduct in the Police Disciplinary Code has been defined as: 'committed when a member (of a police force) acts in a disorderly manner or in any manner prejudicial to discipline or reasonably likely to bring discredit on the reputation of the (force) or of the (police service)'.

What is not disgraceful to an ordinary person may be disgraceful to a professional person.

Criminal convictions, findings in civil proceedings and hearings by other professional bodies

The Association may exercise its discretion to take disciplinary proceedings against a member who is convicted of a criminal offence or who has civil or professional findings against them that ought to have been declared on entry into membership or arising during membership.

Notice

References

Alberti, R.E. and Emmons, M.L. (1982) *Your Perfect Right: a Guide to Assertive Living*, 4th edn, Impact Publishers, San Luis, California.

Alexander, F.M. (1969) *Resurrection of the Body*, University Books, New York.

Andersen, H. and MacElveen-Hoen, P. (1988) Gay clients with AIDS: new challenges for hospice programs. *Hospice Journal: Physical, Psychosocial and Pastoral Care of the Dying*, 4, 2, 37–54.

Argyle, M. (1975) *The Psychology of Interpersonal Behaviour*, Penguin, Harmondsworth.

Ashton, J. and Seymour, H.J. (1988) *The New Public Health*, Open University Press, Milton Keynes.

BAC (British Association for Counselling) (1989a) *Invitation to Membership*, BAC, Rugby.

BAC (British Association for Counselling) (1989b) *Code of Ethics and Practice for Counselling Skills*, BAC, Rugby.

(BACP) British Association for Counselling and Psychotherapy (2004) *What is counselling?* http://www.bacp.co.uk/education/whatiscounselling.html

Ball, B. (1984) *Careers Counselling in Practice*, Falmer Press, London.

Bancroft, J. (1983) *Human Sexuality and its Problems*, Churchill Livingstone, Edinburgh.

Bandler, R. and Grinder, J. (1975) *The Structure of Magic, Volume I: a Book About Language and Therapy*, Science and Behavior Books, California.

Bandler, R. and Grinder, J. (1982) *Reframing: Neuro-Linguistic Programming and the Transformation of Meaning*, Real People Press, Moab, Utah.

Bannister, D. and Fransella, F. (1986) *Inquiring Man*, 2nd edn, Penguin, Harmondsworth.

Barnett, R. (1994) *The Limits of Competence*, SRHE and Open University Press, Buckingham.

Barrett-Lennard, G.T. (1981) The empathy cycle – refinement of a nuclear concept. *Journal of Counselling Psychology*, 28, 91–100.

Barrett-Lennard, G.T. (1993) The phases and focus of empathy. *British Journal of Medical Psychology*, 66, 3–14.

Beane, J. (1981) 'I'd rather be dead than gay: counselling gay men who are coming out.' *Personnel and Guidance Journal*, 60, 4, 222–6.

Beck, A., Rush, A., Shaw, B. and Emery, C. (1979) *Cognitive Therapy of Depression*, Wiley, Chichester.

Berger, C.R. (1992) Communicating under uncertainty. In: W.B. Gudykunst and Y.Y. Kim (eds) *Readings on Communicating with Strangers*, McGraw Hill, New York.

Berne, E. (1964) *Games People Play*, Penguin, Harmondsworth.

Berne, E. (1972) *What Do You Say After You Say Hello?*, Corgi, London.

Bodley, J.H. (2000) *Cultural Anthropology: Tribes, States, and the Global System*. 3rd edn, Mountain View, Mayfield, California.

Bor, R. (1991) The ABC of AIDS counselling. *Nursing Times*, 87, 1, 3–25.

Bor, R., Miller, R., Perry, L. *et al.* (1989) Strategies for counselling the 'worried well' in relation to AIDS. *Journal of the Royal Society of Medicine*, 23, 218–20.

Bor, R., Miller, R. and Salt, H. (1989) *Secrecy Related Problems in AIDS*. Routledge, London.

Bowen, D. (1990) *Shaking the Iron Universe*, Hodder and Stoughton, London.

Bowlby, J. (1975) *Separation*, Penguin, Harmondsworth.

Bradshaw, A. (1997) Teaching spiritual care to nurses: an alternative approach. *International Journal of Palliative Nursing*, 3, 1, 5–17.

Brandes, D. and Phillips, R. (1984) *The Gamester's Handbook*, Vol. 2, Hutchinson, London.

Brown, P. and Levinson, S. (1987) *Politeness: Some Universals in Language Usage*, Cambridge University Press, Cambridge.

Brown, R. (1986) *Social Psychology*, 3rd edn, Collier Macmillan, New York.

Buber, M. (1948) *Tales of Hasidism: the Later Masters*, Schocken, New York.

Buber, M. (1958) *I and Thou*, 2nd edn, Scribner, New York.

Buber, M. (1966) *The Knowledge of Man: a Philosophy of the Interhuman* (ed. M. Freidman) (trans. R.G. Smith), Harper and Row, New York.

Bugental, E.K. and Bugental, J.F.T. (1984) Dispiritedness: a new perspective on a familiar state. *Journal of Humanistic Psychology*, 24, 49–67.

Bugental, J.F.T. (1980) The far side of despair. *Journal of Humanistic Psychology*, 20, 49–68.

Burnard, P. (1985) *Learning Human Skills*, Heinemann, London.

Burnard, P. (1987) Self and peer assessment. *Senior Nurse*, 6, 5, 16–17.

Burnard, P. (1995) *Counselling Skills for Health Professionals*, 2nd edn, Chapman and Hall, London.

Burnard, P. (1996) *Acquiring Interpersonal Skills: a Handbook of Experiential Learning for Health Professionals*, 2nd edn, Stanley Thornes, Gloucester.

Burnard, P. (1997) *Effective Communication Skills for Health Professionals*, 2nd edn, Stanley Thornes, Gloucester.

Burnard, P. and Morrison, P. (1987) Nurses' perceptions of their interpersonal skills. *Nursing Times*, 82, 43, 59.

Burnard, P. and Naiyapatana, W. (2004) *Culture and Communication in Thai Nursing*, University of Wales College of Medicine, Cardiff.

Calnan, J. (1983) *Talking With Patients*, Heinemann, London.

Campbell, A. (1984a) *Paid to Care?*, SPCK, London.

Campbell, A. (1984b) *Moderated Love*, SPCK, London.

Carkuff, R.R. (1969) *Helping and Human Relations, Volume 1: Selection and Training*, Holt, Rinehart and Winston, New York.

Chapman, A.J. and Gale, A. (1982) *Psychology and People: A Tutorial Text*, British Psychological Society and Macmillan Press, London.

Claxton, G. (1984) *Live and Learn: an Introduction to the Psychology of Growth and Change in Everyday Life*, Harper and Row, London.

Clift, J.C. and Imrie, B.W. (1981) *Assessing Students, Appraising Teaching*, Croom Helm, London.

Coles, R. (1992) *The Spiritual Life of Children*, Harper Collins, London.

Coltart, N. (1993) *How to Survive as a Psychotherapist*, Sheldon Press, London.

Connor, S. and Kingman, S. (1989) *The Search for the Virus: the Scientific Discovery of AIDS and the Quest for a Cure*, Penguin, Harmondsworth.

Cook, A., Fischer, G., Jones, E. *et al.* (1988) *Preventing AIDS Among Substance Abusers: a Training Manual for Substance Abuse Treatment Counsellors*, The Center for AIDS and Substance Abuse Training, Falls Church, VA.

Cooper, P., Murray, L., Wilson, A. and Romanuik, H. (2003) Controlled trial of the short and long term effect of psychological treatment of post partum depression. *British Journal of Psychiatry*, 182, 412–19.

Cooper, R. and Cooper, N. (1991) *Culture Shock! Thailand*, Kuperard, London.

Cox, M. (1978) *Structuring the Therapeutic Process*, Pergamon Press, London.

Crompton, M. (1992) *Children and Counselling*, Edward Arnold, London.

Crowley, J. (1997) Education: therapeutic teaching and the education of student midwives, *British Journal of Midwifery*, 5, 3, 159–62.

Crystal, D. (1987) *The Cambridge Encyclopedia of Language*, Press Syndicate of the University of Cambridge, Cambridge.

Davies, D. (1987) *Counselling in Psychological Settings*, Open University Press, Buckingham.

Davis, H. and Fallowfield, L. (eds) (1991) *Counselling and Communication in Health Care*, Wiley, Chichester.

Dennis, H. (1991) Getting the message, *Nursing Standard*, 5, 17, 55–6.

Dewey, J. (1966) *Democracy and Education*, Free Press, London.

Dewey, J. (1971) *Experience and Education*, Collier Macmillan, London.

Dilley, J.W., Pies, C. and Helquist, M. (1989) *Face to Face: a Guide to AIDS Counselling*, AIDS Health Project, University of California, San Francisco, California.

DiMarzo, D. (1989) Double jeopardy: haemophilia and HIV disease. In: M. Donoghue, G. Stimson and K. Dolan, Sexual behaviour of injecting drug users and associated risks of HIV infection for non-injecting sexual partners. *AIDS Care*, 1, 51–8.

DiScenza, S., Nies, M. and Jordan, C. (1996) Effectiveness of counselling in the health promotion of HIV positive clients in the community. *Public Health Nursing*, 13, 3, 209–16.

Dodd, C.H. (1991) *Dynamics of Intercultural Communication*. 3rd edn, Brown, Dubuque.

Dorn, F.J. (ed.) (1986) *The Social Influence Process in Counselling and Psychotherapy*, Thomas, Springfield, Illinois.

Dryden, W., Charles-Edwards, D. and Woolfe, R. (eds) (1989) *Handbook of Counselling in Britain*, Routledge, London.

Dryden, W., Horton, I. and Mearns, D. (1995) *Issues in Professional Counsellor Training*, Cassell, London.

D'Zurilla, T.J. and Goldfried, M.R. (1971) Problem solving and behavior modification. *Journal of Abnormal Psychology*, 78, 107–26.

Egan, G. (1982) *The Skilled Helper*, 2nd edn, Brooks/Cole, Monterey, California.

Egan, G. (1990) *The Skilled Helper: a Systematic Approach to Effective Helping*, 4th edn, Brooks/Cole, Monterey, California.

Egan, G. (2002) *The Skilled Helper: a Problem-management and Opportunity-developing Approach to Helping*, 7th edn, Brooks/Cole, Monterey, California.

Ellis, A. (1962) *Reason and Emotion in Psychotherapy*, Lyle, Stuart, New Jersey.

Ellis, A. (1987) The evolution of rational-emotive therapy (RET) and cognitive behaviour therapy (CBT). In: J.K. Zeig (ed.) *The Evolution of Psychotherapy*, Brunner/Mazel, New York.

Ellis, A. and Dryden, W. (1987) *The Practice of Rational-emotive Therapy*, Springer, New York.

Ellis, R. and McClintock, A. (1994) *If You Take My Meaning: Theory into Practice in Human Communication*, 2nd edn, Edward Arnold, London.

ENB (1982) *Syllabus of Training: Professional Register – Part 3: (Registered Mental Nurse)*, English and Welsh National Boards for Nursing, Midwifery and Health Visiting, London and Cardiff.

Epting, T.R. (1984) *Personal Construct Counselling and Psychotherapy*, Wiley, Chichester.

Erikson, E. (1959) *Identity and the Life Cycle*, International Universities Press, New York.

Ernst, S. and Goodison, L. (1981) *In Our Own Hands: a Book of Self-Help Therapy*, The Women's Press, London.

Fairburn, C.G., Dickerson, M.G. and Greenwood, J. (1983) *Sexual Problems and their Management*, Churchill Livingstone, Edinburgh.

Faltz, B.G. (1989) Strategies for working with substance abusing clients. In: J.W. Dilley, C. Pies and M. Helquist *Face to Face: a Guide to AIDS Counselling*, AIDS Health Project, University of California, San Francisco, California.

Farrelly, A. and Brandsma, J. (1974) *Provocative Therapy*, Meta, Cupertino, California.

Faulkner, A., Webb, P. and Maquire, P. (1991) Communication and counselling skills: educating health professionals working in cancer and palliative care. *Patient Education and Counselling*, 18, 1, 3–7.

Fay, A. (1976) *Making Things Better by Making Them Worse*, Hawthorne, New York.

Fay, A. (1986) Clinical notes on paradoxical therapy. *Psychotherapy: Theory, Research and Practice*, 18, 1, 14–22.

Feldenkrais, M. (1972) *Awareness Through Movement*, Harper and Row, New York.

Feltham, C. (1995) *What is Counselling?* Sage, London.

Feltham, C. and Dryden, W. (1993) *Dictionary of Counselling*, Whurr, London.

Ferguson, E. (1998) Once more – with feeling. *The Observer*, 30th August.

Fiedler, F.E. (1950) The concept of an ideal therapeutic relationship. *Journal of Consulting Psychology*, 14, 239–45.

Fordham, F. (1966) *An Introduction to Jung's Psychology*, Penguin, Harmondsworth.

Frankl, V.E. (1959) *Man's Search for Meaning*, Beacon Press, New York.

Frankl, V.E. (1960) Paradoxical intention: a logotherapeutic technique. *American Journal of Psychotherapy*, 14, 520–35.

Frankl, V.E. (1969) *The Will to Meaning*, World Publishing Co, New York.

Frankl, V.E. (1975) *The Unconscious God*, Simon and Schuster, New York.

Frederickson J. (2003) The eclipse of the person in psychoanalysis. In: R. Frie (ed.) *Understanding Experience: Psychotherapy and Postmodernism*, Routledge, London.

Frie, R. (ed.) (2003) *Understanding Experience: Psychotherapy and Postmodernism*, Routledge, London.

Fullilove, M.T. (1989) Ethnic minorities, HIV disease and the growing underclass. In: J.W. Dilley, C. Pies and M. Heliquist *Face to Face: a Guide to AIDS Counselling*, AIDS Health Project, University of California, San Francisco, California.

Gallia, K.S. (1996) Teaching spiritual care: beyond content. *Nursing Connections*, 9, 3, 29–35.

George, H. (1989) Counselling people with AIDS, their lovers, friends and relations. In: J. Green and A. McCreaner (eds) *Counselling in HIV Infection and AIDS*, Blackwell, London.

Gislason, J.S. (2004) *The Book of Existence and the Human Mind* http://www.alpha store.org/Merchant2/merchant.mvc?Screen=PROD&Store_Code=med& Product_Code=BOHEATM

Gostin, L.O. (1990) The AIDS Litigation Project: a national review of court and human rights commission decisions. Part II: Discrimination. *Journal of the American Medical Association*, 263, 2086–93.

Grant, A., Mills, J., Mulhern, R. and Short, N. (2004) *Cognitive Behavioural Therapy in Mental Health Care*, Sage, London.

Green, J. and Davey, T. (1992) Counselling with the 'worried well'. *Counselling Psychology Quarterly*, 5, 2, 213–20.

Gudykunst, W.B. and Kim, Y.Y. (eds) (1992) *Readings on Communicating with Strangers*, McGraw Hill, New York.

Hall, C. (1954) *A Primer of Freudian Psychology*, Mentor Books, New York.

Halmos, P. (1965) *The Faith of the Counsellors*, Constable, London.

Hammersley, D. (1995) *Counselling People on Prescribed Drugs*, Sage, London.

Hanvey, R.G. (1979) Cross-cultural awareness. In: E.C. Smith and L. Fiber Luce (eds) *Towards Internationalism*, Newbury House, Rowley, MA.

Harris, M. (1999) *Theories of Culture in Postmodern Times*, AltaMira Press, Walnut Creek, CA.

Harris, T. (1969) *I'm OK, You're OK*, Harper and Row, London.

Harrow, J. (2004) *Working with Models: Theories of Counseling*
http://www.draknet.com/proteus/models.htm

Harvey, P. (1990) *An Introduction to Buddhism: Teachings, History and Practices*, Cambridge University Press, Cambridge.

Haydn, H. (1965) Humanism in 1984. *The American Scholar*, 35, 12–27.

Hayward, J. (1975*) Informative: a Prescription Against Pain*, Royal College of Nursing, London.

Hein, K. (1989) Commentary on adolescent acquired immunodeficiency syndrome: the next wave of the human immunodeficiency virus epidemic? *Journal of Pediatrics*, 114, 144–9.

Hellweg, S.A., Samovar, L.A. and Skow, L. (1991) Cultural variations in negotiation styles. In: L.A. Samovar and M. Porter *Intercultural Communications: a Reader*, Wadsworth, Belmont, California.

Helman, C.G. (1990) *Culture, Health and Illness*, 2nd edn, Butterworth Heinemann, Oxford.

Henggeler, S.W., Melton, G.B. and Rodrigue, J.R. (1992) *Pediatric and Adolescent AIDS: Research Findings from the Social Sciences*, Sage, Newbury Park, California.

Herbert, J.T. (1996) Use of adventure-based counselling programs for persons with disabilities. *Journal of Rehabilitation*, 62, 4, 3–9.

Heron, J. (1970) *The Phenomenology of the Gaze*, Human Potential Research Project, University of Surrey, Guildford, Surrey.

Heron, J. (1973) *Experiential Training Techniques*, Human Potential Research Project, University of Surrey, Guildford, Surrey.

Heron, J. (1977a) *Catharsis in Human Development*, Human Potential Research Project, University of Surrey, Guildford, Surrey.

Heron, J. (1977b) *Behaviour Analysis in Education and Training*, Human Potential Research Project, University of Surrey, Guildford, Surrey.

Heron, J. (1978) *Co-Counselling Teacher's Manual*, Human Potential Research Project, University of Surrey, Guildford, Surrey.

Heron, J. (1981) Philosophical basis for a new paradigm. In: P. Reason and J. Rowan *Human Inquiry: a Sourcebook of New Paradigm Research*, Wiley, Chichester.

Heron, J. (1986) *Six Category Intervention Analysis*, 2nd edn, Human Potential Research Project, University of Surrey, Guildford, Surrey.

Heron, J. (1989) *Helping the Client*, Sage, London.

Hesse, H. (1927) *Steppenwolf*, Penguin, Harmondsworth.

Hesse, H. (1979) *My Belief*, Panther, St Albans.

Hobbs, T. (1992) Skills in communication and counselling. In: T. Hobbs (ed.) *Experiential Training: Practical Guidelines*, Routledge, London.

Hoffman, E. (1989) *Lost in Translation*, Dutton, New York.

Hofstede, G. (1994) *Culture and Organisations: Software of the Mind*, McGraw Hill, London.

Homans, G.C. (1961) *Social Behaviour in its Elementary Forms*, Harcourt Brace, New York.

Hopkins, G.M. (1953) *Poems and Prose* (ed. W.H. Gardner), Penguin, Harmondsworth.

Hopper, L., Jesson, A. and Macleod Clark, J. (1991) Progression to counselling. *Nursing Times*, 87, 8, 41–3.

Hopson, B. (1985) Adult life and career counselling. *British Journal of Guidance and Counselling*, 13, 1, 49–59.

Howard, A. (1990) Counselling PLC. *Counselling: The Journal of the British Association for Counselling*, 1, 15–16.

Howard, G.S., Nance, D.W. and Myers, P. (1987) *Adaptive Counselling and*

Therapy: a Systematic Approach to Selecting Effective Treatments, Jossey-Bass, San Francisco.

Howe, J. (1989) AIDS – the rights approach. *Professional Nurse*, 5, 3, 156–9.

Hurt, R.D., Dale, L.C., Fredrickson, P.A. *et al.* (1994) Nicotine patch therapy for smoking cessation combined with physician advice and nurse follow up: one-year outcome and percentage of nicotine replacement. *Journal of the American Medical Association*, 271, 8, 595–600.

Hurtig, W. and Fandrick, C. (1990) The nursing student and the psychiatric patient with AIDS: a case study. *Nurse Education Today*, 10, 2, 92–7.

Hutchinson Encyclopaedia (2000) Helicon Publishing, Oxford.

Jackins, H. (1965) *The Human Side of Human Beings*, Rational Island Publishers, Seattle, Washington.

Jackins, H. (1970) *Fundamentals of Co-counselling Manual*, Rational Island Publishers, Seattle, Washington.

Jackson, P.L. and Vessey, J.A. (1992) *Primary Care of the Child with a Chronic Condition*, Mosby Year Book, St Louis.

James, M. and Jongeward, D. (1971) *Born to Win: Transactional Analysis with Gestalt Experiments*, Addison-Wesley, Reading, Mass.

James, W. (1890) *The Principles of Psychology*, Henry Holt, New York.

Jerrett, M. and Evans, K. (1986) Children's pain vocabulary. *Journal of Advanced Nursing*, 11, 403–8.

Jourard, S. (1964) *The Transparent Self*, Van Nostrand, Princeton, New Jersey.

Jung, C.G. (1978) *Selected Writings*, (ed. A. Storr) Fontana, London.

Kagan, C., Evans, J. and Kay, B. (1986) *A Manual of Interpersonal Skills for Nurses: an Experiential Approach*, Harper and Row, London.

Kahn, R.L. and Cannell, C.F. (1957) *The Dynamics of Interviewing*, Wiley, New York.

Kalisch, B.J. (1971) Strategies for developing nurse empathy. *Nursing Outlook*, 19, 11, 714–17.

Kelly, G. (1955) *The Psychology of Personal Constructs*, Vols. 1 and 2, Norton, New York.

Kelly, G. (1963) The autobiography of a theory. In: D. Bannister and J.M.M. Mair (eds*) The Evaluation of Personal Construct Theory*, Academic Press, London.

King, M., Sibbald, B., Ward, E. *et al.* (2000) Randomised controlled trial of non-directive counselling, cognitive-behavioural therapy and usual generic practitioner care in the management of depression as well as mixed anxiety and depression in primary care. *Health Technology Assessment*, 4, 9.

Kluckhohn, C. (1969) *Mirror For Man: the Relation of Anthropology to Modern Life*, McGraw Hill, New York.

Kluckhohn, C., Murray, H.A. and Schiener, D.M. (eds) (1953) *Personality in Nature, Society and Culture*, Knopf, New York.

Kolb, D. (1984) *Experiential Learning*, Prentice Hall, Englewood Cliffs, New Jersey.

Kopp, S. (1974) *If You Meet the Buddha on the Road, Kill Him!: a Modern Pilgrimage Through Myth, Legend and Psychotherapy*, Sheldon Press, London.

Korzenny, F. (1991) Relevance and application of intercultural communication theory and research. In: L.A. Samovar and M. Porter *Intercultural Communications: a Reader*, Wadsworth, Belmont, California.

Lago, C. and Thompson, J. (1989) Counselling and race. In: W. Dryden, D. Charles-Edwards and R. Woolfe (eds) *Handbook of Counselling in Britain*, Routledge, London.

Laing, R.D. (1959) *The Divided Self*, Penguin, Harmondsworth.

Langer, N. (1997) Training for retirement counselling in a Master of Arts in social gerontology curriculum. *Gerontology and Geriatrics Education*, 18, 2, 87–95.

Langley, T. (1995) Training staff to provide a continence helpline. *Professional Nurse*, 11, 2, 121–4.

Lansdown, R. (1992) Coping with child death: a child's view. *Nursing*, 2, 43, 1263–6.

Lazarus, A.A. (2000) Towards better research on stressing and coping. *American Psychologist*, 55, 665–73.

Leininger, M. (1991) Nursing, health and culture. In: S.M. Dobson (1991) *Transcultural Nursing*, Scutari Press, London.

Leininger, L.S. and Earp, J.A.L. (1993) The effect of training staff in office-based smoking cessation. *Patient Education and Counselling*, 20, 1, 17–25.

Leukefeld, C.G. (1988) AIDS counselling and testing. *Health and Social Work*, 13, 3, 167–9.

Lewis, H. and Streitfield, H. (1971) *Growth Games*, Bantam Books, New York.

Licavoli, L. and Hahn, N.I. (1995) Dietetics goes into therapy: nutrition therapists replace rules with understanding. *Journal of the American Dietetic Association*, 95, 7, 751–2.

Linton, R. (1945) Present world conditions in cultural perspective. In: R. Linton (ed.) *The Science of Man in World Crisis* (pp. 201–21), Columbia University Press, New York.

Lourea, D.N. (1985) Psychosocial issues related to counselling bisexuals. *Journal of Homosexuality*, 11, 12, 52–62.

Lowen, A. (1967) *Betrayal of the Body*, Macmillan, New York.

Lowen, A. and Lowen, L. (1977) *The Way to Vibrant Health: a Manual of Bioenergetic Exercises*, Harper and Row, New York.

Luft, J. (1969) *Of Human Interaction: the Johari Model*, Mayfield, Palo Alto, California.

MacCaffrey, E.A. (1987) Counselling AIDS patients: a unique approach by Shanti therapists. *AIDS Patient Care*, 1, 2, 26–7.

Macleod Clark, J., Hopper, L. and Jesson, A. (1991) Progression to counselling. *Nursing Times*, 87, 8, 41–3.

Macquarrie, J. (1973) *Existentialism*, Penguin, Harmondsworth.

Maguire, P. and Faulkner, A. (1988) Improving the counselling skills of doctors and nurses in cancer care. *British Medical Journal*, 297, 847–9.

Malinowski, B. (1922) *Argonauts of the Western Pacific: an Account of Native Enterprise and Adventure in the Archipelago of Melanesian New Guinea*, Routledge, London.

Malinowski, B. (1923) The problem of meaning in primitive languages. In: C.K. Ogden and I.A. Richards (eds) *The Meaning of Meaning: a Study of the Influence of Language Upon Thought and the Science of Symbolism*, Routledge & Kegan Paul, London.

Marriage Guidance Council (1983) *Aims, Beliefs and Organisation*, The National Marriage Guidance Council, Rugby, Warwickshire.

Masson, J. (1990) *Against Therapy*, Fontana, London.

Masson, J. (1992) *Final Analysis: the Making and Unmaking of a Psychoanalyst*, Fontana, London.

May, R. (1983) *The Discovery of Being*, Norton, New York.

Mayeroff, M. (1972) *On Caring*, Harper and Row, New York.

McClain, M. and Mandell, F. (1994) Sudden infant death syndrome: the nurse counselor's reponse to bereavement counselling. *Journal of Community Health Nursing*, 11, 3, 177–86.

McCreaner, A. (1989) Pre-test counselling. In: J. Green and A. McCreaner (eds) *Counselling in HIV Infection and AIDS*, Blackwell, London.

McGough, K.N. (1990) Assessing social support for people with AIDS. *Oncology Nursing Forum*, 17, 1, 31–5.

McLaren, M.C. (1998) *Interpreting Cultural Differences: the Challenge of Intercultural Communication*, Peter Francis, Norfolk.

McLeod, J. (1993) *Introduction to Counselling*, Open University Press, Buckingham.

McLeod, J. (1998) *An Introduction to Counselling*, 2nd edn, Open University Press, Buckingham.

Mehrabian, D. (1971) *Silent Messages*, Wadsworth, Belmont, California.

Miller, C. (1990) *The AIDS Handbook*, Penguin, Harmondsworth.

Miller, D. (1987) *Living With AIDS and HIV*, Macmillan, London.

Miller, G. and Sunnafrank, M. (1982) All is for one but one is not for all: a conceptual perspective on interpersonal communication. In: F. Dance (ed.) *Human Communication Theory*, Harper and Row, New York.

Miller, R. and Bor, R. (1990) Counselling for HIV screening in women. In: J. Studd (ed.) *Progress in Obstetrics and Gynaecology*, Churchill Livingstone, Edinburgh.

Miller, R., Goldman, E., Bor, R. *et al.* (1989) Counselling children and adults about AIDS/HIV. *Counselling Psychology Quarterly*, 2, 65–72.

Morris, D. (1978) *Manwatching: a Field Guide to Human Behaviour*, Triad/Panther, St Albans.

Morrison, P. and Burnard, P. (1997) *Caring and Communicating: the Interpersonal Relationship in Nursing*, 2nd edn, Macmillan, Basingstoke.

Moskowitz, E. and Jennings, B. (1996) Public health policy forum. Directive counselling on long-acting contraception. *American Journal of Public Health*, 86, 6, 787–90.

Mullins, J., Roessler, R., Schriner, K., Brown, P. and Bellini, J. (1997) Improving employment outcomes through quality rehabilitation. *Journal of Rehabilitation*, 63, 4, 21–31.

Munro, A., Manthei, B. and Small, J. (1989) *Counselling: Skills of Problem Solving*, Routledge, London.

Murgatroyd, S. (1986) *Counselling and Helping*, British Psychological Society and Methuen, London.

Murgatroyd, S. and Woolfe, R. (1982) *Coping with Crisis: Understanding and Helping Persons in Need*, Harper and Row, London.

Murphy, G. and Kovach, J.K. (1972) *Historical Introduction to Modern Psychology*, 6th edn, Routledge & Kegan Paul, London.

Myerscough, P.R. (1989) *Talking With Patients*, Oxford Medical Publications, Oxford.

Nelson-Jones, R. (1995) *The Theory and Practice of Counselling*, Cassell, London.

Nelson-Jones, R. (2002) *Theory and Practice of Counselling and Therapy*, 3rd edn, Continuum, London.

Nemetz Robinson, G. (1985) *Crosscultural Understanding: Processes and Approaches for Foreign Language, English as a Second Language and Bilingual Educators*, Pergamon, London.

O'Connor, F. (1998) Good country people. In: R. Ford (ed.) *The Granta Book of the American Short Story*, Granta, London.

O'Driscoll, M. (1997) Let's talk about sex: providing both sex education and sexual health education to young people. *Nursing Times*, 93, 49, 34–5.

Off Pink Collective (1988) *Bisexual Lives*, Off Pink Collective, London.

Ornstein, R.E. (1975) *The Psychology of Consciousness*, Penguin, Harmondsworth.

Pakta, F. (ed.) (1972) *Existential Thinkers and Thought*, Citadel Press, Secaucus, New Jersey.

Parkinson, F. (1993) *Post-trauma Stress*, Sheldon Press, London.

Patton, M.Q. (1982) *Practical Evaluation*, Sage, Beverly Hills, California.

Pearce, B. (1989) Counselling skills in the context of professional and organizational growth. In: W. Dryden, D. Charles-Edwards and R. Woolfe (eds) *Handbook of Counselling in Britain*, Routledge, London.

Perls, F. (1969) *Gestalt Therapy Verbatim*, Real People Press, Lafayette, California.

Perls, F., Hefferline, R.F. and Goodman, P. (1951) *Gestalt Therapy: Excitement and Growth in the Human Personality*, Penguin, Harmondsworth.

Pfeiffer, J.W. and Jones, J.E. (1974) *A Handbook of Structured Exercises for Human Relations Training*, University Associates, La Jolla, California.

Polyani, M. (1958) *Personal Knowledge*, University of Chicago Press, Chicago.

Pring, R. (1976) *Knowledge and Schooling*, Open Books, London.

Prosser, G. (1985) Communication as social interaction. In: A. Braithwaite and D. Rogers (eds) *Children Growing Up*, Open University Press, Milton Keynes.

Prusak, L. (2003) *Storytelling in Organisations* http://www.creatingthe21st century.org/Larry-IID-bonding.html

Reddy, M. (1985) *The Manager's Guide to Counselling at Work*, British Psychological Society/Methuen, London.

Redmond, M. (1998) *Wondering into Thai Culture*, Redmondian Insight Enterprises, Bangkok.

Reich, W. (1949) *Character Analysis*, Simon and Schuster, New York.

Riebel, L. (1984) A homeopathic model of psychotherapy. *Journal of Humanistic Psychology*, 24, 1, 9–48.

Rogers, C.R. (1951) *Client-centred Therapy*, Constable, London.

Rogers, C.R. (1957) The necessary and sufficient conditions of therapeutic personality change. *Journal of Consulting Psychology*, 21, 95–104.

Rogers, C.R. (1967) *On Becoming a Person: a Therapist's View of Psychotherapy*, Constable, London.

Rogers, C.R. (1983) *Freedom to Learn for the Eighties*, Merrill, Columbus, Ohio.

Rogers, C.R. (1985) Toward a more human science of the person. *Journal of Humanistic Psychology*, 25, 4, 7–24.

Rogers, C.R. and Dymond, R.F. (1978) *Psychotherapy and Personality Change*, University of Chicago Press, Chicago.

Rogers, C.R. and Stevens, B. (1967) *Person to Person: the Problem of Being Human*, Real People Press, Lafayette, California.

Rolf, I (1973) *Structural Integration*, Viking Press, New York.

Ross, L.A. (1996) Teaching spiritual care to nurses. *Nurse Education Today*, 16, 1, 38–43.

Rowe, D. (1987) Introduction. In J. Masson (ed.) *Against Therapy*, Fontana, London.

Ryle, G. (1949) *The Concept of Mind*, Peregrine, Harmondsworth.

Said, E. (1979) *Orientalism*, Random House, New York.

Sapir, E. (1948) Culture, language, genuine and spurious. In: D.G. Mandelbaum (ed.) *Edward Sapir: Culture, Language, and Personality: Selected Essays* (pp. 78–119), University of California Press, California.

Sartre, J-P. (1956) *Being and Nothingness*, Philosophical Library, New York.

Sartre, J-P. (1965) *Nausea*, Penguin, Harmondsworth.

Sartre, J-P. (1973) *Existentialism and Humanism*, Methuen, London.

Schulman, D. (1982) *Intervention in Human Services: a Guide to Skills and Knowledge*, 3rd edn, C.V. Mosby, St Louis, Missouri.

Searle, J.R. (1983) *Intentionality: an Essay in Philosophy of the Mind*, Cambridge University Press, Cambridge.

Sennott-Miller, L. and Kligman, E.W. (1992) Healthier lifestyles: how to motivate older patients to change. *Geriatrics*, 47, 12, 52–9.

Shaffer, J.B.P. (1978) *Humanistic Psychology*, Prentice Hall, Englewood Cliffs, New Jersey.

Shapiro, L. (1984) *The New Short-term Therapies for Children: a Guide for the Helping Professions and Parents*, Prentice-Hall, New Jersey.

Simon, S.B., Howe, L.W. and Kirschenbaum, H. (1978) *Values Clarification*: revised edition, A and W Visual Library, New York.

Sketchley, J. (1989) Counselling people affected by HIV and AIDS. In: W. Dryden, D. Charles-Edwards and R. Woolfe (eds) *Handbook of Counselling in Britain*, Routledge, London.

Smith, C.E., Haynes, K., Rebeck, S.L. *et al.* (1998) Patients as peer preceptors for orthopedic oncology rehabilitation patients. *Rehabilitation Nursing*, 23, 2, 78–83.

Smith, E.W.L. (ed.) (1976) *The Growing Edge of Gestalt Therapy*, Citadel Press, Secaucus, New Jersey.

Smith, M. (2003) The fears of the counsellors: a qualitative study. *British Journal of Guidance and Counselling*, 31, 2.

Stedeford, A. (1989) Counselling, death and bereavement. In: W. Dryden, D. Charles-Edwards and R. Woolfe (eds) *Handbook of Counselling in Britain*, Routledge, London.

Steil, L. (1991) Listening training: the key to success in today's organisations. In: D. Borisoff and M. Purdy (eds) *Listening in Everyday Life*, University of America Press, Maryland.

Stewart, V. and Stewart, A. (1981) *Business Applications of Repertory Grid*, McGraw Hill, London.

Stokes, P. (2003) Exploring the relationship between mentoring and counselling. *British Journal of Guidance and Counselling*, 31, 1, 26–38.

Storr, A. (ed.) (1983) *Jung: Selected Writings*, Fontana, London.

Street, E. (1989) Family counselling. In: W. Dryden, D. Charles-Edwards and R. Woolfe. (eds) *Handbook of Counselling in Britain*, Routledge, London.

Sumner, W.G. (1906) *Folkways*, Ginn, Boston.

Swain, J., Griffiths, C. and Heyman, B. (2003) Towards a social model approach to counselling disabled clients. *British Journal of Guidance and Counselling*, 31, 1, 137–52.

Tatar, M. and Bekerman, Z. (2002) The concept of culture in the contexts and practices of professional counselling: a constructivist perspective. *Counselling Psychology Quarterly*, 15, 4, 375–84.

Tennen, H., Rohrbaugh, M., Press, S. and White, L. (1981) Reactance theory and therapeutic paradox: a compliance-defiance model. *Psychotherapy: Theory, Research and Practice*, 18, 1, 14–22.

Theroux, P. (1977) *The Great Railway Bazaar*, Penguin, Harmondsworth.

Tillich, P. (1952) *The Courage to Be*, Yale University Press, New Haven, Connecticut.

Triandis, H.C. (1972) Collectivism v. individualism. In: W.B. Gudykunst and Y.Y. Kim (eds) *Readings on Communicating with Strangers*, McGraw Hill, New York.

Triandis, H.C. (1994) Cultural syndromes and emotion. In: S. Kitayama and H.R. Markus (eds) *Emotion and Culture: Empirical Studies of Mutual Influence*, American Psychological Association, Washington, DC.

Triandis, H.C., Brislin, R. and Hui, C.H. (1991) Cross-cultural training across the individualism–collectivism divide. In: P. Samovar and D. Porter *Individual communication: a reader*, 6th edn, Wadsworth, Belmont, CA

Truax, C.B. and Carkuff, R.R. (1967) *Towards Effective Counselling and Psychotherapy*, Aldine, Chicago.

Truell, R. (2001) The stresses of learning counseling: six recent graduates comment on their personal experience of learning counseling and what can be done to reduce harm. *Counselling Psychology Quarterly*, 14, 1, 67–89.

Tschudin, V. (1991) *Counselling Skills for Nurses*, Balliere Tindall, London.

Tyrrell, M. (2004) *Client Centred Therapy* http://www.uncommon-knowledge.co.uk/psychotherapy/client_therapy.html

Valdes, J.M. (1986) *Culture Bound: Readings for Writers*, St Martin's Press, New York.

Varner, I. and Beamer, L. (1995) *Intercultural Communication in the Global Workplace*, Irwin, Chicago.

Vonnegut, K. (1968) *Mother Night*, Cape, London.

Wallis, R. (1984) *Elementary Forms of the New Religious Life*, Routledge & Kegan Paul, London.

Wanguri, D.M. (1996) Diversity, equity and communicative openness. *Journal of Business Communication*, 33, 4, 443–57.

Watkins, J. (1978) *The Therapeutic Self*, Human Science Press, New York.

Watzlawick, P. (1984) *The Invented Reality: How Do We Know What We Know? Contributions to Constuctivism*, Norton, New York.

West, W. (2002) Some ethical dilemmas in counselling and counselling research. *British Journal of Guidance and Counselling*, 30, 3.

West, W. (2003) An introduction to the symposium on counselling and armed conflicts. *British Journal of Guidance and Counselling*, 31, 4.

Wheeler, D.D. and Janis, I.L. (1980) *A Practical Guide for Making Decisions*, Free Press, New York.

Wilkinson, J. and Canter, S. (1982) *Social Skills Training Manual: Assessement, Programme Design and Management of Training*, Wiley, Chichester.

Williams, D. (1997) *Communication Skills in Practice: a Practical Guide for Health Professionals*, Jessica Kingsley, London.

Wilson, C. (1955) *The Outsider*, Gollancz, London.

Winbolt, B. (1997) Just words away from harm: counselling and the breaking of bad news. *Therapy Weekly*, 23, 26, 6.

Woodruff, R.C. (2002) Pastoral counselling: an American perspective. *British Journal of Guidance and Counselling*, 30, 1.

Wright, J. (2002) Online counselling: learning from writing therapy. *British Journal of Guidance and Counselling*, 30, 3, 285–98.

Youll, J. and Wilson, K. (1996) A therapeutic approach to bereavement counselling. *Nursing Times*, 92, 16, 40–2.

INDEX

Essential Theory for Social Work Practice

Chris Beckett

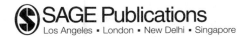

SAGE Publications
Los Angeles • London • New Delhi • Singapore

First published 2006

Reprinted 2006, 2007

SAGE Publications Ltd
1 Oliver's Yard
55 City Road
London EC1Y 1SP

SAGE Publications Inc.
2455 Teller Road
Thousand Oaks, California 91320

SAGE Publications India Pvt Ltd
B 1/I 1 Mohan Cooperative Industrial Area
Mathura Road
New Delhi 110 044

SAGE Publications Asia-Pacific Pte Ltd
33 Pekin Street #02-01
Far East Square
Singapore 048763

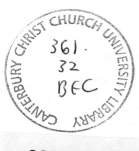

British Library Cataloguing in Publication data

A catalogue record for this book is available from the
British Library

ISBN 978-1-4129-0873-3
ISBN 978-1-4129-0874-0 (pbk)

Library of Congress Control Number: 2005931508

Typeset by C&M Digitals (P) Ltd., Chennai, India
Printed on paper from sustainable resources
Printed in Great Britain by The Alden Press, Oxford

Contents

About this book

This is an introductory text about social work practice and the kinds of ideas that inform it. It is primarily intended as a resource for social work students undertaking qualifying courses and for their teachers, both in an academic context and in the field.

Although it is an introductory text, this is not simply a tour of the existing literature. It represents a personal attempt on my part to think through what we mean by theory and practice in a social work context. I have not been afraid to do a little theorising of my own and I have tried to be true to my own belief in the importance of *realism* in social work discourse. In my view theory is only useful if it equips social workers to do a better job in the conditions that actually exist. There is no point in designing social work for an ideal world, for in an ideal world there would be no need of social workers.

As in my other introductory textbooks I have interspersed the text with a number of 'exercises'. These invite the reader to apply the ideas discussed to various problems, usually based on case scenarios. They are followed by some comments of my own, which anyone working on these exercises would be advised not to look at until they have gathered their own thoughts on the problem in question. These exercises could be used in various ways. They could be extracted and used for teaching purposes, for instance. Those readers (probably the majority) who don't want to pause and work on them as tasks should simply read through the exercises and my comments, because I refer to them in the subsequent text.

I have also introduced what I call 'practice notes' in text boxes (marked with ✕) in Parts II and III of this book. These provide some brief thoughts, in relation to the ideas and/or methods under discussion, about the skills that are required to apply them, the ethical considerations that they raise and the real world constraints that need to be taken into account.

Text-boxes marked with ↗ are asides from the main argument of the text are provided which add further information, suggest alternative angles or make connections with other ideas.

Finally, two brief notes on terminology.

He or she: I find it cumbersome to use 'he or she' all the time, so I have tended to say one or the other. In referring to social workers I tend to use 'she' simply because the majority of social workers are women.

Service users: As well as the term 'service user', I also use the more old-fashioned term 'client' for brevity and variety. I don't myself subscribe to the view that there is anything derogatory or demeaning about the word 'client', which is used without any negative connotations by lawyers, business people and others. I avoid the word 'user' on its own because 'user' in common parlance refers to a manipulative person who selfishly uses other people – I think this *is* a decidedly negative connotation.

Acknowledgements

I owe a large debt to my students, my present and former colleagues and my former clients for helping me to develop the thinking which I have presented in this book. Thanks to Bridget McKeigue for many entertaining discussions about social work rhetoric and social work reality. Thanks too to Vivienne Crawford and Sally Horsnell for ideas that I've included. And thanks to my dear wife Maggie who, among many other things, is a much better social worker than me.

Part I   THEORY AND PRACTICE

Introduction

Given the title of this book it may seem an odd thing to say, but in some ways I wish we did not use the phrase 'social work theory'. It seems to me to conjure up the idea of social work as a completely distinct activity with its own distinct theoretical framework to guide it. In fact social work consists of a rather diverse range of activities, most of which overlap with activities carried out by members of other professions and occupational groups, and the ideas which are used to guide these activities are likewise diverse and often originate from outside of social work itself.

But there is no doubt that social workers do need to be equipped with ideas about what their job is and how to do it. Social work can have such far reaching implications for people's lives that it is essential that it is done on a clearly thought-out basis.

Part I attempts to provide some foundations for the rest of the book by looking at what it is that social workers do (Chapter 1) and considering what they need to have in their toolkit in order to do it well (Chapter 2). Among the things that they need are the kinds of ideas that are normally described as 'theory'. Defining theory as 'a set of ideas or principles used to guide practice, which are sufficiently coherent that they could if necessary be made explicit in a form which was open to challenge', Chapter 3 will look at the nature of theory and how it relates to practice.

I What is social work?

Blue pills

You have been having dizzy spells. You go to a doctor and she writes you out a prescription with the words 'I really have no idea why, but today I just feel like prescribing *blue pills*!'

You would probably not feel very confident in the doctor's prescription. On the other hand suppose the doctor, after asking you some questions about your symptoms, said something like:

> I believe that the reason you are getting dizzy spells is that your body is short of iron. I think that what we need to do now is to build up the levels of iron in your blood. I suggest I give you a prescription now for some iron tablets to see if that will help and then you come back again in two weeks time.

In this case, I think you would feel more reassured, for the doctor is not simply offering a response to your problem, but indicating that she has a thought-out basis for doing so. After all, the reason why you went to your doctor in the first place was that you thought she might *know* something about why people have dizzy spells and what can be done about them.

The premise of this book is that social workers too should have a 'thought-out basis' for what they do. Social work is a very different kind of activity from medicine and I really do not wish to suggest by the above example that we should see social workers as being 'like doctors' (they are no more like doctors than they are, say, like teachers or policemen or housing officers) but one thing that social workers *do* have in common with doctors is that their actions may have enormous consequences for other people. If you are an elderly person who needs help with her care, or a child whose parents are mistreating her, or a person with schizophrenia who has violent delusions and may be a danger to others, then the decisions that social workers make could change the whole course of your life. Like a doctor's patients, the users of social work services are entitled to expect that those services are offered on as sound and solid a basis as is feasible. A social worker should know what her job is and how to carry it out.

This book will not offer you detailed prescriptions as to how to deal with particular situations such as these, but it will invite you to explore the nature of the social worker's role and invite you to consider what kind of thinking is – or ought to be – entailed in it.

To think about this we need first to consider what we mean by 'social work'.

Defining social work

Exercise 1.1

Try and define the following jobs in a way that includes the various tasks that they carry out, while clearly differentiating them from other occupations:

- Dentist
- Plumber
- Social worker

Comments

Dentist and plumber are pretty easy. You could probably come up with reasonable one-sentence definitions for each:

- *A person who deals with problems with teeth.*
- *A person who installs and repairs systems of water pipes.*

Social work is harder. You may well have thought of a better definition but the best I can come up with is something like:

- *Professional with special responsibility for people who are in some way vulnerable, excluded or disadvantaged in society, whose job is to promote the ability of people in these groups to meet their own needs and reach their potential.*

The problem with my definition of a social worker is that, even though it is already longer than my definitions of dentists and plumbers, it is still not specific enough. My definition could still include health visitors, psychiatric nurses, special needs teachers and probably a good many other groups too. Essentially the same problem exists, I think, with the definition of social work adopted by the International Federation of Social Workers (IFSW) in 2000:

> The social work profession promotes social change, problem solving in human relationships and the empowerment and liberation of people to enhance well-being. Utilising theories of human behaviour and social systems, social work intervenes at the points where people interact with their environments. Principles of human rights and social justice are fundamental to social work. (International Federation of Social Workers, 2000: www.ifsw.org)

I think you will agree that, if you didn't know already what social workers did, then the above definition would not help you very much. Imagine someone asking you at a party what you did for a living and you replying: 'I promote social change, problem-solving in human relationships and the empowerment and liberation of people to enhance well-being'. Would this enlighten them? (And wouldn't it sound rather pious?) Actually the above is only the beginning of the IFSW definition, which continues:

> Social work in its various forms addresses the multiple, complex transactions between people and their environments. Its mission is to enable all people to develop their full potential, enrich their lives, and prevent dysfunction. Professional social work is focused on problem solving and change. As such, social workers are change agents in society and in the lives of the individuals, families and communities they serve. Social work is an interrelated system of values, theory and practice.

And the IFSW definition then goes on to discuss values, theory and practice, giving the following account of 'practice':

> Social work interventions range from primarily person-focused psychosocial processes to involvement in social policy, planning and development. These include counselling, clinical social work, group work, social pedagogical work, and family treatment and therapy as well as efforts to help people obtain services and resources in the community. Interventions also include agency administration, community organisation and engaging in social and political action to impact social policy and economic development.

This is a long list of different kinds of intervention, but you will probably be able to think of forms of social work practice that it does not cover. Likewise, you will see that many, if not all, of the forms of practice listed are not exclusive to social work but are shared with other professions: *counselling, group work* and *administration* being three obvious examples.

The truth is that the term 'social work' is used to describe a rather diverse group of activities that have various things in common with one another, but also have a lot in common with activities carried out by other occupational groups. Although this is part of the reason why social work is so hard to define; it is only a part. The other reason is that, as Neil Thompson (2000: 12) puts it, 'social work is a political entity and so, of course, how it is defined, conceptualised and implemented is therefore a contested matter'. Social work is also hard to define, in other words, because there is *disagreement* about what it is or ought to be. Again, this is not unique to social work. The provision of health care, education and policing are also highly political and highly contested areas. And yet the basic functions of a doctor, a teacher or a policeman do not seem to be in dispute in the same way as those of a social worker. Social work is a profession the very *nature* of which is contested. Are social workers (many of whom are employed by the state) primarily agents of state control or are they allies of the socially excluded against the system? Is real social work, at its heart, akin to therapy and counselling, or is social work mainly about practical problem solving? Should social workers intervene more into private lives in order to protect vulnerable people, or do social workers already intervene far too much? Should social workers have more professional autonomy, or should they be subject to more scrutiny and control?

Some of these questions will re-emerge later in this book, but for the moment, let us consider the many different activities that are lumped together under the heading of 'social work'.

The diversity of social work

Social work practice is extremely diverse in a number of ways. First of all, and most obviously, social workers deal with a very diverse range of service users. There are social workers who specialise in working with children and families, young offenders, and elderly people, and with adults or children who have physical disabilities, learning disabilities or mental health problems. There are social workers who specialise in working with sexual offenders, people with drinking or drug problems, homeless people, migrants, transsexuals, people in hospital and their families, people with HIV, military personnel ... and many other groups, in various combinations. There are also social workers who are generalists. In the UK, following the Seebohm reforms of the 1970s, which brought together the various different 'welfare' departments of local authorities into generic social service departments, there was a period during which many social workers offered a generic service based on geographical area rather than client group specialisation. In recent years, the trend in Britain has been in the other direction, towards increasingly narrow specialisms. Social workers in the children and families field, for instance, may be subdivided into subgroups such as: 'intake' workers, who only carry out initial assessments; long-term workers, who deal with cases which are thought to require some input over a long period of time; and looked-after children (LAC) workers who specialise in working with children and young people in public care.

Another way in which social workers differ from one or another is in the nature of the organisations that they work for. Many social workers are employed by the state and perform functions defined by laws and government regulations. But many work for voluntary organisations of one kind or another, and some for private companies or on a self-employed basis. Increasingly, in the UK, social workers operate within consortia, trusts or interagency teams, which bring together several different agencies and involve working closely alongside other professionals. Another trend in the UK has been for increasing numbers of social workers to be employed by private employment agencies, which then sell on their services to the public sector.

Social workers also differ in the kind of 'setting' that they work in. Many social workers work in fieldwork settings where they are based in an office and visit people in their own homes, or in clinical settings where service users normally come to see them. Some are attached to non-social work agencies or are based in institutions such as hospitals. Many social workers work in residential settings providing 24-hour care for service users, or in day centres of various kinds. Within these settings social workers may also work with individuals, with groups, with families or with communities. Trevithick (2000: 17) uses the term *practice approaches* to describe these different levels of working.

Perhaps the most profound way in which social work differs between one context and another lies in the different *roles* they play. Some social workers are primarily involved in sorting out practical care arrangements, for instance, while others carry out a role that is more akin to that of a counsellor or therapist. Some work with people who voluntarily seek out their services, others work with people who may have no desire at all to have a social worker in their lives, but are forced by the law to do so. A good many social workers do not normally deal directly with service users at all but are involved in developing or maintaining services which others will draw upon.

Actually few social workers perform just one single function. Even within a single job description, most carry out various combinations of different roles. A social worker in the mental health field for instance may move from working on practical problems such as housing or finance, to offering a form of counselling, to (at least in the UK) making decisions about whether or not a particular service user should be detained compulsorily in a mental hospital. These roles sometimes sit together uneasily, sometimes complement each other well.

Social work's many roles

A very basic way of looking at the variety of activities that social workers become involved in, would be to look at the actual tasks they perform. Thus, in the course of an average day, a field social worker, for example, may be involved in:

- interviewing service users;
- recording interviews;
- travelling;
- completing assessment forms or reports;
- meeting with other professionals;
- making telephone calls to other professionals.

However, looking at social work in terms of these tasks actually tells us very little about what social workers are actually *doing* for those on the receiving end of their services. A social worker may interview service users for a whole variety of reasons, from helping them to come to terms with past events, to collecting information that will be used to determine their eligibility for a service and to determining whether they can safely be entrusted with the care of a child. So to understand the job a social worker is doing in a particular situation we need to look at what the interview is intended to achieve – and how, and why – and at what it in fact *does* achieve. If you ask a social worker what she has been doing and she replies 'interviewing a client' or 'recording', what she is describing is a sort of

Figure 1.1   Roles played by social workers

```
┌─────────────────────────────────────────────────┐
│                  Advocacy roles                   │
│                                                   │
│   Direct advocate                                 │
│   Indirect advocate                               │
├─────────────────────────────────────────────────┤
│             Direct change agent roles             │
│                                                   │
│   Counsellor/therapist                            │
│   Mediator                                        │
│   Educator                                        │
│   Catalyst                                        │
├─────────────────────────────────────────────────┤
│                  Executive roles                  │
│                                                   │
│   Almoner                                         │
│   Care Manager                                    │
│   Responsibility holder                           │
│   Control agent                                   │
│   Co-ordinator                                    │
│   Service developer                               │
└─────────────────────────────────────────────────┘
```

container or box. What is interesting and important is what is *inside* the box: what the interview is for and how it was done; what the recording was for and how it was done.

If the social worker is herself not clear what the purpose of an interview is (or for that matter, what the purpose is of a piece of recording, or of assessment forms, or of meetings with other professionals) then the piece of work in question is rather unlikely to achieve anything useful. It is also usually unlikely to be useful if the *service user* doesn't understand what is going on – it is certainly very disempowering for service users if the social worker knows what is happening but they do not. In my experience, much bad practice results simply from lack of clarity about what role a social worker ought to be playing. Clarity about what role or function you are performing – or should be performing – in any given situation, is a necessary precursor to good practice. So it is worth thinking about the nature of those roles.

My suggestion is that the roles that social workers perform can be divided into three broad groups: *advocacy* roles, *direct change agent* roles and *executive* roles. I illustrate this in Figure 1.1 where I have further subdivided the advocacy role into *direct* and *indirect advocacy*, the direct change agent role into *counsellor/therapist, mediator, educator* and *catalyst* and the executive role into *almoner, care manager, responsibility holder, control agent, co-ordinator* and *service developer*. I will now look at these roles in more detail.

Advocacy roles

A social worker is acting as an advocate when she helps give a service user a voice, either by speaking on behalf of the service user or by helping the service user to speak for him or herself. This is an important facet of the role of a social worker in most contexts, though it is not unique to social work by any means. Many other professionals are also involved in advocacy, and some people are employed specifically as advocates. I will not go into this any further here because this role will be explored later on in Chapter 8, but in Figure 1.1. I have subdivided advocacy roles into *direct advocacy* (that is speaking on behalf of the service user) and *indirect advocacy* (that is helping service users to advocate on their own behalf).

Direct change agent roles

I will use the term 'direct change agent' to refer to the professional use of self, through some form of structured conversation or interaction with individual service users or groups of service users, as a facilitator of change. All social work involves some use of self as a communicator, listener, negotiator and supporter. Many social workers would see themselves as performing a somewhat more specific role than this, akin to the work of a professional counsellor or therapist. Some social workers (for example, those attached to Child and Adolescent Mental Health clinics) perform a quite specific therapeutic or counselling role, for example, by acting as a systemic family therapist. Many other social workers incorporate at least some therapeutic and counselling techniques into their interactions with service users.

This is probably the role that is most 'theorised' in books about social work. Doubtless this is partly because ready-made theory lies to hand in the literature on counselling, psychotherapy, clinical psychology and so on, but many would also see this role as the essential core of social work itself, even though it is not a role which is unique to social work. It is not uncommon to hear practitioners who do not have time to work in this way complaining that they don't get to do 'real social work' any more:

> ... there is an embracing perception that all administrative regulation detracts from the 'real' work of visiting consumers .... In the area office, administrative work is perceived as an intrusion and higher management the culprits of this diversion from 'real' work. (Pithouse, 1998: 18)

Part II will look at 'ideas about change' and will draw on ideas from psychology and various schools of psychotherapy and counselling. I myself do not subscribe to the view a social worker who does not do much work as a direct change agent is somehow not a 'real' social worker. However real social work is certainly about *change* and whether a social worker is operating as a direct change agent, or whether she is making plans in which others will be the primary change agents, it is essential that she should have given thought to the question of change in human life and what helps or hinders it. That is why 'ideas about change' are the subject of Part II of this book.

Counselling and therapy are not the only models for a direct change agent role. Sometimes the direct change agent role may take the form of mediating between individuals in order to resolve conflict or to generate new solutions to problems. Sometimes it may be more about teaching new concepts and skills. So I have suggested *mediator* and *educator*, as alternative direct change agent roles, as well as *counsellor/therapist*. These roles do merge into each other somewhat, but I have also added *catalyst* to describe the kind of function that a social worker might perform in a group work or community work context. I will return to this in Chapter 6.

Executive roles

The executive roles are concerned with making things happen in a practical sense. They could actually also be called *indirect* change agent roles, since they are about bringing about change not as a result of a personal interaction, but by recruiting external resources of one kind or another, whether they be material resources, legal powers or the services of others.

In my opinion, it is the executive roles in particular that most clearly distinguish social work from other caring professions. A multi-professional group may jointly make plans for what to do in a given situation, but it will typically be the social worker in that group to whom falls the task of pulling things together, sorting out practical arrangements and co-ordinating the efforts of the other professionals. If there are matters to resolve that do not fall clearly within the brief of other professions then the social worker will typically be the professional to whom falls, by default, the task of resolving them (money, housing, tracing relatives, getting legal advice, arranging care). If one member of the multi-professional group is to be given the job of keeping the service user informed about the overall plan (even if different professionals separately talk to the service user about their own particular roles), then it will typically be the social worker who takes on that job. And, if the agreed plan requires that a court be asked to make an order, then the social worker will typically be the professional whose job it is to make this happen. I do not suggest that any of these jobs are exclusively done by social workers, but they are *characteristic* of social work and (at least in the UK) are quite often specifically assigned to social workers by law.

The following are some more specific roles that characteristically form part of the overall 'executive' role.

The almoner

Hospital almoners were one of the precursors in the UK of the modern profession of social work. The word almoner means 'distributor of alms'. Since distributing material resources is still one of the functions carried out by many social workers, it seems appropriate to give the historic name of 'almoner' to this particular function.

Under some circumstances social workers provide money and other material resources directly. Social workers are also often involved both in collecting information that is used to determine how resources should be allocated and in the decision-making process itself. Social workers carrying out assessments and making judgements about levels of need or risk are taking part in a system for allocating limited resources as fairly as possible to where they are most needed. Indeed informing such decisions is one of the main purposes served by social work assessments.

The role to which I have given the name of almoner is another role that, while quite characteristic of social work, is certainly not unique to it. Housing officers, benefits officers and indeed a whole range of public employees and welfare professionals are involved in similar kinds of activity.

The care manager

The care manager role involves assessing the need for, organising and overseeing a variety of services provided by workers other than the social worker herself. In the UK this term (American in origin) is most often used to describe the task undertaken by field social workers providing services to adults, whose primary job is typically to put together a 'package' of care to meet the social care needs of service users. However, it forms a major part of the role of many social workers in the children and families field also, who are often also in the business of organising 'packages' of services. Indeed, in the UK context many social workers bemoan the fact that this is largely what they do and that they have little or no time left for more direct work with service users.

Care management has not always been known by this name but it is a distinctive social work role that has been part of social work practice from the beginning. Some of the tasks that social workers undertake as care managers include: seeking the views of service users, carers and other professionals, completing assessment reports, negotiating for resources, liasing with other agencies including care providers and arranging reviews.

This role will be discussed in more detail in Chapter 9.

The responsibility holder

Both residential and field social workers are frequently involved in performing a variety of tasks – arranging doctor's appointments, taking service users from A to B, providing emotional support – that are analogous to those performed in families by parents or other carers for people who are unable to take full responsibility for themselves. Social workers may delegate many of these tasks to other carers such as foster parents or care assistants (leaving the social worker with a 'care manager' role in relation to them) but it often happens that a social worker (particularly, but not only, in the case of residential social workers) is the most appropriate person to perform them.

In respect of children in public care, but also in respect of some adults whose own decision-making capacity is limited (such as old people with dementia or adults with severe learning difficulties), social workers may have the task of protecting the best interests of clients in decision-making arenas such as courts (the role of the 'children's guardian' in the courts of England and Wales is a case in point), making plans on their behalf or, depending on their level of understanding, advising them in making their own plans. Other professionals too may of course have a hand in this but it is a characteristic social work function that is not performed to the same extent by any other professional group and which is sometimes specifically given to social workers by law. In the UK, for instance, it is only social work agencies who are given parental responsibility for children in state care under a care order (Children Act, 1989, s33(3)).

The control agent

The role I am calling 'control agent' is that which regulates and enforces boundaries of behaviour in order to protect vulnerable people either from being harmed themselves or from harming others. This function requires the use of legal powers if necessary, or otherwise the use of the implicit authority that comes from the possession of such powers. In England and Wales social workers with the elderly and social workers with children may go to court to obtain legal powers under, respectively, the National Assistance Act, 1948 and the Children Act, 1989. Approved Social Workers (ASWs) in England and Wales are given powers under the Mental Health Act, 1983, which are, in a sense, even greater, since they do not have to ask a court to make an order but may themselves sign applications under which people can be detained for assessment or compulsory treatment. This can only be done on the recommendation of medical practitioners but the final decision rests with the ASW alone. Social workers working with young offenders are another group with a 'control agent' function, as they are expected to monitor compliance with court orders and refer cases of non-compliance back to court.

The control agent role is not unique to social work. Indeed, if a 'control agent' role is associated with one professional group in particular, that group would surely not be social workers but the police and for that reason the 'control agent' role could also be described as 'policing', a term that Steven Walker and myself previously used (Walker and Beckett, 2003: 54). Allocation of this role is also culture specific: duties that are given to social workers in one country may be given in other countries to the police, court officials or doctors. The role given to social workers in Britain under the Mental Health Act, 1983, for instance, is not necessarily given to social workers in other countries. Nevertheless, the control agent role is part of social work internationally and the combination of a control agent role with other roles, such as the direct change agent role, is quite characteristic of social work.

In my view there is often a certain squeamishness in social work discourse about the control agent role. Books about social work have a tendency to mention it only briefly or in passing, and government guidance has a tendency to pass over it. For example, the *Framework for the Assessment of Children in Need and their Families* (Department of Health, 2000), which at time of writing is the government's principal guide to social work assessments in the children and families field in England and Wales, rightly places great emphasis on working in partnership with parents and children, but gives very little advice on situations in which social workers might feel that parents' views have to be overruled or parents' reports questioned. Yet I would hazard a guess that in the UK, half or more of all the work undertaken by children and families social workers is on cases where a control agent role is a central component of what they are doing.

Chapter 10 focuses in particular on the control agent role.

The co-ordinator

Social workers are often required to co-ordinate the activities of a group of professionals. This is different from care management, because the work of the professionals involved is not commissioned or controlled by the social worker concerned, but the social worker is required to facilitate communication and joint planning. A good example of this in the UK context is the 'key worker' within the child protection system, who, under the *Working Together* arrangements (Department of Health, 1999a) must always be a social worker. The key worker is:

responsible for making sure that the outline child protection plan is developed into a more detailed interagency plan ... [and] for acting as lead worker for the interagency work ... . S/he should co-ordinate the contribution of family members and other agencies to planning the actions that need to be taken, putting the child protection plan into effect and reviewing progress ... . (Department of Health, 1999a: 57)

In the mental health field in England and Wales a somewhat similar role is played by 'care co-ordinators' under the *Care Programme Approach*, though this role may be played by other professionals and not just social workers (Department of Health, 1999b). In fact social workers in all specialisms can find themselves playing a co-ordinating role, though it may not always be formalised in the way that it is in these two examples.

The service developer

Social workers are also involved in a variety of ways in *developing* or *maintaining* services as distinct to delivering them. Social workers in many specialisms will have a component of their job that is about service development as well as service delivery. An obvious example would be those social workers who specialise in recruiting, training and supporting foster-parents or adoptive parents, but really any social worker who moves into a supervisory or management position could be described as playing a service development role.

Combining roles

I argued above that it is the executive roles (and not, as is sometimes suggested, the direct change agent roles) that are actually the roles most distinctive to or characteristic of social work. Perhaps what is even *more* characteristic of social work is the way in which so many very different roles are combined within a single job. This can be very challenging when different roles seem to pull in different directions as Exercise 1.2 may help to illustrate.

Exercise 1.2

From your knowledge of social work, which of the above roles are carried out by social workers in the following contexts. Can you see any possible clashes between the roles that they play?

(1) Field social work in a multi-agency team set up to meet the care needs of adults with disabilities living at home.
(2) Social work for a voluntary organisation supporting adults with long-term mental health problems in group homes.
(3) Field social work in a children and families initial assessment team.
(4) Residential social work in a specialist unit, run as a private company, for adolescents with severe behaviour problems.
(5) Social worker employed by a local voluntary organisation, to set up a befriending and advocacy scheme for adults with learning disabilities.

(Continued)

(Continued)

Comments

I would suggest that the following are the roles that might predominate in each of these different contexts:

(1)   *Care manager, almoner, advocate, co-ordinator. The most obvious possible clash of roles here is between almoner and advocate. (Can you take responsibility for sharing out the agency's limited resources and yet at the same time be a whole-hearted advocate for your own client?)*
(2)   *Co-ordinator, advocate, responsibility holder, direct change agent.*
(3)   *Care manager, almoner (carries out assessments which are used to make decisions on resource allocation), control agent, co-ordinator. Also direct change agent, responsibility holder, advocate. There are a number of possible clashes of roles here, notably between the control agent role on the one hand and the advocate and direct change agent roles on the other. (Can a professional who can take you to court and seek an order to remove your children, also be your supporter?)*
(4)   *Responsibility holder, direct change agent, control agent (though in this context, this is arguably part of the responsibility holder role). Also advocate and co-ordinator.*
(5)   *Service developer, care manager, co-ordinator.*

A note on words

I want to conclude this chapter with two warnings about the use of language in social work. The first warning relates to the way that words are used differently in different places. In the above discussion, I have suggested that the jobs done by social workers can be divided up according to: (1) *specialism;* (2) *type of agency;* (3) *setting;* and (4) *roles.* I then suggested three different kinds of role, namely *advocacy, direct change agent* and *executive* – and a number of subdivisions of each.

Naturally, I hope you find these useful as an aid to your thinking but I must stress that this is my own personal classification. Writers on social work use many different terms and divide things up in many different ways. They may also use the same words with various different meanings. Trevithick (2000: 17) for instance, points out that the word 'method' is used in several quite distinct ways in the social work literature. Andrew Maynard and I (Beckett and Maynard, 2005: 158–9) have likewise observed that the words 'anti-oppressive' and 'anti-discriminatory', while used very frequently in social work texts, don't always mean the same thing, some writers making a clear distinction between the two, others using them almost interchangeably.

Variations in the way that language is used and ideas categorised may be frustrating, but it is an inevitable reflection of the 'contested and ambiguous nature' (Parton and O'Byrne, 2000: 37) of social work, and the fact that social work is very much a 'socially constructed' entity. What I mean by this is that, when we talk about social work, we are not describing something that exists 'out there' – such as butterflies or orchids – but something that we ourselves are inventing and reinventing. Scientists all over the world are able to broadly agree on how to categorise butterflies or orchids, albeit with a few fierce disputes here and there. But this level of agreement will never be reached in social work.

This means that when reading social work texts it is important to understand the way that the writer is using language. Likewise, when writing about social work you need to spell out the way in which you are using terms, rather than assuming that your reader will necessarily understand them in the way you mean.

More generally – and this is something that I will return to in Chapter 11 under the heading of 'rhetoric and reality' – the contested nature of social work means it is important to be *sceptical* about the language used in social work, just as you might be sceptical about the language used by a politician or by a lawyer in a courtroom. There may be another side to the story, and what things are called, or are supposed to be, doesn't necessarily reflect the way they actually are. Just because something is called a 'needs-led assessment' does not necessarily mean that it is led by needs. Just because a social worker describes herself as 'working in partnership' with a client, doesn't necessarily mean that is how a client sees it. And just because something is printed in a social work textbook such as this one, doesn't necessarily mean that it is necessarily an accurate reflection of the way things are.

Chapter summary

The following are the main headings within this chapter, along with a very brief summary of what was covered under each:

- **Blue pills:** Why social workers, like other professionals need a clear rationale for what they do.
- **Defining social work:** What do we mean by social work and why is it so hard to pin down?
- **The diversity of social work:** Different groups of service users, different contexts and settings, different 'roles'.
- **Social work's many roles:** More about the main 'roles' that social workers play.
- **Advocacy roles:** Getting the voice of a service user heard: direct and indirect advocacy.
- **Direct change agent roles:** Roles in which social workers use their interactions with service users as a means of bringing about or facilitating change: counsellor/therapist, mediator, educator and catalyst.
- **Executive roles:** Roles in which the social worker draws on other external resources as a means of bringing about or facilitating change: almoner, care manager, responsibility holder, control agent, co-ordinator, service developer.
- **Combining roles:** How different roles can clash with one another and pull us in different directions.
- **A note on words:** A warning that terminology is not used consistently in writing about social work and a discussion of the reasons for this. An additional warning to maintain a degree of scepticism about language used in social work.

The next chapter will look further at what a social worker needs in order to do the job properly, in particular at knowledge, skills and values.

2 | The social work toolkit

- What makes a good social worker?
- Knowledge, skills and values
- More on knowledge
  - Research findings
  - Policies and procedures
  - Theory
- More on skills
- More on values
- Realism

Having considered what social work consists of in Chapter 1, I want now to consider what a social worker needs in order to do a good job. A good place to start is therefore to think of an actual task that a social worker might be required to do, and consider what the social worker needs, to be able to do it well.

Exercise 2.1

Susan is a child of six, who has spent two years of her life – including the first three months – in various foster homes, due to the difficulties her mother Frances has had in coping as a parent. The difficulties were due to Frances' mental health problems and her ambivalent feelings towards Susan, who was the child of a rape. The current fostering episode has been going on for four months and Frances has come to a decision that she cannot care for Susan and that she wants to give her up for adoption.

(Continued)

(Continued)

The social worker required to follow through on this request is called Tom.
What would Susan and Frances want and need from Tom?

Comments

Placing older children in permanent families is difficult and carries a high risk of failure (research suggests that the chances of an adoption breakdown are in excess of 10 per cent for a child placed at Susan's age [PIU, 2000]). Susan has been experiencing changes of carer and ambivalence from her mother all her life so far. She is very unlikely to settle easily into an adoptive home. She will find it hard to trust or commit herself to new carers. She will find it hard to let go of her mother sufficiently much to make room in her heart for new carers. She may well behave in ways that are hurtful and difficult for her adopters.

Frances will of course also find the whole process extremely difficult. She may have further changes of heart. She may show her ambivalence again by simultaneously asking for Susan to be adopted and undermining the plan when it is actually happening.

Adopters will be hard to find for a child of this age, and yet it is important to find the right adopters – adopters who will be able to stay the course. There will be a lot of legal and procedural steps to go through. There will be questions about future contact between Susan and Frances. There will be other professionals with strong views about a very emotive case.

You may have come up with other ideas but here is a list, in random order, of ideas that occur to me about what Susan and Frances will need from Tom:

- *Ability to listen.*
- *Knowledge of the adoption process.*
- *Unflappability and an ability to inspire confidence.*
- *Firmness: an ability to stick to his guns.*
- *Ability to convey that he is not passing judgement and to convey what Carl Rogers (1967) called 'unconditional positive regard'.*
- *Ability to work with children.*
- *Able to cope with the distress of others in a sensitive way without being overwhelmed by it.*
- *Strong commitment to meeting the needs of children.*
- *Ability to communicate.*
- *Realism: a determination to build a plan that will work rather than a plan that looks good but will fall apart in practice.*
- *Knowledge of children's needs – and in particular knowledge of children's needs in this kind of situation and the effects on children of inconsistent parenting and parental rejection.*
- *Awareness of the needs of parents giving their children up for adoption.*
- *Some understanding of the effect of mental health problems.*
- *Understanding of the needs of adoptive parents.*
- *Understanding of the emotional dynamics of the adoption process.*
- *Understanding of the dynamics of child placement.*
- *Knowledge of techniques for working with children and helping them come to terms with loss and distressing experiences.*
- *Ability to 'grasp the nettle' and make difficult, perhaps unpopular decisions, where these are in Susan's best interests.*
- *Ability to network and recruit help.*

What makes a good social worker?

I am sure there are many other things that could have been added to the list above. The point I want to make now, though, is that the kinds of qualities that are needed by the social worker in Exercise 2.1 fall into several categories. Some of them are about *knowledge*: knowledge of the adoption system, knowledge of the effects of parenting on child development, understanding of the placement process, knowledge of techniques for working with children and so on. Some of them are about *skills*: ability to network and recruit help, ability to listen, ability to work with children, ability to inspire confidence and so on. Some again are about *values*: commitment to meeting the needs of children, non-judgemental attitude and so on.

You might feel that some of the points in my list are not about knowledge, skills *or* values, so much as about *personal qualities* (unflappability, for example). I suggest, though, that what we call personal qualities are really either skills or values that have become part of ourselves and that we bring to the job. 'Unflappability' is really a skill – the ability to remain calm in difficult situations – although it is true that people with very anxious temperaments may find it hard to acquire; rather in the same way that ball control in football is a skill, but some people have a natural aptitude for it and some do not.

Another point that you might make is that some of the most important things that Susan and Frances might need from Tom are not to do with him personally, but to do with the context in which he operates. Whatever his knowledge, skills and values, Susan and Frances would need him to be properly supervised and supported, to have adequate time, to have good administrative support and so on. At the end of this chapter, under the heading 'realism', I will come back to the issues raised by the real-world context in which social work is practiced, where resources are limited and practice is necessarily constrained as a result.

Knowledge, skills and values

For reasons that I will discuss shortly, it is important to be clear that knowledge, skills and values are three different things. The nature of the difference between them can be illustrated by analogy with driving a car. The *knowledge* component of driving is information. To drive a car you need to know what the steering wheel, brake and accelerator do. But anyone who has ever learnt to drive a car with a manual transmission will know that there is a vast difference between knowing what you are *supposed* to do when you change gear and operate the clutch and actually being *able* to do so in a fluent way. (Or consider learning to ride a bicycle, swim, play a musical instrument or touch type. In all these cases, knowing what is required is a vastly different thing from actually being able to do it.) The actual ability to do something is a *skill*, and it is something quite distinct from knowledge. In fact it is possible to develop a skill without possessing knowledge. Each of us has learnt a whole range of skills in early childhood, such as the ability to speak our native language, simply by trial and error without ever having been told how, and without ever having to learn the principles involved.

[handwritten margin note, left side top: Beckett uses the analogy of driving a car]

[handwritten margin note, left side bottom: Slide Heading]

Values are something else again, for you could possess all the knowledge and the skills required to drive a car and *still* be a bad driver, in the sense that you could drive dangerously or in a way that was inconsiderate to other road users. If someone is caught driving at twice the speed limit in a built up area, it is unlikely to be because they don't know what the accelerator does or because they can't find the brake, nor is it likely to be because they lack the necessary skills to use these controls. It is more likely to be because, at least at that particular moment, they chose to give priority to something other than sticking to the rules or considering the safety of themselves or others. It is about their values.

Knowledge can tell us what our choices are and what their consequences might be. Skills set limits on what choices are practicable. But when it comes to making the choice itself, this will be determined by values.

There are different kinds and levels of knowledge and skills, and there are different levels at which it is necessary to think about values. To return to my driving analogy, a degree of knowledge is required by those of us who use a car, but we do not really need to know how a car engine works. A different level of knowledge is required by those who actually repair cars. The ordinary driver also requires some skills, but not the same level of skills as are required in a rally driver or a police driver who is expected to engage in high-speed car chases as part of their job. In much the same way Tom, the social worker in Exercise 2.1, will need to apply knowledge and use skills far in excess of those that are normally needed in day to day life. His system of values will also need to be more highly developed in respect of his professional role in the sense that his job will face him with ethical dilemmas that he might never encounter in other contexts.

Life is always more complex than any theory or model. To divide the qualities required by a good social worker into knowledge, skills and values is somewhat rough-and-ready and you may be able to think of finer distinctions or identify difficult grey areas that cannot neatly be assigned to one or other of these categories. But I think it is a useful division all the same because it helps us to be clear what is at issue in any given situation. Confusion and misunderstanding can occur when we are not clear in a given situation whether we are talking about knowledge, skills or values.

One common source of confusion is between *knowledge* and *skills*. It is easy to forget that merely knowing something is not the same as being able to put it into practice. Knowing that Mrs X could do with some counselling is not the same thing as being a skilled counsellor. Knowing that the Y family are making a scapegoat of one of their children is a very far cry from having the skills needed to help the family move away from this destructive pattern of behaviour.

Another source of confusion is between *knowledge questions* and *value questions*. Knowing the degree of risk posed to Z in a given situation is one thing. Deciding what degree of risk is *acceptable* is quite another. The first is about knowledge; the second is about values.

Before looking at knowledge, skills and values separately you may like to consider the kinds of knowledge, skills and values that are needed in another area of social work.

Exercise 2.2

Alice Young is 88. A former librarian, she lives on her own in a detached house. She is physically rather frail and has on three recent occasions had falls and been unable to get up: on one occasion this was in the garden, on another she was in the hallway and was able to attract the attention of a passer-by by shouting, on another it was in the back of the house and it was sheer luck that her nephew, David, happened to be visiting the same day. David visits weekly. Alice has no other relatives in the area and she avoids contact with the neighbours. She can be quite aggressive if people approach her. The house is dirty and in a very poor state of repair. She has no central heating and lives most of the time in a downstairs room piled with books and papers where there is an electric fire. David has several times tried to persuade her to have some help in the home but she has always adamantly refused.

A neighbour has contacted the social services department, saying that Miss Young is not safe living on her own, because of the risk of further falls and also, it is suggested, a fire and health risk. The neighbour, Mrs Thomas, is a forceful woman who was once a magistrate and the headmistress of a local school. She insists that she represents the general opinion of the whole street when she says that Miss Young needs to be found a home where she will be with others and can be looked after. She considers that Miss Young is mentally confused and not capable of making judgements herself. She cites a retired doctor, a university professor and a solicitor as other neighbours who support her and would also like to be consulted. Mrs Thomas suggests that the role of the social services department is to kindly but firmly insist that Miss Young go into residential care.

The social worker dealing with this is Fatima. If you were Miss Young, what qualities would you want and need Fatima to have?

Comments

Powerful, forceful people such as Mrs Thomas can be quite hard to stand up to. A group of powerful people whose social position leads them to expect to have their own way can be really formidable. Therefore, among the qualities I think Fatima would need would be the ability to stick to her guns and stand up to pressure. This is partly a question of skill and partly a question of values. Fatima needs to be committed to the idea that her client is Alice Young and that it is Alice Young's best interests that she should be thinking about.

On the other hand, the neighbour's concerns are genuine and understandable and the neighbours need to be listened to and then helped to feel comfortable with whatever the outcome of the assessment is. So skills of empathic listening, tact, diplomacy and assertiveness are all necessary.

Such skills will also be necessary in dealing with Miss Young herself. This will be a difficult task as it sounds as if Miss Young may well be suspicious of — and resistant to — any sort of social work involvement. Fatima will need to be able to cope if Miss Young is aggressive and she will need to be able to find a way of conveying reassurance. She will also need to be able to enlist support from whatever network Miss Young has — her nephew and her GP, if no one else — and perhaps involve other professionals.

The qualities I have discussed so far are mainly to do with skills and values, but Fatima needs knowledge too. The neighbours suggest that Miss Young is 'mentally confused' and incapable of making her own decisions, but people often assume that elderly people are mentally confused

(Continued)

(Continued)

when in fact they are not, particularly if they are 'difficult' or eccentric. Although Fatima will need to obtain medical advice on Miss Young's mental state, she needs to have a good understanding herself of the effects and symptoms of different kinds of dementia (Alzheimer's disease and arterio-sclerotic illness are two of the commonest causes) and how to distinguish between these and, say, the effects of isolation or of personal eccentricity.

She will also need to have a good idea of what services are available – and what services her agency would be able to fund – so that she can discuss these knowledgeably with Miss Young. (The last thing Miss Young needs is to be offered services which turn out not to be available!)

In the event that Miss Young agreed to having some support at home, Fatima would also need the skills and knowledge that are required to be a good care manager, something we will come back to in Chapter 9 (always assuming that Fatima would continue to work with the case and would not have to pass it on to another worker.)

More on knowledge

Out of knowledge, skills and values, knowledge is the easiest to write about. In principle you can acquire knowledge from a book but in respect of skills and values, a book can only ever provide pointers and suggestions.

Earlier on in this chapter, when I used the analogy of driving a car to explain the difference between knowledge, skills and values, I suggested that the knowledge part of driving a car is knowing about the controls and how they work. Of course there is not much comparison between the fairly basic knowledge that is needed to drive a car and the range of knowledge that is available in social work. Social work is not a machine with a single, agreed set of controls. (No one disputes that the brake pedal is what you use to stop a car moving, but social workers can and do disagree about which approaches are helpful and which are not.) Nevertheless knowledge in social work, as in driving a car, consists of information which, when skilfully and ethically applied, allows us to do a competent job.

The following are some of the kinds of information, over and above local factual knowledge and life experience, that are available to us:

- Research findings
- Policies and procedures
- Theory

I will now briefly consider these in turn.

Research findings

We hear a lot at the moment about the importance of 'evidence-based' practice. What this means is practice the principles of which are derived from research. It would be naïve to suggest that 'research' represents a unified, uncontentious body of knowledge. The interpretation of research findings is often a matter of debate and the methodology is frequently open to question. It is often the case that research findings can be produced in support of several different – and even opposite – courses of action. Nevertheless, research findings represent a body of accumulated thought and knowledge, which can greatly expand and enhance the knowledge that we possess as the result of our own experience. This is for the following reasons. (In order to illustrate my points I will refer to one particular piece of research which I happen to be familiar with: the research study by Gibbons et al. [1995] on the long-term effects of physical abuse.)

(1) *It greatly increases the amount of information placed at our disposal in terms of quantity.* That is: it often draws on a much larger number of cases than we could have encountered in our own experience. Thus Gibbons et al. (1995) looked at *170 cases* of children who had been physically abused and compared them with another group of 170 children who had not been physically abused but were carefully matched with the abused group in other respects.

(2) *It greatly increases the amount of information placed at our disposal in terms of range.* Research can provide us with information about situations that we may ourselves never have encountered before or may offer us a perspective that we could not have obtained from our own experience. Gibbons et al. look at the effect of abuse 10 years on. Few social workers are in a position to systematically follow up on abuse cases after that period of time and none are in a position to make comparisons with a matched control group of non-abused children.

(3) *The more rigorous methodology used in formal research challenges assumptions and biases that inevitably creep in when we attempt to evaluate our own experience.* Human beings tend to look for evidence to confirm their pre-existing theories. Thus, if we believe that abuse has such-and-such an effect on child development we will tend to notice evidence that seems to confirm this, while unconsciously discounting evidence to the contrary. Good research methodology is designed to eliminate these kinds of unconscious biases. In the Gibbons et al. study, the researchers who compared the data collected from abused and non-abused children did so 'blind', which means that when rating a particular case they did not know which group it came from (a process analogous to the way that wine enthusiasts sometimes go in for 'blind tastings' so as not to be influenced by preconceptions based on reading the labels on the bottles.)

The kind of research that can be used to inform social work practice falls into a number of categories. It may provide information about the extent of a problem. It may provide pointers that can be used to identify situations where problems are more likely to occur (risk indicators). It may help with our understanding of a problem by exploring its causes or its effects. Research also commonly looks at outcomes of different types of intervention or evaluates different approaches. It can also give voice, in a systematic way, to the perspectives of people other than the professionals themselves – including, crucially, the perspectives of service users and carers – by collecting and publishing their views. And, in so far as researchers try to systemise or draw out their findings in the form of explanations or suggestions for action, the findings of research become a source of *theory*.

Policies and procedures

Policies and procedures exist at a number of levels. At the highest level there is the law of the land, which sets out the legal duties and responsibilities of social workers in various areas. Among the key pieces of legislation in England and Wales, for instance, are:

- The NHS and Community Care Act, 1990 (laid down the framework for the provision of personal care to adults).
- The Children Act, 1989 (provides the framework for social work with children and families).
- The Mental Health Act, 1983 (sets out the powers and duties of ASWs).

All three of these pieces of legislation represented major turning points in provision for these three client groups, although all have been modified or added to by subsequent legislation and will in due course be supplanted altogether. There are of course many other pieces of legislation which are relevant to social work in the UK, including the Human Rights Act, 1998, which incorporates the European Convention on Human Rights into British Law.

As well as legislation, social workers also need to be aware of government guidelines.

↗ Examples of government guidelines

In the field of services for older people, the British government provides a multi-agency assessment framework: *Single Assessment Process for Older People* (Department of Health, 2002).

In the children and family field, the key British government guidelines (at time of writing, though likely soon to be revised) are *Working Together to Safeguard Children* (Department of Health, 1999a), which sets out the framework of the interagency child protection system in England and Wales and the *Framework for the Assessment of Children in Need and their Families* (2000).

In addition to legislation and government guidance, employers also have specific policies and laid-down procedures that define how you are supposed to do your job and specify who within the organisation is responsible for what.

Familiarity with these documents is important because:

- If you don't follow prescribed guidelines you are likely to find that you are acting illegally and in breach of your contract with your employers.
- One of the things that service users need from you is that you 'know your way around the system'. You need to be able to give service users accurate information in response to questions like: How will their request for a service be dealt with? Who will make the decision? Why has such-and-such a meeting got to take place? Indeed, you need to be able to anticipate these questions and provide the information that they need without them having to keep asking for it. Giving service users accurate information about the system is a basic, but very important way

of empowering them. (You may well know yourself from personal experience how frustrating it can be dealing with large organisations where no one seems to be able to tell you what is going on.)

- Guidelines and procedures set basic standards and can help ensure consistency and clarity. Ignoring them can result in the opposite: absence of standards, inconsistency and confusion.

So knowledge of the relevant legislation, government guidance, and agency policies and procedures is an important part of social work knowledge. This is not to say that a social worker is required to believe that everything that is laid down in the form of guidelines and procedures is necessarily helpful. Any thoughtful social worker will find many things to disagree with in the rules she is expected to follow – sometimes laws and guidelines are impossible to implement in practice, are self-contradictory or have negative consequences – and I would suggest that one of the responsibilities of a conscientious social worker is to give honest, assertive feedback when this is the case. But ignorance of the procedural framework is not an acceptable option.

Theory

The third kind of knowledge is what can be loosely called *theory*. Since theory and its application to practice is the subject of the rest of this book, I will not discuss it further here except to say that, if research provides us with information on which to act and policies and procedures provide us with rules, theory provides us with ideas and models which we can use to make sense of the situations we find ourselves in and/or to help us shape our responses.

More on skills

Practice techniques can be learnt from books but the actual business of applying them is something that can only be learnt through *doing*. It is rather like learning to ride a bicycle. One could write down what you need to do to ride a bicycle – hold the handlebars, turn the pedals, adjust your body weight from side to side so as to maintain balance and so on – but the skill of balancing on a bicycle is one that everyone has to learn by trial and error. It is a matter of acquiring useful patterns of responses which, with repetition, become almost automatic.

In Parts II and III I will include, at intervals, what I will call '*practice notes*' (indicated by 🛠) in which I discuss the application of the various ideas and methods under discussion. In these notes I will include comments on 'skill requirements' in which I will refer to the kinds of skills that you would need to possess or develop in order to be able to make effective use of the ideas under discussion. Different people come to the job with differing levels of skill in specific areas. It is important to be aware of the level of your own strengths and weaknesses in the area of skills so that you (1) know what you need to work on and (2), as far as possible, work in ways that utilises your strengths. Exercise 2.3 invites you to look at your current skills.

Exercise 2.3

The following is a list of some of basic, non-specialist skills which are helpful in most areas of social work practice. (You will probably be able to think of many others.)

You may find it helpful to look through this list and divide the skills up under the following headings:

- *Confident now* – those skills which you are confident you possess.
- *Confident for the future* – those skills which you are not sure you possess now but which you feel you could acquire with practice.
- *Not confident* – those skills which you suspect you may always find difficult.

(1) Ability to stay calm in the face of anger and distress.
(2) Ability to say difficult things to people (that is, to give people messages which may distress them in a way that is both clear and honest and sensitive to their feelings).
(3) Competence at expressing yourself clearly in writing.
(4) Ability to stand up for what you believe is right in the face of pressure to change your mind.
(5) Analytical ability (that is, the ability to get to the 'nub' of a problem, ability to see a pattern).
(6) Ability to get on the right wavelength with people you are talking to (children, people with disabilities, people from different cultural or class backgrounds).
(7) Ability to think on your feet (that is, to respond appropriately to situations which you had not planned for in advance).
(8) Competence at multi-tasking (keeping track of several different jobs at the same time).
(9) Ability to avoid panic in stressful situations.
(10) Ability to prioritise (that is, to choose between competing demands on your time, perhaps at short notice).
(11) Ability to assimilate information quickly.
(12) Organisational skills.
(13) Ability to 'read' human situations.
(14) Ability to convey empathy.
(15) Ability to accept criticism.
(16) Ability to use authority.
(17) Ability to follow through plans to completion.
(18) Ability to challenge the behaviour of other people without being aggressive or judgemental.
(19) Ability to choose the right words when talking with people.
(20) Ability to operate effectively in meetings and in groups.
(21) Ability to enthuse and motivate others.
(22) Ability to admit to your limitations and seek the help of others.

Comments

I obviously cannot guess how you may have answered this but I have included in this list skills which, in my own case, would fall into each of the three categories.

(Continued)

(Continued)

> You may like to consider how the skills you are confident in and those you are unconfident in seem to group together. For instance, if you are less confident in (1), (5), (11) and (12) it looks as if the area you need to work on is to do with organising and presenting information. If you are less confident about (2), (4), (15), (16) and (18), then the area you are finding difficult would seem to be to do with assertiveness.
>
> It is important to get the perspective of others, though, because others may well see you as having skills which you yourself were not sure that you possessed. For a social worker, after all, it is often the viewpoint of others that is most important. (If your service users think you are good at conveying empathy then you are, even if you yourself doubt it. By the same token if your service users think you are not good at it, then you aren't, even if you thought you were.) This means that you should not necessarily always assume that you can accurately assess your own skills. But an awareness of areas which you find difficult and a willingness to be honest about this is important for good, reflective social work practice.

More on values

Some commentators have criticised social work education for being too preoccupied with values at the expense of knowledge and skills:

> Values in particular have come to occupy a strangely central position, with CCETSW [*Central Council for the Education and Training of Social Workers was the body responsible for the training of social workers in Britain until the advent of the GSCC*] appearing to believe that they can be substitute for knowledge and understanding (Jones, 1996: 190–1).

Values in themselves are certainly *not* enough. Good intentions are of little use, or even harmful, if you do not possess the skills or the knowledge to express those values in practical terms. Consider the case of the heart surgeon who was a very good man – and very well-versed in medical ethics – but had no understanding of anatomy and did not know how to use a scalpel.

But, although values may not be very useful without skills and knowledge to put them into practice, it is certainly *also* the case that knowledge and skills are not much use without values. This is because, as Downrie and Telfer (1980: 22) very concisely put it: 'No amount of knowledge of what is the case can ever establish for us what we ought to do about it'. Think about the case of Alice Young, the elderly woman in Exercise 2.2 whose neighbours wanted her put in a residential home for her own safety. It would be desirable to gather as much information as you could about the possible risks to Miss Young in her own home and about Miss Young's capacity to make decisions. But let us imagine for a moment that you had infinite knowledge and were able to calculate the *precise* risks to Miss Young of staying in her own home and the *precise* level of her cognitive functioning. This would be very helpful but it would still not actually answer the question for you as to whether Miss Young should be allowed to make her own decisions about the risks she takes. For the value questions remain:

- When is a person's right to make her own choices in life, including risky choices, outweighed by her right to be protected by others?
- How much does a person's thinking capacity have to be impaired to tip the balance in favour of protection?
- How great does the risk have to be to tip the balance in favour of protection?

I think that social workers sometimes get confused about this and imagine that, if only they gathered enough information these difficult decisions would somehow solve themselves as if they were purely technical problems.

In the '*practice notes*' in Parts II and III, I will summarise some of the issues about values which seem to be raised by the various ideas and techniques which I discuss, under the heading 'ethical considerations'. You will probably disagree with me about some of these, and will probably think of other important values questions which I have failed to mention.

Realism

In Chapter 1, I alerted you to the fact that, in social work (as in social policy more generally), rhetoric is often a very different thing from reality. What social work claims to do, or is asked to do, or feels it ought to do, is often quite different from what it does or can do in fact. It seems to me that, since social work has a real effect on the lives of real people, one of the ethical duties of a social worker is to attempt to deal with reality rather than with fantasy. In other words, social workers should spend their time doing things that will actually improve the lives of service users, rather than things whose main benefit is that they create illusions which make social workers themselves feel good, or their managers feel good or politicians look as if they are doing something, or ease the consciences of the general public. Andrew Maynard and I (Beckett and Maynard, 2005: 98) spoke of this principle as the 'duty of realism':

> As social workers we should not inflict interventions on service users which have a low chance of success or are likely to do more harm than good, in order to meet our own need to feel that we are 'doing something'. Nor should we pretend that the likely outcomes of our interventions are more positive than they really are in fact.

Part of the duty of realism is recognising the constraints that social workers operate under in terms of time, material resources, knowledge, skills, training and support. If you are provided with inadequate resources to do your job you can and should challenge this – realism is *not* about accepting things as they are without complaint; it is about refusing to pretend that things are better (or worse) than they actually are – but the fact remains that it is irresponsible to go ahead with a plan of action if the resources at your disposal mean that it will be impossible to carry the plan through, just as it would be irresponsible (for instance) for a doctor to carry out a surgical procedure if she lacked the appropriate equipment or expertise.

Because this principle is important, and not often enough discussed in the social work literature, I will include notes on 'real-world constraints' under the '*practice notes*'. I will also return to the theme of realism in a broader way in Chapter 11.

Chapter summary

This chapter has considered the various ingredients that go to make good social work practice. The topics covered have been:

- **What makes a good social worker?** The things that a service user would want and need from a social worker and suggested that these could be divided into knowledge, skills and values.
- **Knowledge, skills and values:** The difference between knowledge, skills and values and some confusions that can occur.
- **More on knowledge:** The kinds of knowledge available to social workers including *research findings, policies and procedures* and *theory*.
- **More on skills:** The skills involved in social work.
- **More on values:** The role of values in social work.
- **Realism:** Realism should be a basic principle in social work.

In the next chapter I will discuss what is meant by 'theory' in the context of social work, and how it relates to practice.

3 | What do we mean by 'theory'?

- The basis for action
- Practice and theory
- Assessment and intervention
- Thinking theoretically
- Thinking about intervention
- Eclecticism

In the previous chapter, I discussed what the social work 'toolkit' should consist of – what a social worker needs to do a good job – and I proposed that the components of that toolkit could, roughly speaking, be divided into 'knowledge', 'skills' and 'values'. 'Theory', I suggested, was one kind of knowledge. This chapter will explore what is meant by the word in the context of social work. To start to think about that, it may be helpful to consider an example of the kind of practical problem which social workers are asked to deal with.

Exercise 3.1

Candice Jones, a 20-year-old lone mother, has referred herself to a social work agency for help in managing her four-year old son Carl. She says that he is completely outside of her control and won't do anything she says. If she attempts to challenge him or discipline him, he begins to scream and shout and sometimes hits her or runs out and away down the road, where he is at risk from traffic. Candice says she has never hit him but she is exhausted and he is making her very angry and frustrated and she wants help before she does something stupid.

(Continued)

(Continued)

If you were asked to follow up on this referral, what further questions might you want to ask Candice or Carl? Write down a few. (Please note: I mean by this, questions which *you yourself* think would be useful to ask and not simply questions which you feel you might be required to ask under agency rules.)

Having written down this list, consider the following question in relation to each item on it: *Why* would it be helpful to know this?

Comments

Of course I don't know what questions you may have come up with, but I would guess that they may have included some of the following:

(1)   Is Carl suffering from a medical condition?
(2)   Has Carl suffered some kind of distressing event in his life?
(3)   Where is Carl's father? What is Carl's and Candice's relationship with him?
(4)   What is Candice's family background?
(5)   How does Carl get on at school?
(6)   Does Candice suffer from depression?
(7)   Have any professional agencies had any concerns about Carl or Candice or about Candice's care of Carl?
(8)   Does Candice have the support of friends and family?
(9)   What are Carl and Candice's living conditions and economic circumstances?
(10) Was Carl a wanted child?
(11) What were the circumstances of Carl's birth and how did Candice relate to him as a baby?
(12) When does Candice feel she copes well with Carl?
(13) When are Carl and Candice happiest together?

The list could go on and on of course, but for the present purposes the interesting thing is to consider why you chose the particular questions you did, because this will reveal your underlying theoretical ideas.

For instance, if you chose questions like (10) and (11), it suggests that you think that problems like these may be caused by poor attachment between mother and child from an early stage. If you chose questions like (1) or (2) this suggests that you think that Carl's problems may be caused by factors outside his relationship with his mother.

All of the questions from (1) to (11) are about exploring the history and circumstances of these two people, and if your questions were all of this kind, it suggests that you think you need to explore possible explanations for the problem in order to know how to respond to it (which is the thinking behind current UK government guidelines on assessment of families and children, see Department of Health [2000]), and/or that you think that it is likely to be helpful to Candice or Carl to talk about things that are difficult in their life. (Which of these do you think is the more important?)

If on the other hand your questions were more like (12) and (13), it would suggest that you feel it is more important to try and build on strengths than to get to the bottom of why a problem occurred in the first place.

My point is that, whether you are consciously guided by a theoretical framework or not, your choice of questions is shaped by theories.

The basis for action

In fact it would be impossible to know *what* to do in a situation like that described in Exercise 3.1 unless you had some sort of theory or theories about the nature of the problem and/or about what helps people who experience themselves as having problems. I do not mean by this that it is necessary in every case to be able to apply a theory with a name that comes out of a book. In many situations social workers rely on their own theories, which may be built up from experience, from discussion with other social workers and from many other sources apart from formal academic ones. It is not my intention to suggest that you need to have a formal academic theory to justify every action you perform. But I *do* suggest that every action you perform must be based on ideas about:

(1)   What are the core issues in this situation which I need to address?
(2)   What is likely to be helpful and why?

I would add to this that as a professional person you should be able to state what those ideas are ('I am asking questions about how Candice found Carl as a baby because I believe difficulties in establishing a good relationship at an early stage often lie behind problems of this kind').

What is more, in the case of more major decisions, you should also be able to explain the *basis* of your thinking ('My reason for believing this is that …' – and here you might refer to research findings, or to your own professional experience, or to advice you received from someone with special expertise in this area). Practice should be thought-out – and you should be able to explain your thinking. As a general rule practice that is not thought-out will tend to be bad practice. Your clients are not likely to experience you as helpful, for instance, if you ask them a lot of questions without any idea why you are doing so.

Practice and theory

The word 'practice' as used in a professional context means, in essence, 'how you go about doing your job'. The *New Oxford Dictionary of English (NODE)* (2001) includes the following in its definition: 'The actual application or use of an idea, belief or method as opposed to theories about such application or use …', 'The customary, habitual, or expected procedure or way of doing something …', 'The carrying out or exercise of a profession …'.

The term 'theory' is harder to pin down and, as I commented in the introduction to this part of the book, is actually a little confusing because it is used in several different ways, as the following examples illustrate:

- Einstein's *theory* of relativity.
- Labelling *theory*.
- Attachment *theory*.
- 'Harriet says that John isn't interested in her, but my *theory* is that he is playing hard to get.'
- 'In *theory* this ought to work, but I don't know whether it will work in practice'.

The first three examples are instances of what I am going to call (following Sibeon, 1989) *formal* theories. I mean by this that they are systems of ideas which have been described in detail in published form. Einstein's theory is also a *scientific* theory. In the 'hard' sciences the word 'theory' is used in a very specific sense. It means not only a system of ideas, but a system of ideas which is *testable*. Einstein's theory can be tested by using it to make precise predictions about the way that physical objects will behave in certain situations and by seeing whether the predictions are accurate.

Labelling theory (Becker, 1996) and attachment theory (see Chapter 4) derive from the social sciences: the former from sociology; the latter from psychology. Theories in the social sciences such as these are also to some extent testable against the evidence, but their predictions rarely achieve anything like the same degree of precision as theories in the hard sciences, so that it is a much more debatable and contestable matter as to whether a theory is supported by the evidence or not. This is not because social scientists are less clever than physicists, but because the social sphere is vastly more complex than the physical one. For one thing there are far more variables to take into account. (Even the physical sciences cannot make precise predictions when there are many variables: we all know from experience, for instance, that science cannot be relied upon to offer precise predictions of the weather even only a single day ahead.) For another thing many of the phenomena under study in the social sciences are not directly observable (as are, say, planets) but are things that exist in the human mind and in human culture. As a result they are:

(1) Much harder to precisely define. Suppose, for instance, you were going to do a piece of research on 'aggressive behaviour' and wanted to compare your findings with other research on the same thing. How confident could you be that what you meant by 'aggressive behaviour' was precisely the same as what other researchers meant?

(2) Often contentious and debatable. For example, views differ on what constitutes 'child abuse', as public debate on smacking indicates.

(3) Themselves change over time and/or vary from one cultural context to another. For example, ideas about what precisely is meant by 'marriage' are not the same now as they were 100 years ago, and are not the same in the UK as they are in, say, Pakistan.

Since social work operates essentially in the psychological and social spheres, the kinds of formal theories that are available to us in social work have the same quality as theory in the social sciences generally: they are debatable and contestable. They are useful to make sense of things and to help us organise our thinking, but they rarely have the quality of precision that would remove any element of doubt or remove the possibility of argument. (And of course, as I pointed out in the previous chapter, even precise knowledge does not take away the difficult *value* questions that are involved in making decisions.)

What *formal* theories in the hard sciences and in the social sciences have in common is that they are sets of ideas, which help us to make sense of things. But this is true also of *informal* theories, theories that we come up with ourselves or that are part of 'common knowledge'. In my example above – 'Harriet says that John isn't interested in her, but my theory is that he is playing hard to get' – the speaker is offering an informal theory, a way of making sense of John's behaviour.

One confusion that is caused by the word 'theory' is that many people understand the word to mean something that resembles a scientific theory. In fact that is not really what is meant by theory in a social work context. It is almost never possible to be able to state with certainty what precisely caused a given situation or to be able to predict with certainty what will occur in the future. At the beginning of this book I used the example of a patient going to a doctor suffering with dizzy spells and the doctor forming the hypothesis that this was the result of iron deficiency and prescribing iron tablets. Medicine is far from being an exact science itself, of course, but social work is very much less so. In social work it is rarely possible to pinpoint the cause of a problem in that way and it is rarely possible to come up with such a straightforward remedy.

Another confusion, which I will come back to shortly, is caused by the idea that a theory must be, if not a scientific theory, then at any rate a *formal* theory to count. This too is a mistake. If you look at dictionary definitions of the word 'theory', they suggest a rather looser meaning. The *NODE* (2001) offers: 'A supposition or a system of ideas intended to explain something, especially one based on general principles independent of the thing to be explained …', 'A set of principles on which the practice of an activity is based …' and 'An idea used to account for a situation or justify a course of action …'.

Social workers are entitled to develop their own theories, as well us to use theories developed by other people, but this is not to say that any sort of rationalisation for a course of action is equally valid. For the purposes of this book, therefore, I am going to suggest a working definition of the word 'theory', which embraces both formal and informal theories but sets a certain minimum standard as to clarity and coherence. My definition is as follows:

> Theory: a set of ideas or principles used to guide practice, which are sufficiently coherent that they could if necessary be made explicit in a form which was open to challenge.

This definition includes two components. First, as per the dictionary definitions given earlier, it includes the idea of theory as being a set of ideas which are used to guide practice. But second, I have added the idea that the set of ideas should be possible to define with sufficient clarity that someone else could challenge them by offering objections or counter-arguments. 'I'm doing X because I have a hunch that it will work' *is not* a theory, because it isn't open to challenge: you can only either share or not share the hunch. On the other hand 'I'm doing X because I believe that the difficulty here is Y, and that X is likely to reduce this difficulty', *is* a theory in my terms, because two explicit statements are made to explain the choice of X as a course of action. These two statements are:

(1) 'the difficulty here is Y'; and
(2) 'X is likely to reduce this difficulty'.

Because they are made explicit, both of these statements are open to challenge, by which I mean that someone who did not agree could offer evidence to suggest that either that the difficulty was not Y, or that X is not necessarily helpful even when Y is the difficulty.

Assessment and intervention

Various distinctions can be made between different kinds of theory; over and above the formal versus informal distinction which I've already drawn. Sibeon (1989) proposed a three-part distinction between 'theories of what social work does', 'theories of how to do social work' and 'theories of the client world', each of which in turn can be subdivided into 'formal' and 'informal'. A reviewer who looked at an early outline of this book suggested that one important distinction that I needed to make was between theories the function of which is to *explain* things, and theories that are about how to bring about or facilitate change. Attachment theory, which I'll discuss in the next chapter, is, for instance, a good instance of an explanatory theory. In contrast, the body of ideas in the social work literature about 'empowerment' (to be discussed in Chapter 8) is an example of theory directed at how social work should be practised rather than at explaining the way things are. Explanatory theories are what we need at the stage of assessment, in order to decide (1) what information we need to collect and (2) how to interpret that information when we obtain it. Ideas about how to bring about change, conversely, are needed when we come to decide on how to 'intervene' (to use that slightly ugly word that is used in social work to refer to the things social workers actually *do* to make a difference.)

However, I see a difficulty in making a hard and fast distinction for two reasons. First, most explanatory theories are associated with specific approaches to intervention. For example, behaviourist psychology offers tools for understanding why people behave as they do but it also offers tools for changing the way that people behave – the latter having been developed in the helping professions into a number of techniques; including cognitive behavioural therapy. It would be unusual to use one set of theoretical assumptions as a tool for assessment and then use another completely different set for the purposes of planning an intervention. (In some psychotherapeutic approaches the assessment and the intervention may be almost the same thing.)

Second, even ideas about intervention such as 'empowerment' are built upon implicit ideas about human psychology and human society, which do in fact form a kind of explanatory theory, even if it is never actually set out as such. In the case of 'empowerment' this theory could be summarised in terms something like this:

> The difficulties experienced by many people are the result of their oppression by society, which in turn results in making them feel powerless to influence events or to resolve things for themselves. Conventional 'help' – for example, medication prescribed by a psychiatrist – may simply confirm their powerlessness and the powerfulness of others. Real change requires that the oppressed take power for themselves or become more aware of the power which they do in fact already possess.

In fact a 'theory' of intervention that was not embedded, either explicitly or implicitly, in some sort of explanatory theory, would not merit the name of 'theory', even on my own relatively loose definition of the term given earlier, for it would be on a par with the thinking of the fictional doctor in the first chapter of this book, who prescribed blue pills just because she felt like it. It just happens that some theoretical approaches place more emphasis on looking in detail for explanations, while others don't.

In the same way an 'assessment' that is not informed by any kind of theory would merely be a random collection of facts and observations. You need to have some sort of theory, some kind of idea as to what the purpose of the assessment is and what needs to be thought about in order to achieve that, even just to determine what kind of kind of things to discuss in an assessment. (Is a person's early childhood relevant? The circumstances of their birth? Their favourite colour? The names and occupations of their grandparents? The kind of neighbourhood they live in? Their sex life? Their birth sign?) And you need more theory to make sense of that discussion and to know how to use it.

Thinking theoretically

The list of questions below was given to me by a social worker who used them in a real piece of work. This social worker was responsible for the case of a child who had been brought into public care because, in the view of the authorities, she was seriously neglected by her mother, who was unable to attend to her child's needs when they conflicted with her own. However, after a period of time the child's mother said that things had now changed and that she wanted the decision to be reconsidered. The social worker sat down with her supervisor to think about how to go about exploring with the mother whether or not she really had made changes that were likely to last. She came up with the following set of questions to ask the mother:

Parental interview re change

(1)   What is your understanding of why the children were taken into care?
(2)   What is your understanding of the impact of this on the children?
(3)   If the children returned what support have you now got?
(4)   What were the concerns highlighted in the parenting assessment and what are your thoughts on specific points?
(5)   What do you feel has changed since the children left you?
(6)   What changes do you feel that you would need to make?
(7)   What has happened to make these changes possible?
(8)   How would you describe your relationships within the family?
(9)   How do you now see your relationship with Social Services?

(Questions devised by Sally Horsnell and reproduced with her kind permission)

These questions do not in themselves constitute a theory of course, but underlying them is a fairly clear and consistent theoretical approach.

Exercise 3.2

What ideas about change – and about how to test out change – underlie Sally Horsnell's questions? (That is, what would seem to be her theory about change?)
   Can you see any limitations or difficulties with this as a theory?

Comments

The theory about change that I notice here could be summed up something like this:

   Changes in behaviour are unlikely to be permanent unless they are accompanied by changes in the way we understand things – and unless we are able to take some responsibility for our own actions.

(Continued)

(Continued)

> The questions seem to me to be designed to explore whether the mother has some insight into why there were concerns about her parenting in the past and whether she takes some responsibility for it. The questions are based on the assumption that if she is really going to be able to parent differently in the future, she would need to be able to understand, and take some responsibility for, the fact that there were problems with her parenting in the past. By asking the mother to describe how she saw the problems, and what she sees the changes as having been (rather than, for example, by the social worker describing the problems and asking the mother if she agrees), the social worker aims to get some sense of the extent to which the mother really understands what the problem was in the past.

Because the theory can be made explicit in this way, it is open to challenge. Here are three possible limitations of this approach that I can see:

(1)   *The approach presupposes that the decision to remove the child into public care was justified in the first place. If in fact the child had been removed from the mother without good reason, then of course there would be no reason why the mother should feel the need to change. (In rather the same way, prisoners who have been wrongly convicted may fail to get early discharge because they are unable to demonstrate remorse for crimes which they did not commit.) So this approach would not be appropriate where there was reasonable cause for doubt about the original decision.*

(2)   *I personally believe that it is necessary to have some insight and to be able to take responsibility in situations of this kind. However, one might question whether it is always necessary to have insight and to take responsibility in order for change to occur. Probably we can all think of changes that occurred in our life without much conscious reflection. In which case, the theory implied by these questions is not universally applicable to all kinds of personal change.*

(3)   *You might also argue that, even though insight is important, it is not necessarily sufficient. Many of us can probably think of shortcomings of our own into which we do have some insight, but which we find it hard to change.*

For more thoughts on assessing capacity to change you might look at Howarth and Morrison (2000), or the work of DiClementi (1991) on which they draw.

I hope this exercise has demonstrated that using theory in practice does not necessarily mean using a *formal* theory in the sense of using a theory out of a book with a specific name. It means being clear about the ideas that guide your practice and thinking through how you are going to approach each task. Formal theory can augment and inform this process of thinking things through, but it cannot ever be a substitute for thinking for yourself.

Thinking about intervention

Exercise 3.2, just given, was about assessment. I now want to consider the way in which theory underlies intervention.

Exercise 3.3

In Exercise 3.1, Candice Jones was asking for help with her small son Carl. Assuming a social work agency judged that the situation was sufficiently serious to merit some form of intervention, the kinds of service that might be offered, in my experience, could include one or more of the following:

(1) Candice is invited to attend a family centre with Carl where staff will work with her on parenting skills.
(2) Carl is referred for psychiatric assessment, with the possibility of drug treatment if he is diagnosed as suffering from a recognised syndrome, such as ADHD.
(3) Respite day care is arranged for Carl, to allow Candice some time out on her own and/or to provide Carl with opportunities for stimulation and socialisation (overnight respite care with a specialist foster carer is also offered in some situations, for example where children have disabilities).
(4) Candice is offered some form of counselling.
(5) Candice is offered the support of a worker from the social work agency or from a voluntary agency, such as Homestart in the UK, to visit her at home regularly and offer her support with parenting Carl. The support might include practical assistance, moral support and perhaps an element of advice or instruction.

What might be the rationale for choosing each one of these options? (In other words, what might be the theory behind it, *formal* or *informal*?)

Can you think of reasons that might exist for avoiding choosing some of these? (What theoretical objections might exist to them?)

Comments

The theory behind (1) is that problems like Candice's are the result of gaps in her knowledge and/or skills in respect of parenting. This sounds obvious, but it seems to me that parenting skills training is sometimes offered without consideration as to whether the problem really is about skills. If I drive badly it might mean that I am lacking in skills, but it could equally well mean that I am lacking in motivation, preoccupied, under the influence of drugs or alcohol, unwell or very tired. Sending me on a driving skills course would only be helpful if the problem was indeed to do with skills and not about one of these other things. The same is true of parenting. In fact, being offered training in skills that you already possess can be counter-productive, demoralising and alienating. Perhaps Candice possesses all the knowledge and skills necessary to be a good parent, but is too depressed to use them?

Suppose that option (2) is followed and drug treatment is offered. The theory here would be that there is an organic reason for Carl's difficult behaviour; a reason to do with biochemistry. Some parents are actually quite keen to have explanations like this for their children's difficult behaviour and an objection to going down this road would be that, by locating the cause of the problem at the level of biochemistry, this option may prevent other difficulties from being explored. Another objection might be that to give a child a psychiatric 'label' at such a young age is a very serious matter and could have long-term consequences for him. Here you could refer to a formal theory. Labelling theory is all about the long-term influence of such labels on the way that people are perceived.)

(Continued)

(Continued)

In the case of option (3) there might be various theories behind offering respite, but one theory might be that Candice is under stress as a result of caring for Carl and needs relief from that stress. This might well be an entirely valid theory. Caring for small children can be extremely stressful. But respite care on its own could mask other problems. For example, if Candice has never been able to love Carl and his behaviour is a symptom of insecure attachment on his part (to refer to another formal theory), then frequent separations of Carl and Candice will not in themselves get to the root of the problem at all, and could make Carl feel even more abandoned and desperate. Nor would it help with Candice's parenting skills if that in fact was the issue.

You could doubtless think of similar theoretical advantages and disadvantages for options (4) and (5).

In my experience social work agencies can respond badly to situations in one of several ways:

- Failing to offer any kind of help at all other than some sort of bureaucratic brush-off.
- Offering a particular service not because it necessarily fits well with the needs of the service user, but because it happens to be available or because it is always offered in cases of this kind (this is called a service-led as opposed to a needs-led approach; see page 146).
- Overwhelming the service user by 'throwing the book at them' and putting in all the available services at once. (In my experience this is particularly prone to happen in child protection cases and may result from the need of professionals to feel that they are doing everything possible in response to child abuse or neglect.)

Offering no service at all is of course usually unhelpful, though it is often unavoidable if an agency simply does not have the resources to meet all the demands that are made of it. Offering the wrong service or throwing the book at the service user, however, can actually be *worse* than doing nothing, because ill-chosen interventions can, for the sorts of reasons discussed in the commentary on Exercise 3.3, do more harm than good. In fact, I would suggest that any intervention from a social work agency is, on balance, likely to do more harm than good if it is not carried out for clearly thought-out reasons, for as the word itself suggests, a social work 'intervention' (like a surgical one or a military one) is a serious intrusion; disruptive by its very nature. Action should be based on a proper, coherent theoretical basis, though (to repeat myself) this does not necessarily have to be a formal theory.

Eclecticism

'Eclecticism' refers to the practice of 'mixing and matching' ideas from a variety of different sources. I think that this is what social workers in practice almost invariably do (though they may not always be aware of the sources they are drawing from). In fact I would go as far as to say that it is what they *inevitably* do since there is certainly no single global theory that provides you with a blueprint for understanding and dealing with every aspect of every situation.

The example in Exercise 3.3 illustrates, I hope, that it is important to think and that it is important to be clear what your theories are (whether those theories are purely informal or are derived from formal theories or are a mixture of the two.) What I think it also illustrates is that what seems a good idea from one perspective can be a bad idea from another: respite care may be good for parental stress but bad for a child's sense of security; drug treatment for behaviour problems may look like a good idea from a purely medical angle, but less so from a social one. This is one reason why it is so important to be clear about the thinking behind your actions and to be able to spell it out in a form that is open to challenge, so as to allow debate. By and large the best course of action does not flow from dogmatically applying one particular approach but by weighing up the merits of different approaches as a way of dealing with the situation at hand.

Exercise 3.4

Peter Brown is a man of 59 who suffers from schizophrenia. He lives in a ground floor flat.

He is reported by his neighbours to be up all night pulling up his floorboards and knocking the plaster off his walls. He tells them that the building is to be demolished in order to build a motorway. In preparation for this he has had his gas and electricity disconnected and has broken up his furniture as firewood (it is mid-winter). Although Mr Brown is generally liked by his neighbours, they fear for the structure of the building and their own safety. He has already begun removing some bricks.

You are an ASW in England or Wales working under the Mental Health Act, 1983, which gives you the job of deciding whether Mr Brown should be compulsorily detained in a mental hospital for assessment under Section 2 of the Act. The legal grounds for this are that the person in question must be 'suffering from mental disorder of a nature or degree which warrants the detention of the patient in a hospital for assessment (or for assessment followed by medical treatment) for at least a limited period' and that 'he ought to be so detained in the interests of his own health and safety or with a view to the protection of other persons'.

Mr Brown himself has no interest in going into hospital and professes himself to be entirely happy. Two doctors, one a psychiatrist, one Mr Brown's GP have recommended in writing that he should be detained for assessment, on the ground that he is clearly suffering from schizophrenia and he is clearly putting other people in the building at risk as a result of his schizophrenic delusions, but the law gives you the final decision.

I asked an experienced ASW what sort of things he would want to think about if faced with this situation. His comments were as follows:

(1) 'I would think about whether there are any relatives/neighbours in contact. What sort of contact does the GP have? Is this man involved in any care network? What does the CPN (Community Psychiatric Nurse) think? Is this a first episode or have there been concerns in the past? Is he on medication? Is he taking it? Has there been a recent upheaval in his life?'

(2) 'It is also relevant to take account of the time of day this referral came in at and how near the weekend it is. Recent years have seen the development of weekend services but the support available could be quite variable.'

(3) 'Could a relative come to stay? Could visiting care workers restart the medication and monitor? Is admission to temporary residential care a possibility?'

What underlying ideas do you notice behind the social workers response?

(Continued)

(Continued)

Comments

These responses sound very pragmatic and not particularly theoretical at all, and yet there is a set of underlying ideas behind them:

- *A person's mental illness is only one of the factors that may predispose them to behave in ways that endanger themselves or others. Other things, in particular the availability of support from other people, are also important.*
- *The insights of people who know a person as an individual may be as relevant to thinking about that person's state, responsiveness and likely behaviour as are insights derived from specialist knowledge of psychiatric illnesses.*
- *The ASW's job is to look at this bigger picture, rather than simply at the medical diagnosis, prior to making a decision. The ASW therefore provides a check on adopting a purely medical model when thinking about how to manage people's mental health problems.*

In the example above, the social worker's job seems to be in part to temper a purely medical approach and to open up possibilities based on the idea that mental health can be looked at in social terms as well as medical ones. The contrast between medical and social models of mental health provide an example of the way in which the same phenomenon can be looked in different, but not necessarily mutually exclusive ways. There are many other possible examples. For instance in the next chapter, I will discuss psychodynamic approaches, which place a lot of emphasis on understanding the causes of things in the past, and behaviourist approaches, which look for explanations in the present. In Chapter 5 I discuss other approaches again which suggest that looking for the causes of things is not necessarily the point anyway. In Chapter 6 I will introduce yet another way of looking at things by introducing the idea of 'circular causation' (in which A causes B, but B simultaneously causes A) and I also introduce the idea that it may be better to work with people in families or groups rather than as individuals.

One of the advantages for a social worker of being familiar with some *formal* theory, as well as the informal theory that we all use, is that this provides a means of *naming*, and thereby sharing and contrasting, different approaches. The psychodynamic and behaviourist approaches discussed in the next chapter, for instance, both contain ideas that are in a sense common knowledge; theories that everybody uses whether or not they have ever heard of Pavlov or Freud. But the advantage of giving these different approaches names – making them *formal* – and consciously contrasting them, is it allows us to think more clearly about what approach we are using and why. As Malcolm Payne (1997: 57) puts it:

> Formal theory is used in adapted and eclectic form in actual practice. However … consideration of the precise requirements of a practice theory, the debate about it and distinctions from comparators [that is other theories] makes clear the issues which face social workers in practice, which are otherwise indistinct in the whirlwind of daily practice.

This is a theme I will return to in the final chapter. In the meanwhile, in the discussion of various theoretical ideas and approaches that follows in Part II of this book, I will try not just to draw attention to possible applications of these approaches in social work but also to point to distinctive insights which each of these ideas contain. These insights may be useful and important even in situations where it is not practicable to apply the whole approach from which they are derived.

Chapter summary

The following are the headings used in this chapter:

- **The basis for action:** A theory of some kind is almost always implicit in any kind of action.
- **Practice and theory:** Definitions of 'practice' and 'theory'. The distinction between 'formal' and 'informal theories'.
- **Assessment and intervention:** Other possible distinctions between different kinds of theory. The role of theory in assessment on the one hand and intervention on the other.
- **Thinking theoretically:** How we apply theory to practice. Noticing the theory which is implicit in different approaches.
- **Thinking about intervention:** The theories that guide intervention, whether we are conscious of them or not.
- **Eclecticism:** How different theoretical approaches may challenge or complement one another.

This ends Part I. Part II will look at a range of ideas about *change*.

Part II IDEAS ABOUT CHANGE

Introduction

Social work is about change. Social workers attempt to provide services that will bring about positive change or to support services users with the process of bringing about changes themselves in their own lives. In many situations, social workers are required also to try and estimate what changes might occur *in the absence of* social work intervention. For example, if you are a social worker in England or Wales assessing need under the Children Act, 1989, you are working on a definition of need which is defined as something, which if not met, will have long-term development consequences: 'health or development ... likely to be significantly impaired, or further impaired ...'. In other situations social workers are involved in trying to assess a person's *capacity* to change. In all areas of social work, one or more of the following are key questions:

- How do I bring about, or support, change and/or how do I help to prevent changes for the worse?
- How will this situation develop (change) if I don't intervene?
- What, if any, changes (positive and negative) might result as the result of the various courses of action open to me? (How can social work change things for the better and avoid changing things for the worse?)
- What are the limits to this person's capacity to change?

In some situations common sense – and knowledge of the available services – is all that is required to answer the question. If the change required is that an elderly person be enabled to have a regular bath again, or to have a hot midday meal, then you do not need a complicated theory to tell you what sort of things might be done about it, though this is *not* to say that imagination and skill is not required to meet such needs in the best way possible. But there are many situations where common sense is simply not enough. Common sense cannot explain why people self-harm, for example, or why some parents mistreat their children. The question is, what kinds of ideas do you apply to situations of this kind in order to decide what to do?

The following chapters are a mixed bag of contrasting ideas that may be useful in thinking about change. Chapter 4 considers ideas that look for the psychological causes of problems in order to decide how to change things in the future.

Chapter 5 looks at approaches that do not get involved in seeking causes, but instead emphasise strategies for promoting a client's own capacity to change. Chapter 6 examines change at different levels, in families, groups and communities, and introduces the idea of 'circular causality'. Chapter 7 looks at the very pragmatic approach to change that constitutes Task Centred Casework and at approaches that exploit the potential for change and growth that exists in times of crisis.

4 | Cause and effect

- Explanations in the past and the present
- Past-orientated approaches: psychodynamic models

  - Importance of the past
  - Idea of the unconscious
  - Idea of transference
  - Importance of insight and meaning

- Attachment theory
- Applications of psychodynamic models
- Present-orientated approaches: behaviourism
- Cognitive-behavioural therapy
- Applications of behaviourist ideas
- Contrasting past- and present-based approaches

If my car develops a problem and I take it to a garage, my expectation is that a mechanic will, first, try to find out what is causing the problem and, second, having established the cause, put it right. Similarly, if I were to develop a rash on my skin and went to a doctor, I would assume that the doctor would start by identifying possible causes for the rash and would then provide a treatment accordingly. If the rash was caused by fungal infection, for instance, she might prescribe a fungicidal cream; if the rash was caused by an allergy, she might advise me as to the allergens that I would need to avoid. I would be alarmed if the mechanic was to replace part of the car engine without first identifying where the problem lay, or if a doctor were to write a prescription, like the imaginary doctor at the beginning of this book, without first trying to establish the nature of the problem that needed treating.

This probably sounds very obvious, but that is really my point. Because we are accustomed, in many areas of life, to solving problems by first looking for explanations, it makes intuitive sense to use a similar approach to the kinds of problems that are presented in social work. It seems almost self-evident that we should start by carrying out an assessment and then, on the basis of that assessment, choose an intervention. Actually, as the next chapter will discuss, looking for explanations is *not* necessarily the only starting point for thinking about how to bring about change. But it is certainly one starting point and it is the one I will discuss in this chapter.

Sometimes looking for explanations may suggest solutions for problems that are essentially practical. If a service user's problems seem to be the consequence of isolation, a social worker might try to change things by linking the service user up with a club or support group, for instance. If a service user was unable to get out of her front door due to the step being too high, a social worker might try to arrange for a ramp to be provided. However, the causes of feelings and behaviour are typically rather harder to pin down than the causes of rashes or of mechanical problems in cars. They are particularly puzzling when people seem to behave in ways that are harmful to their own interests or to carry on doing things which they themselves say they would like to stop: why do people with anorexia refuse to eat? Why do some people long for an intimate relationship yet find it impossible to stay in one? Why do some people become drug addicts or become addicted to other things, such as gambling? This chapter will not answer these questions, I am afraid, but it will sketch out two alternative sets of approaches by which you might begin to think of possible answers.

Both these sets of approaches, by the way, operate at the level of individual psychology. Of course there are other levels – biological, sociological, political – at which we can look for explanations. I will not be considering them in this chapter, but I will come back to some of them in Chapter 6.

Exercise 4.1

- Julie, a 15-year-old in foster care, is cutting her arms with razor blades.
- Jacob, a 52-year-old learning disabled man living in a group home, is attracting hostility from the neighbours by exposing himself in the street.
- Lucy, a 21-year-old lone parent, admits that she finds it difficult to bring herself to cuddle her two-year-old daughter. 'I do love her,' she says, 'but I just can't bear to touch her. It gives me the creeps.'

What sort of explanations do you think there might be to Julie and Jacob's behaviours and Lucy's feelings?

Comments

It is quite likely that neither Julie or Jacob will be able to say precisely why they are doing things, just as most of us would be hard put to explain our own particular habits, likes, dislikes and fears. However, my guess is that you are quite likely to have thought of historical factors such as distress caused by previous experiences (perhaps Lucy experienced abuse as a child?) or you might have thought of more immediate factors (perhaps Julie gets some feeling of relief of tension by cutting herself or perhaps it allows her to distract herself from other feelings?) The two are of course not necessarily mutually exclusive.

Explanations in the past and the present

When looking for explanations do we delve into the past to try and find out how things *got* this way? Or do we look at present circumstances and explore what *keeps* things this way? These two alternative approaches to the business of explaining things might be called past- and present-orientated approaches.

Suppose, for instance, you were trying to help someone who was having difficulty giving up smoking. A *past-orientated* approach might be to look at what in a person's past history makes them feel the need to smoke. For instance, a Freudian psychoanalyst might look at smoking as a form of oral gratification and see the habit of smoking as an instance of *fixation* in the oral stage. Perhaps the smoker's mother did not respond to him quickly as a baby when he was hungry and he learnt to comfort himself and cope with the anxiety by sucking on his own fingers. Perhaps cigarettes are a breast substitute?

A *present-orientated* approach would not concern itself with the distant past, but would explore the current circumstances. It might consider what it is in the 'here and now' that makes smoking so rewarding, and so difficult to give up. Behaviourists would argue that *whatever* caused the problem behaviour in the past, there must be something happening now to keep it going.

Past-orientated approaches: psychodynamic models

Freudian theory is the obvious example of an approach that places a great importance on exploring past experience as a way of resolving problems in the present. Indeed emotional problems in the present, in the Freudian view, are almost invariably the result of 'unresolved' issues from the past. Although, there must be very few social workers who attempt to apply Freudian ideas in anything like a pure form, nevertheless Freudian theory has had an immense effect on the helping professions and on our culture generally, to the point that the past-orientated approach has become part of everyday thinking. Think of the books you have read or films you have seen which involve a character trying to discover or come to terms with some aspect of his or her past, or think of the way that Freudian terminology has entered the language: 'he is very *anal* about his CD collection'; 'I think she is *in denial* about her marriage'; 'John's problem is his *unresolved grief* which he really needs to *work through*'.

Freudian psychology has spawned a range of different approaches which we can loosely group together as 'psychodynamic'. What these approaches have in common are as follows.

Importance of the past

- Early childhood experiences lay down long-term patterns, which last into adulthood and may be difficult to change.
- Serious problems in the present are typically the result of traumas in the past, which have been unresolved.
- Relationships with parents or carers are prototypes for our relationships with others later in life.

Idea of the unconscious

- People repress things from their conscious minds when they seem too much to bear or seem too dangerous to acknowledge.
- People have a whole armoury of defences to protect themselves against realities that they find hard to bear and against feelings that they find hard to own.
- Behaviours that seem inexplicable, perhaps even to ourselves, are the result of forces of which we are not consciously aware.

Idea of 'transference'

- People in psychoanalysis or therapy tend to displace onto the therapist strong feelings – positive and negative – which they had for previous figures in their life.

Importance of insight and meaning

- Understanding ourselves, bringing things into consciousness and confronting and 'working through' issues, which we may have left unresolved in the past, are central to recovery from psychological difficulties.

↗ **'Working through'**

Originally the process by which a patient in analysis discovers piecemeal over an extended period of time the full implications of some interpretation or insight. Hence, by extension, the process of getting used to a new state of affairs or of getting over a loss or painful experience. In this extended sense, mourning is a process of working through, since it involves the piecemeal recognition that the lost object is no longer available ... Rycroft (1995: 200)

Traditional psychodynamic approaches tend to involve an extremely lengthy process of personal exploration, involving a very intense working relationship with the analyst or therapist. This is simply not practicable in many situations, and certainly not in social work that (1) typically involves fairly time-limited interventions and that (2) involves a hybrid of different roles (Chapter 1) which usually preclude the possibility of the social worker operating as a therapist in the pure sense. Many would also question whether even full psychoanalysis, carried out by fully trained analysts and involving intensive input over many years, is necessarily very successful.

Nevertheless, the various psychodynamic approaches have introduced into our culture generally – and the helping professions in particular – an impressive range of ideas, which I believe do help to make sense of human behaviour, including concepts such as *repression, denial, splitting, transference and counter-transference,* and *projection.* I think it is worth familiarising yourself with concepts such as these not because they in themselves will provide you with definitive explanations of things, but because they add to the range and sophistication of your thinking about human psychology.

Attachment theory

One valuable insight, that psychodynamic ideas have provided, is the recognition that children develop their own idiosyncratic psychological strategies for making sense of the world and helping them cope and that these strategies can – especially when developed in extreme situations – in the long run create difficulties. Attachment theory, which develops this idea, is an important offshoot of psychodynamic theory with a relatively strong empirical base. Anyone interested in child and family social work should, in my opinion, be familiar with attachment theory and should be able to avoid some of the elementary mistakes that are sometimes made in its application (such as failing to distinguish between a *strong* attachment and a *secure* attachment). The single concept in attachment theory, which I personally find the most generally useful, is the idea of the *internal working model*, because it helps to make sense of the ways in which people seem to have different characteristic stances in their relationships with others (some expect rejection, some constantly seek to be the centre of attention, some always seem to put others' needs before their own) and to explain why these patterns are so resistant to change.

Attachment theory is a good example of a body of theory (backed up by a good deal of empirical evidence) that identifies causes in the past as explanations for the present behaviour of individuals; including their ability to cope with change. It remains very influential in social work (see Howe et al. [1999], for example, for an attempt to translate attachment theory into a model for social work practice). It is particularly relevant to fostering and adoption work where social workers are involving in moving children to new carers and in some cases are attempting to help the children to put down permanent roots in new families.

The basic elements of attachment theory are as follows:

(1) A human child, like many other animals, is biologically programmed to seek a relationship with a carer – or a limited number of carers – who will provide a source of security and support while the child learns about the world.

(2) In humans a child starts to form such selective attachments at about the age of five or six months. As the child gets older, the child grows increasingly capable of spending time away from her attachment figures, but the need for attachment figures is lifelong.

(3) The child's relationship with her primary care givers during the formative period when attachments have first formed, becomes a template for the child's relationship with others and the wider world (the internal working model.) This is well supported by empirical evidence in humans (for example studies of children raised in institutional care) and seems to be true also of other primates too (Harlow, 1963).

(4) Early attachment relationships can affect many aspects of development including mental health in adult life, parental ability in later life, the ability to form friendships and to establish satisfactory sexual relationships. While some of these connections between early childhood experience and later life can be overstated, or stated too deterministically, there is plenty of good empirical evidence that these early relationships – both in humans and in other primates – do have long-term implications for mental health, social functioning and parenthood in later life.

Where there is an insecure attachment (that is, an attachment which is not fully meeting a child's needs for security and safety in the relationship or not meeting them at all) this presents an anxious situation for a child – and sometimes a terrifying one. The proposal of attachment theory is that a child will attempt to protect themself against this anxiety – and against the sense that all is not as it should be – by a variety of psychological manoeuvres, which result in the child developing what Bowlby (1998) called a 'faulty working model' of themselves, others and of human relationships generally. To maintain a faulty working model, a child needs to use 'defensive exclusion' (a concept that is obviously related to Freud's 'denial' and 'repression') in order to shut out contrary evidence from consciousness, and to avoid recognising feelings and desires which might threaten the child's precarious stability. As a result, the faulty working model tends to resist being modified in the light of later experience.

Actually the word 'faulty' is slightly misleading. These models, when they are first developed, represent the child's best way of coping with a bad situation. For some children it may be quite true, for example, that 'the only way to get any attention is to be very naughty and get beaten and told off, and to cry for a long time, because then I get a cuddle'. The models *can* be regarded as faulty, however, in two senses. First, they involve suppressing information that the child is unable to cope with; so that they may be in a factual sense inaccurate. (Some children may cope with their fears about being abandoned, for instance, by telling themselves that their parents are always available when really needed, even in situations when an outside observer would quickly come to the conclusion that this really isn't so.) Second, they may not work well when the child – or the adult that the child becomes – continues to apply them in new situations. Consider the child who has learnt to get attention by creating a scene and making people angry – and imagine that child continuing to apply that principle to their relationships as an adult.

↗ Working models and theories

It occurs to me that the notion of 'working models' is closely linked to the question of 'theory' and its relation to practice which is the subject of this whole book. What attachment theory really says is that children form *theories* about the world on the basis of the information available to them. These theories, once established, are resistant to change, even when the original situation no longer applies and even when contrary evidence is available. We all know from experience that this is true of theories in general.

One of my aims in this book is to encourage you to keep an open mind about the theories you apply and to be prepared to modify your theories in the light of new information.

One of the aims of social work, and of therapeutic work based on attachment theory or other psychodynamic approaches, is to help people to modify the working models – the theories – that they apply to their relationships with others, if those working models are no longer helpful.

If children do form models of personal relationships based on their own experience and then try and apply the models in the way that they deal with subsequent relationships, we would expect there to be certain characteristic patterns that arise from different kinds of childhood experience. Building on the pioneering work of Mary Ainsworth (Ainsworth et al., 1978) several characteristic patterns of attachment have been identified. The ones that are usually given in the literature on attachment are listed below (although various refinements and modifications have been proposed: see, for example, Crittenden [2000]):

- Secure attachment
- Insecure-anxious-avoidant attachment
- Insecure-anxious-ambivalent attachment (also known as resistant)
- Insecure-disorganised attachment
- Non-attachment

Applications of psychodynamic models

I cannot think of many social work contexts in which it would be feasible or appropriate for social workers to carry out full-scale psychodynamic psychotherapy. Social work rarely if ever allows the time for it and in any case social workers are usually performing a complex mix of roles that precludes the kind of relationship which is generally thought to be required for in-depth therapy. (If one of those roles is, for instance, the 'control agent' role, then therapy sessions would really need to begin with a warning that 'anything you say may be taken down and used in evidence'.) Nor do social work qualification courses, broad and eclectic as they are, provide sufficient training. And, since all psychodynamic approaches emphasise *depth* – and the complexity and uniqueness of each individual's system of meanings and defences – I think one should be wary of trying to apply psychodynamic methods in scaled-down form, which is perhaps a bit like trying to play a symphony on a penny whistle.

That said, there is no reason why ideas originating in psychodynamic theory should not be used by social workers to help them to think about their work. Familiarity with the concept of transference, for instance, allows us to recognise that our own emotional responses to service users (the fact that they make us feel angry, afraid, maternal or bullied) may constitute important information not only about ourselves but about the world of that service user. In any case, psychodynamic ideas are now so pervasive that, whether we are aware of them or not, we do in fact use them in our everyday thinking and ought to be aware of where those ideas originate in order for us to be able to use them critically rather than unthinkingly. It is possible to argue – and this is my own personal view – that psychodynamic models are often rather over-elaborate and that they include valuable insights but also contain a lot of speculation which has been hardened into a kind of dogma that cannot really be supported by empirical evidence.

Attachment theory has a rather stronger empirical base than some other branches of psychodynamic theory. It offers a framework for gaining an understanding of family relationships and for understanding the different assumptions and expectations that people bring to relationships (for more on this see Howe et al., 1999). But perhaps its most important application in social work is in work with children in public care. An important use of explanatory models in general is that they provide a frame not only for understanding how things got to be as they are but, by extension, for thinking intelligently about likely developments in the future. Attachment theory provides a powerful framework for thinking about issues to do with placement planning and for raising questions, such as those relating to parental contact. Exercise 4.2 illustrates the kinds of issues that can arise.

Exercise 4.2

Consider the following case study of the Faye children, which I think is fairly typical of the kinds of situation that come before the courts as a result of concerns about the ability of parents to provide adequate care.

* * *

10 April: The two Faye children Tammy (two years) and Jacob (four months) are taken into public care on an Emergency Protection Order when it has found that their mother Gill (aged 18) left them with two 14-year-old babysitters and then did not return for three days. It seems she felt she could no longer cope and had gone to stay with friends in another town. Gill had no family in the area. There had been previous concerns expressed by Jacob's father, Danny (age 20) who had heard rumours about Gill leaving the children on their own and from Tammy's father, Howell (24) who had heard the same thing.

The two children are placed with short-term foster parents, the Bryces. Care proceedings are initiated and the children are placed on an Interim Care Order [*for readers outside the English/Welsh jurisdiction, this is a court order which places them in public care for a limited time*] while an assessment is carried out of Gill's parenting and her capacity to change.

12 July: After three months it is agreed that Gill has made good progress, attending a family centre regularly for contact with the children and working well with centre staff on parenting skills. The centre staff report that both children have a 'strong attachment' to her and they have particularly been struck by the fact that Tammy is very clingy to Gill and very distressed every time she has to say goodbye to her mother.

The children are returned to Gill, though are still under an Interim Care Order.

30 July: After two weeks, however, Gill says that she cannot cope with Tammy's behaviour, that she realises that she is too young to be a mother, and that she wants both children adopted. The Bryces do not feel able to have both the children back. (Tammy was very demanding and caused some difficulty with their own five-year-old daughter: they would be happy to have Jacob on his own.) They are placed temporarily with the Smiths.

13 August: After two weeks there, Jacob is moved to the Bryces while Tammy is moved to another foster home, the Youngs. Although Gill now supports the local authority's adoption plan, a new factor now arises in that Tammy's father, Howell, has asked to be joined to the proceedings and indicated his intention to apply for Tammy to live with him. (He has had only occasional contact with Tammy over the past year, but says this was because Gill made contact difficult.)

1 September: Jacob's father, Danny, then also comes forward and states his own wish to care for Jacob; as this is preferable to adoption.

(Continued)

(Continued)

10 September: New three-month assessments of the parenting capacity of both fathers are now set in train at the family centre, involving each child being brought to the centre three days a week. In addition, weekly contact is arranged between Jacob and Tammy, because the local authority's preference is to place them for adoption together.

8 October: Tammy's behaviour is reported by the Youngs to be becoming more difficult. She has numerous tantrums, she is hard to settle at night, she is clingy yet unresponsive and 'difficult to love'. The Youngs indicate that they will need her to move within three months (8 January) as they are moving house and don't feel she can move with them.

1 November: Howell, Tammy's father admits to not finding it easy to re-establish a relationship with his daughter who is restless and fractious in his company, but he suggests that this is the result of her neglect by Gill and says that Tammy needs 'psychiatric help'. He seeks the approval of the court for a psychiatric assessment.

3 November: A psychiatric assessment is jointly agreed by all parties. A hearing is set for 22 February to consider the psychiatrist's report and the outcome of the assessment of the parenting assessment of both fathers.

* * *

What issues arise in this case about the children's needs and about possible long-term harm to them?

How might attachment theory help to inform our thinking about a case like this?

Comments

A decision has to be made here about the long-term future of both children, whether they return to their mother, to their fathers or are placed separately or together in an adoptive family. Issues about contact with their parents and one another would also arise depending on that decision.

The evidence suggests that placing Tammy is going to be hard and it would appear that she has developed a way of getting attention (part of her 'internal working model') that causes carers and potential carers to feel unable to cope with her, this could result in a vicious spiral in which she is exposed to more and more rejection and her own desperate behaviour gets more and more extreme. (She has already moved through three public care placements and is facing another move. Sadly this is not that untypical: see Beckett and McKeigue [2003].) So there is real urgency to reach a decision in her case. There is also an urgent need for her to be given an opportunity to make sense of what is happening to her and to be helped to think about all this loss and rejection in a way that is not too destructive to herself and her 'working model' of the world (this is where ideas such as those of Vera Fahlberg [see below] may be useful).

Although Jacob seems to present less worry and difficulties to his carers, there is an urgent need for a resolution in his case too. He was only four-months old when he came into public care, but as of November he is 10-months old and well into the age at which human babies naturally form specific attachments to carers (at about five or six months), so moves, changes and uncertainty will be increasingly difficult for him also.

The moves and changes and uncertainty about the long-term future, which the Faye children are experiencing, would be distressing for any child. It is precisely at times of distress that children most

(Continued)

(Continued)

need the security of a dependable attachment figure, but that is the one thing that cannot be provided for these children until some resolution is reached.

One further point: the family centre staff spoke of a 'strong attachment' between Tammy and her mother. People often confuse a 'strong attachment' with a secure or happy attachment. In fact children who are insecure in their attachments may display much more 'attachment behaviour' (such as clinging) than children who are securely and happily attached, precisely because they are unconfident of the availability of their attachment figure, and/or because the needs that they want their attachment figure to meet in fact continue to be unmet. Harry Harlow's cruel monkey experiments (mentioned earlier) showed that baby monkeys would cling tenaciously to stuffed toy monkeys if that was the only attachment figure available to them.

I hope Exercise 4.2 makes clear that, as well as helping to inform planning for children, attachment theory can also inform the equally important *detail* of work with children who have to move and provide a way of thinking about a child's needs in terms of direct work to help children make sense of changes around them in ways that are not too destructive to themselves and minimise the harm caused by moves and changes of carer (Fahlberg, 1981, 1994.) It can help with thinking about how to work with children to help them change, or better understand, their 'working models' in a way that will allow them to accept love and care (Delaney, 1998.)

This theoretical framework can also help social workers inform their work in a care management or service development role when they are providing support to carers who are in direct contact with children. Understanding how a child's behaviour may be a pattern established long ago in different circumstances may help carers to be able to hang on in situations where they might otherwise assume that they had failed.

Practice notes

Attachment theory and other psychodynamic ideas

Skill requirements

- If you are going to use attachment theory as an assessment tool, you need to be well-versed in the theory, possess good observational skills and skills in asking questions and listening.
- If you are going to apply the sort of therapeutic techniques for working with children suggested by writers such as Fahlberg or Delaney, you need to be confident in working directly with children. Until you are familiar with the techniques, you will need to ensure you have good support and supervision from someone who is. Good supervision is important even when you *are* more experienced.

(Continued)

(Continued)

- Application of any theoretical framework like attachment theory requires a certain 'lightness of touch'. It is not helpful to try and make everything fit neatly into the theory and it is not helpful to suggest to others that your knowledge of the theoretical model makes you necessarily the exclusive 'expert'.
- In-depth psychotherapeutic work is not something to be attempted without adequate training and adequate support.

Ethical considerations

- It is important not to claim more expertise than you really have; for this is to claim more power or influence than is really justified. Attachment theory is useful, as are ideas from other branches of psychodynamic theory, but we should not claim that it is more of an exact science than it is.
- The conventional western nuclear family is not the only way in which a child's attachment needs can be met. The fact that different parents (from different ethnic or class backgrounds for instance) have different priorities for their children doesn't mean that they are necessarily less attached to them.
- Some early manifestations of attachment theory are quite sexist, in that they assumed that the primary carer of a child had to be the mother.
- It is irresponsible to initiate intensive therapeutic work yourself unless you are sure: (1) you are adequately prepared and supported for it; (2) you are the right person to do it; and (3) it is the right time to do it.
- But it is also very irresponsible to move children around without doing adequate direct work to help them to make sense of it and without trying to minimise emotional harm.
- All psychodynamic models incorporate the idea that people are not always aware of their own reasons for doing things. While this may be true, it may result in a therapist deciding that they know, *better than the client himself*, what a client wants and needs and/or assuming that the 'presenting problem' offered by the client is merely a symptom for a deeper problem which may perhaps also seem more interesting to the therapist. This can result in very arrogant and oppressive behaviour.

Real-world constraints

- The ability to recognise the existence of a problem should not be assumed to be the same thing as the ability to provide a solution. The social engineering that is involved in removing children from their families and placing them elsewhere is an extreme measure carrying considerable risks. While attachment theory confirms the desirability of placing children in permanent placements where they can put down secure roots, it is also the case, as June Thoburn (2002) has pointed out, that so-called 'permanent' placements often do not in fact provide 'permanency', particularly in the case of older children, where over a third of 'permanent' placements break down.

(Continued)

(Continued)

- Likewise, however much an individual would seem to be in need of therapeutic 'help', it is not necessarily the case that therapy will be 'helpful'. This requires that the individual is ready for help and fully signed up to it, and that the kind of help that is available is actually suited to their needs.
- Social workers with an interest in working in a therapy role should be very clear about the ways in which their job is different from that of a therapist or counsellor and should be very clear about the different relationship they have with service users. This is particularly the case, perhaps, with those social workers whose work includes a substantial 'control agent' role and whose clients are not necessarily voluntary ones.

Present-orientated approaches: behaviourism

A very influential body of psychological thinking, particularly in the middle of the 20th century, *behaviourism* is also sometimes also known as *learning theory*. In sharp contrast to psychodynamic thinkers, the early behaviourists did not bother themselves at all with speculative theories about what goes on inside people's minds. In fact most of the basic ideas of behaviourism were derived from experiments in which animals were trained to behave in different ways by manipulating the reinforcements they received. Ivan Pavlov famously showed that a dog's natural reflex response of salivating when it smells food, can be 'conditioned' to other stimuli, so that, if a bell is always sounded when food is offered, after a while the dog will salivate when it hears the bell.

The kind of conditioning studied by Pavlov is known as 'classical' (or 'respondent') conditioning and involves conditioning an automatic reflex such as salivation so that it is activated by new stimuli. More relevant to us, though, is another kind of conditioning called 'operant conditioning', which involves conditioning not automatic reflexes but voluntary actions. Key terms in operant conditioning are *stimulus, response* and *reinforcement*. Since the approach originated in work with animals I will use an animal example to illustrate them. Imagine that you have a dog and have trained him to sit when given the command 'sit', and that you have done so by giving the dog a biscuit every time he does as you want. In this example, the *stimulus* is the command 'sit'. The *response* that you are reinforcing is that of sitting down. The *reinforcement* is the biscuit, which increases the likelihood of – and therefore reinforces – the desired response. A biscuit is a *positive* reinforcement, in that it is something pleasant which the dog wants. If you gave the dog an electric shock, which would only stop when he sat down, that would be a *negative* reinforcement, meaning that the reinforcement results from something unpleasant stopping. Not that I am recommending this as a technique either in dog training or social work.

If the negative or positive reinforcement stop, then the behaviour will continue for a while, but will normally gradually reduce in frequency (*extinction*). If the behaviour starts to be reinforced again, however, the behaviour will rapidly revert to its previous high frequency (*spontaneous recovery*), indicating that when a behavioural response to a given stimulus becomes *extinct*, it does not simply disappear but goes, as it were, into abeyance.

Behaviourists such as B.F. Skinner (1974) studied the way in which connections between stimuli and behavioural responses could be manipulated by different schedules of reinforcement. They studied the way that learning could become *generalised* (that is, animals that had learnt to behave in a certain way in response to a certain stimulus – say, the sound of a bell – would tend to behave in that way in response to other similar stimuli), but that animals could also be trained to *discriminate* in a very precise way between different similar stimuli. In some circumstances inaction rather than action can be reinforced and something called *learnt helplessness* can result (Seligman, 1975). *Social learning theory* (Bandura, 1977) takes behaviourism into a social context and incorporates the idea that observing *others* being rewarded or punished for particular behaviours can also result in learning (*observational learning*).

It seems to me that one of behaviourism's most valuable contributions, one of its 'big ideas', is the insight that whatever caused a certain behaviour in the past, there must be something *keeping it going* if it continues into the present. There must be some sort of pay-off for the individual involved, otherwise the behaviour would become extinct.

For example, suppose Mr Jones is so shy that the very idea of going up to someone and starting a conversation makes him feel physically sick. There may be all kinds of reasons why Mr Jones reacts in such a way. If he were to be given help with this problem, a psychodynamic approach would be to probe with Mr Jones into his past in search of the origin of his fearfulness in social situations. Perhaps some traumatic event occurred in his early childhood that made him fearful of approaching people or perhaps his relationship with his parents was such that it taught him to expect ridicule or rejection? However, from a behavioural point of view all that is pointless speculation. The important thing is that he *keeps on* avoiding conversations and that therefore there must be something going on right now that reinforces this pattern of behaviour. (Presumably it is negative reinforcement? Each time Mr Jones avoids a conversation he also avoids the discomfort of a great increase in his anxiety levels and experiences a sense of relief.)

A behaviourist approach would be to find ways of giving Mr Jones the experience of starting conversations and finding out that nothing unpleasant happened as a result. This would reduce the negative reinforcement of his conversation-avoiding behaviour. And if Mr Jones were to find that starting conversations had a pleasurable outcome then the new behaviour of starting conversations would be positively reinforced. There might be a variety of ways of arranging this. For example role play could be used to give Mr Jones the experience in a safe controlled environment. Or he could be given some practical advice about starting conversations that would make him less worried and a positive response more likely. The point is, though, that, regardless of what caused the problem in the beginning, if the pay-off for avoiding conversations is reduced and/or the pay-off for starting conversations is increased then he will start behaving differently.

Exercise 4.3 presents another imaginary scenario for you to consider.

Exercise 4.3

Julian, aged five, is driving his parents frantic with his habit of, for no apparent reason, going to the fridge and emptying its entire contents out onto the floor. The first time it happened, Julian's mother was feeling rather frazzled and had just come in from outside after rushing to get her washing in off the clothes line before a downpour. Finding the food all over the floor, she admits she 'lost it' and screamed and shouted at him until he burst into tears. After that, realising she had gone over the top, she gave him a big cuddle.

She assumed that was the end of it but the next day he did the same thing and she found herself reacting in the same way. And he has done it many times since.

What might be reinforcing Julian's behaviour and what might be a way of changing it?

Comments

Two possibilities suggest themselves to me:

(1) *Even though it isn't pleasant being screamed at, it may be that it was exciting to Julian to elicit such a powerful reaction from his mother (particularly if he normally finds it difficult to get her attention). What was perhaps meant to be negative reinforcement may in fact have provided positive reinforcement.*

(2) *Whether or not being screamed at was in itself positively reinforcing, the cuddles that followed it almost certainly were (particularly, again, if Julian was short on cuddles.) Emptying the fridge may have become associated with a particularly long and lovely cuddle.*

If either or both of these apply then an approach that would work would be:

(1) *To completely ignore fridge-emptying and any behaviour like it.*
(2) *To ensure that other more sociably acceptable behaviours are reinforced with attention and cuddles.*

Cognitive-behavioural therapy

The little boy in Exercise 4.3 might well not consciously know why he kept emptying the fridge. Likewise he wouldn't have to understand *why* his mother was ignoring his behaviour for this method to work. Behaviourism assumes that learnt connections between things can occur without conscious thought, like Pavlov's dogs being conditioned to salivate to the sound of a bell. Cognitive-behavioural therapy (CBT), however, is an approach that draws on ideas from behaviourism but also enlists the thinking and insight of the person who is on the receiving end. The shy man, Mr Jones, who I used as an example earlier, might work with a CBT therapist on exploring his problem and finding ways of encouraging the development of new, more helpful behaviours. He would not simply be 'trained' out of his behaviour without any input from himself; he would be an active participant in training himself to behave differently.

A cognitive behavioural assessment looks at the problem behaviours in concrete here-and-now terms in the best behaviourist tradition. 'The search for the long-lost cause of problems is, in the absence of major trauma, regarded with suspicion' as Sheldon (1995: 112) notes. The overall aim is to establish:

> the *controlling conditions* that surround a given problem ... *where* things tend to happen and not happen; what happens around the client or to him or her just *before* a sequence of the unwanted behaviour occurs; what happens around the client or to him or her during the performance of the behaviour; and what happens after the performance of the behaviour. (1995: 113, original emphasis)

The object here is to identify the *stimuli* which have the effect of making the client feel like behaving (*responding*) in the way under question and to identify the *reinforcement* – or pay-off – that results. If you have ever tried to give up smoking or cut down on comfort eating, you can probably see how this might work. There are certain situations where you are particularly vulnerable to lighting a cigarette or having a snack. Perhaps these are situations in which you are bored, anxious or ill at ease? In these situations the behaviour of snacking or smoking distracts you from your uncomfortable feelings and is thereby negatively reinforced. CBT works with people on finding ways of reshaping the behaviour by themselves recognising and altering the pattern of reinforcement. (The shy Mr Jones was an example of ways in which one might approach this). So it is both an explanatory tool and a technique for intervention.

CBT is widely used and has many attractions in addressing behaviour problems, which can include things such as worrying or having negative thoughts as well as outward behaviour. Its advocates offer empirical evidence that, compared with other kinds of therapy, it has a very high success rate (Sheldon, 1995: 18–24) and versions of it are currently used in a variety of contexts including Youth Offending Teams.

Applications of behaviourist ideas

A pure behavioural approach, based on operant conditioning, can be very useful in helping parents to manage their children's difficult behaviour. The specific techniques of CBT provide a useful tool for tackling behaviours that are causing problems for people – they are used by social workers in some specialist contexts. CBT has the advantage that, unlike some of the more totalitarian proposals that have been made in the past by behaviourists, it requires the co-operation of the service user in identifying the problem behaviour to be addressed and in developing ways to change it.

I do not think social workers (in all but a few specialist contexts) very often apply a pure behaviourist or CBT approach, simply because the job of a social worker, with its many roles, typically does not lend itself to working in these quite narrow and specific ways. But the behaviourist way of thinking is an important part of a social workers mental toolkit and is useful even if not applied in formal behavioural work or CBT. The virtue of behaviourist thinking is that it encourages a practical approach to problem solving. Many problematic behaviours (such as that of Julian in Exercise 4.3) continue because people unintentionally reinforce the very behaviour that they want to stop. Social workers should therefore ask ourselves whether we are unintentionally reinforcing behaviour in our service users, which will be unhelpful to them.

What social workers are trying to do in many situations is something that roughly approximates to what Chris Trotter (1999, 2004) calls a 'pro-social' approach. By this he means an approach intended to promote 'pro-social behaviour', meaning behaviour that is constructive, rather than destructive in a social context: such as treating children in a non-abusive way or avoiding committing violent offences. Among other elements, which I will discuss further in Chapter 10, he suggests this approach should include:

- Clearly identifying pro-social comments and behaviours and rewarding them (with praise and recognition).
- Modelling pro-social behaviour (that is, behaving yourself in the way you are trying to encourage).
- Challenging undesirable comments and behaviours and being careful not to inadvertently reinforce them.

This approach is entirely consistent with behaviourism, and an understanding of behaviourist ideas should help us to do it better and more rigorously: 'Behaviour theory is ... central to, and provides an explanation for, the positive research findings associated with the pro-social approach' (Trotter, 1999: 43).

Another of behaviourism's 'big ideas' is that it isn't primarily talking or thinking that shapes behaviour but *reinforcement*. It is no good telling someone to stop being aggressive, for example, if in fact we allow them to get our attention by being aggressive and fail to give them attention when they are not aggressive: whatever we might say, we are still reinforcing aggression. To give an instance: if Mr Smith is kept waiting for an hour to see a social worker when he sits patiently in the office reception area but is seen almost at once when he is abusive to the receptionist, then he is likely to learn that abusing the receptionist is a good way of getting attention; even if he is told that he shouldn't abuse the receptionist. Trotter gives several examples of ways in which, by our actions, we may inadvertently reinforce behaviour that we actually wish to discourage. For example, in the case of a client on probation who is failing to keep the appointments she is required to attend by a court order:

> if the worker in this instance decides to see the client in McDonald's in the hope that the client will become more cooperative, and this is in some way communicated to the client, then the client can get a sense that her uncooperative behaviour has led to a reward. The uncooperative behaviour is reinforced and is more likely to continue. (Trotter, 1999: 70)

Trotter (citing a doctoral thesis by Patrick Burns, 1994) goes on to note that we may also unintentionally reinforce behaviour through our body-language:

> Burns found that probation officers often inadvertently reinforced anti-social and pro-criminal comments through the use of body language (e.g. smiling). (Trotter, 1999: 72)

The implication of this is that we need to examine not only what we say, but what we *do* when we are dealing with service users to see what behaviours we are in fact reinforcing. And we need to think too about what behaviour of ours may by reinforced, without our realising it by the responses of service users. (Am I saying this to avoid the service user shouting at me? Am I saying this because I want the service user to be pleased with me?) I think social workers very often inadvertently reinforce not only anti-social, aggressive and unco-operative behaviour but also passive, helpless, dependent behaviour – and service users in turn often reinforce over-helpful behaviour on the part of social workers.

Practice notes

Ideas derived from behaviourism

Skill requirements

- If you are going to try and use CBT or any other method derived from behaviourism, you need to be well-versed and well-practised in the techniques involved, so that they come naturally; and/or have the support of someone who is able to supervise you closely.
- The successful use of any therapeutic technique requires presentational skills: you need to be able to convey a confident belief that change is possible.
- Listening skills are also required.
- You need to be able to identify situations where this approach will be useful. This requires knowledge of contexts where the approach has been tried and used successfully, but it also requires that you develop the skill of judgement.

Ethical considerations

- With any therapeutic technique you need to ensure that you have a mandate. Does the service user understand what it is you are trying to do and do they consent to it?
- Some behavioural approaches raise serious issues about the oppressive use of power. (In the 1950s attempts were made to condition gay men out of homosexuality by showing them pictures of naked men and giving them electric shocks.) These issues do not seem to me to arise in situations where the service user is fully informed about what the technique entails – and is consenting. But some issues of this kind may be raised in situations where the service users are involuntary clients.
- It is particularly important not to focus on narrow behavioural issues at the expense of the wider picture. This is a real danger with behavioural approaches. For example, if the child in Exercise 4.3 was emptying the fridge to get attention and cuddles then we need to think not only about training him not to open the fridge, but also about ensuring that he gets enough attention and cuddles in other ways. Otherwise we would be meeting his parents needs for him to stop behaving in a difficult way, but ignoring his own needs.

Real-world constraints

- There are real-world constraints on the use of formal behaviour therapy and cognitive behaviour therapy in many social work contexts. Nevertheless, as discussed, it is possible to think behaviourally in *any* context in which human beings interact.
- Some behaviours are very entrenched and we should not imagine that all behaviours can be easily changed by short-term behavioural intervention.

Contrasting past- and present-based approaches

We should not think of behaviourist-influenced approaches as being the *opposite* of psychodynamic approaches. The two have a lot in common. Both are based, for instance, on the idea of the human being as a biological system, which seeks pleasure and tries to avoid pain. Both offer accounts of the ways that we establish patterns of behaviour without necessarily being conscious of the reasons. And, although I have made a distinction between past- and present-orientated approaches, of course no one really denies that both the past and the present are factors in shaping how we behave: the difference is really one of emphasis. Look at these extracts from a book about self-harming behaviour:

> Through these actions emotional pain becomes physical pain, and therefore easier to deal with ...
> When she cut open her skin, the pain meant that she had something else to think about, and the practical problem of her bleeding arms to deal with ...
> The trigger was often a row within the family or with a friend ... (Gardner, 2001: 17–18)

These explanations, it seems to me, are entirely consistent with behaviourism, and include the idea of *stimulus* (trigger) and *negative reinforcement* (distraction from painful feelings). However, the book is actually written from a psychodynamic perspective. Gardner goes on to say:

> Behind this immediate event [*the trigger just mentioned*] there seemed to lie both anxiety about the young woman's fear of destroying the person because of her unexpressed and usually repressed anger, alongside the loss of any hope of having her needs met and gratified by them. (2001: 18)

We are now very clearly in the territory of psychodynamic rather than behavioural thinking, because we are talking about meanings, about events that occurred in the past, about loss and about the repression of feelings which are too difficult to deal with.

In offering you a contrast between past- and present-orientated approaches in this chapter, I have not been trying to get you to choose between one or the other, but rather to encourage you to incorporate both sets of ideas into your theoretical toolkit. In the next chapter I will introduce yet another way again of looking at things which we might term *future*-orientated.

Chapter summary

These are the headings dealt with in this chapter:

- **Explanations in the past and the present:** Looking for explanations for things is an intuitively obvious starting point when trying to bring about change, though not the only starting point. Two approaches are to look for explanations as to the origins of the thing that we want to change, or to look for explanations as to what keeps it going now.

(Continued)

(Continued)

- **Past-orientated approaches – psychodynamic models:** Brief summary of the psychodynamic approach to psychology.
- **Attachment theory:** Introduction to attachment theory and its applications in social work.
- **Applications of psychodynamic models:** Social workers are unlikely to be well-placed to carry out in-depth psychodynamic interventions, but can use psychodynamic ideas as a useful framework for thinking. Attachment theory has specific applications to thinking about issues about child placement.
- **Present-orientated approaches – behaviourism:** Summary of the basic concepts of behaviourism.
- **Cognitive-behavioural therapy:** Discussion of this approach.
- **Applications of behaviourist ideas:** Specific and more general applications to social work.
- **Contrasting past- and present-based approaches:** Similarities as well as differences.

5 | New possibilities

- Forgetting about causes
- Carl Rogers and client-centred therapy

  - Genuineness, congruence
  - Unconditional positive regard
  - Being a separate person
  - Acceptance

- Rogerian principles in social work
- Solution-focussed brief therapy

  - 'Exceptions'
  - The 'miracle question' and 'scaling questions'

- 'Constructive social work'
- Applications and limitations: constructive approaches
- 'Postmodernist' thinking and social work theory

> In my early professional years I was asking the question, How can I treat, or cure, or change this person? Now I would phrase the question in this way: How can I provide a relationship which this person may use for his own personal growth? (Rogers, 1967: 32)

In the middle of the 20th century the psychodynamic and behaviourist approaches described in the last chapter were bitter rivals. Behaviourists tended to see psychodynamic theory as unscientific, untested mumbo-jumbo, while advocates of the psychodynamic approach tended to see behaviourism as superficial, simplistic and mechanistic. But, as I discussed at the beginning of the previous chapter, both of these schools of thought shared the assumption – along with doctors, garage mechanics and plumbers – that, in order to solve a problem, you had to understand how it works; what caused or is causing it. They differed in that behaviourist approaches tend to be interested in discovering what is maintaining a problem behaviour in the here and now – what is the pay-off that keeps a behaviour going – psychodynamic approaches tend to be more interested in the origins of a problem in the past, and particularly in early childhood.

There was however another strand of thinking that also came to the fore in the middle of the 20th century. This was approach typified by Carl Rogers' (1967)'client-centred therapy' (sometimes called Rogerian or Person-Centred therapy), whose influence can still be felt in social work. As the quote above indicates, Rogers was not convinced that the way to solve problems was necessarily to delve into their causes. Since his starting point was that human beings are free to choose their own lives and are not simply the products of nature and nurture, his ideas obviously could not be used to predict or describe how people will change. What they do instead is suggest ways in which change can be made possible. Workers in both the Freudian and behaviourist traditions – each in their very different ways – set themselves up to some extent as experts *prescribing* what people should do or *explaining* people to themselves. What was different about Rogers' position is that he thought the therapist's role was neither to prescribe nor to explain, but to create an environment conducive to the client thinking things through for herself.

In this chapter I want to discuss a broad 'family' of approaches, which share this sort of assumption, beginning with Rogers and moving on to look at solution-focussed brief therapy (SFBT). I will then look at the concept of 'constructive social work', a term which Nigel Parton and Patrick O'Byrne (2000) have coined to describe a synthesis of ideas derived from SFBT, from narrative approaches to therapy and from constructionist ideas. One of the things that these approaches have in common is that they are not concerned with looking for causal explanations either in the present or the past, but are instead concerned with making it possible to move forward. If we were to describe psychodynamic models as past-orientated and behaviourist approaches as more present-orientated, then the ideas I am going to discuss in this chapter could perhaps be called *future*-orientated. However, there is in fact a causal theory implicit in them that takes a form something like this: 'What prevents people from bringing about change in their lives is their lack of belief that change is possible or their lack of confidence in their own problem-solving ability.' All these approaches are about helping people to believe in the possibility of change.

Forgetting about causes

I began the last chapter by saying that it can seem almost self-evident that to solve a problem we need to understand what caused – or is causing – it, as a doctor does with physical illnesses or a mechanic does with a car. Of course psychological and emotional problems tend to be much more complex than the workings of cars or physical illnesses and it is seldom, if ever, possible to pinpoint the causes of such problems with any degree of precision or certainty. Nevertheless, we tend to think that we have to try to do so with as much precision as we possibly manage, perhaps using ideas such as those described in the previous chapter.

But actually in everyday life there are many problems that we solve without even thinking about looking for causes, and some where looking for causes would just seem silly. For example, suppose my problem was that I could not play the piano but wanted to be able to do so. If I went to a piano teacher she would not begin by carrying out an assessment to find out why I was unable to play the piano already. She would not try and find out what factors in my early childhood had led to my failure to learn the piano or what aspects of my current environment were reinforcing my current non-piano-playing behaviour. She would simply start teaching me the techniques involved.

We tend to adopt medical, mechanical or even military analogies in social work. We use words such as 'treatment', 'intervention' and 'therapy' and sometimes refer to service users as 'damaged' or suffering from 'disorders'. But perhaps helping people to learn to play the piano is as good an analogy for many of the things that social workers are asked to help with? And in fact a pedagogical (that is, educational as opposed to therapeutic) approach does seem to lie behind at least some of the services that social workers in the UK provide – or commission from others – for their service users. (I think for example of parenting skills training of various kinds.) This is why, in Chapter 1, I included 'educator' as one of the 'direct change agent' roles that social workers can play.

However, teaching the piano is still not the right analogy either for the approaches I am discussing in this chapter, for a piano teacher is still an expert in the specific skills she aims to impart to her pupils. The future-orientated approaches I will discuss here are broadly based on the idea that people *already have* the necessary skills to move on in their lives, but may need some encouragement and support to recognise that fact and to get started:

> The individual has within himself the capacity and the tendency, latent if not evident, to move forward towards maturity.... This tendency may become deeply buried under layer after layer of encrusted psychological defences; it may be hidden behind elaborate facades which deny its existence; but it is my belief that it exists in every individual, and awaits only the proper conditions for it to be released and expressed. (Rogers, 1967: 35)

One attraction of such approaches in social work is that, on the whole, they are consistent with the idea of *empowerment*, which I will be discussing more fully in Chapter 8. Professionals using these methods do not need to claim to have superior expertise to their clients and they do not claim to be able to explain or interpret their clients to themselves, they simply help their clients to draw on their own expertise and their own problem-solving capacity. This is a real strength because it is easy to oppress people by forcing them into some explanatory theoretical model, which may be alien to their own experience and may undermine their own confidence in their ability to think things through for themselves. And dispensing with explanations can be quite liberating not only for the client but for the professional helper whose task in some senses also becomes easier. 'Constructive social workers', say Parton and O'Byrne,

> do not assume that they know the answer to any person's problem, nor that they know what the best or better solution might be. This is partly because they do not profess to understand the person's life or the nature of their difficulties. They are 'atheoretical' in the sense that they respect the service user's theory as much as any other and they do not believe that there is a theory that can explain the situation with which they are faced. *They feel they are in the happy position of not needing such an explanation, since explanations of problems are not seen as necessarily linked to the understanding of solutions.* (2000: 66–7, my emphasis)

Carl Rogers and client-centred therapy

> It is possible to explain a person to himself, to prescribe steps which should lead him forward, to train him in knowledge about a more satisfying mode of life. But such methods are, in my experience, futile and inconsequential. The most they can accomplish is some temporary change, which soon disappears ...
>
> The failure of any such approaches ... has forced me to recognise that change comes about through experience in a relationship. (Rogers, 1967: 33)

Carl Rogers' belief that the relationship between therapist and client is itself the crucial factor in a therapeutic relationship is borne out by much research which confirms that the quality of this relationship may be a more significant predictor of success than the theoretical model adopted by the therapist: '...therapist theoretical orientation is not strongly related to treatment outcome', and '... consistent evidence exists to support the assertion (now nearly a "truism") that a warm and supportive therapeutic relationship facilitates therapeutic success' (Beutler et al., 1994: 248, 259).

However, while Rogers avoided mechanical explanations of human behaviour of the kind proposed by the behaviourists, or complex models of the workings of the human personality of the kind developed by Freud and his followers, his ideas do show the influence of both these schools of thought, and do include a kind of explanatory theory as to why people get stuck with their problems.

Having experimented with various approaches, he came to the conclusion that the most useful contribution a person could make to the growth of others – whether as a therapist or in other roles such as that of parent or teacher – was to create an environment in which people would feel safe to be themselves. The elements of an effective helping relationship were, in his view, the following.

Genuineness, congruence

An effective helper needs to be perceived by the person being helped as 'trustworthy', 'dependable' or 'consistent'. Rogers came to realise that this wasn't just a matter of, for example, being punctilious about things such as confidentiality, but about being *genuine*:

> I have come to realise that being trustworthy does not demand that I be rigidly consistent but that I be dependably real. The term 'congruent' is one I have used to describe the way I would like to be .... (Rogers, 1967: 50–1)

This means that the therapist need to both be aware of and to be able to express her own genuine feelings:

> When I am experiencing an attitude of annoyance toward another person but am unaware of it, then my communication contains contradictory messages. My words are giving one message, but I am also in subtle ways communicating the annoyance I feel and this confuses the person and makes him distrustful, though he too may be unaware of what is causing the difficulty. (1967: 51)

The implication of this is that the therapist needs to have achieved a level of personal growth which allows us to be self-aware in order to be able to support the personal growth of others.

Unconditional positive regard

We need to be able to offer and therefore need to be able to genuinely feel positive attitudes towards the client. For a whole range of reasons we are inclined to hold back on our positive feelings. Indeed, he suggests that one of the reasons for the professionalisation and bureaucratisation of the helping professions is that it enables us to keep a distance.

Being a separate person

Rogers proposed that to be effective helpers we need to be have a strong and secure sense of our own identity as a separate person:

> Can I own and, if need be, respect my own feelings as something belonging to me and separate from his feelings? Am I strong enough in my own separateness that I will not be downcast by his depression, frightened by his fear or engulfed by his dependency? Is my inner self hardy enough to realize that I am not destroyed by his anger, taken over by his need for dependance, nor enslaved by his love? (1967: 52)

When starting out in the helping professions it is quite easy to make the mistake of thinking that to be truly caring and empathic we must simply take on board the feelings of others and deny or suppress our own feelings. Rogers' useful insight here is that this is wrong. We actually *need* to have a strong sense of the separateness of our own feelings from those of our client in order to understand and accept the feelings of the other person. If we don't have that sense of separateness then other people's feelings will easily overwhelm us with the result that, instead of attending to them, we will become preoccupied by our own fears of being taken over.

By the same token an effective helper needs to be able to permit the *client* to be separate too: 'Can I give him the freedom to be? Or do I feel that he should follow my advice, or remain somewhat dependent on me, or mold himself after me?' (1967: 53).

Acceptance

The reason that Rogers' approach is called 'client-centred' is that it aims to 'understand the client *as the client seems to himself*' (1946, cited by Rogers 1951: 30, original emphasis). The aim of therapy is to enter into the client's world, and accept it, trying to understand his feelings and personal meanings *as he does*, without evaluating or judging, and to do this in relation to every facet of that person (as opposed to 'only receive him conditionally, acceptant of some aspects of his feelings and silently or openly disapproving of other aspects' (Rogers, 1967: 54).

Related to this is the need to act in a way that will not be perceived by the client as a threat. This is actually quite difficult to do, since when a person is exposing his innermost secrets, the wrong reaction from a therapist can feel very threatening indeed, even if it amounts to no more than a frown, or an overemphatic response. (This is evidenced, Rogers noted, by polygraph tests of people in therapy, which show how a person's anxiety levels can shoot up in response to what seem quite minor comments from the therapist.) Since the aim of the therapist is, in Rogers' view, to create an environment in which the client feels safe to explore every aspect of himself, and particularly those aspects which he finds troubling – 'in the psychological safety of the therapeutic relationship the client is able to permit in his awareness feelings and experiences which ordinarily would be repressed, or denied to awareness' (Rogers, 1967: 237) – it is important that the therapist tries to avoid doing anything that might make the client feel exposed, vulnerable or threatened. As part of this the therapist needs to try and free the client from 'the threat of external evaluation', the 'rewards and punishments of external judgement' (Rogers, 1967: 54).

Finally, Rogers emphasised the importance of seeing an individual 'as a person who is in the process of *becoming*' rather than as someone 'bound by his past and by my past' (1967: 54).

In a way, Rogers' approach requires the therapist to already *be* in the place where the client needs to get to in order to be able to deal with his own problems in his own way. That is, the therapist needs to be self-aware and open to experience (and therefore able to trust his own judgements), not too dependent on the views of others (what Rogers called having 'an internal locus of evaluation' [1967: 119]) and willing to see himself as 'a process' rather as trying to get to some imaginary end-state where everything is perfect. This may seem quite a tall order, though the logic of it is clear: if the therapist is helping the client to get to a point where it becomes possible to deal with his problems, the therapist himself must be able to know and recognise such a place herself. Rogers' assumption is that life is fuller, richer and more satisfying for those who are at such a place and are therefore self-aware and able to deal with the world as they find it:

> It appears that an individual finds it satisfying in the long run to express any strong or persistent emotional attitudes in the situation in which they arise, to the person with whom they are concerned, and to the depths to which they exist. This is more satisfying than refusing to admit that such feelings exist, or permitting them to pile up to an explosive degree, or directing them toward some situation other than the one in which they arose ...
>
> Our clients find that as they express themselves more freely, as the surface character of the relationship matches more fully the fluctuating attitudes which underlie it, they can lay aside some of their defenses and truly listen to the other person. Often for the first time they begin to understand how the other person feels, and why he feels that way ... .
>
> Finally, there is increasing willingness for the other person to be himself. *As I am more willing to be myself, I find I am more ready to permit you to be yourself* ... . (1967: 327, my emphasis)

I think the last sentence encapsulates rather well not only Rogers attitude to personal relationships, but his beliefs about professional helping relationships.

Rogerian principles in social work

Rogers' ideas, and ideas akin to those of Rogers, have had an immense effect on the development and practice of therapy and counselling, an effect that quite possibly equals or exceeds that of Freud. Rogers' big insight is that it is the quality of the relationship between therapist and client, rather than the therapist's explanatory theoretical framework, that is the crucial factor in determining the usefulness of therapy – and this insight seems on the whole to be well supported by research evidence quite. An important part of his insight is that self-awareness on the part of the therapist is necessary in order to establish the kind of relationship which is conducive to growth and change. Since Rogers' thoughts are not focussed purely on therapy, but on all helping relationships (including teaching and parenting), they would seem to be relevant to social workers, at least in situations where the role of a social worker is at least in some small part that of what I have called 'direct change agent', and this applies to a great deal of social work.

Exercise 5.1

(1)   Can you think of ways in which social workers and other professionals, in their dealings with service users, characteristically fail to be 'effective helpers' in Rogers' terms? What are the consequences of this, and why does it occur?

(2)   In what ways do you think you might find it most difficult to meet Rogers' criteria for an effective helper?

Comments

(1)   *Unfortunately, anyone who has any experience of working in the helping professions will have little difficulty in thinking of ways in which the business of 'helping' does in practice fall short of Rogers' criteria for effective helping. In particular, a tendency to hide behind professional or bureaucratic masks seems to be commonplace in every helping profession, with the result that genuineness and acceptance are simply not conveyed.*

Why we hide behind these masks is a complex question. Perhaps in part it arises from a fear that we will be found inadequate if we fully reveal ourselves? Social workers also often anticipate having to give messages that will not be welcomed – for example, that a requested service cannot be funded – and therefore hold themselves back in anticipation of having to deal with the anger or disappointment of the client.

Sometimes it is tempting to try to avoid giving difficult messages. Social workers sometimes minimise or fail to discuss the 'control agent' aspect of their role and attempt to come over as friendly, unthreatening and 'nice'. This can result in a feeling of incongruence and falsity. Honesty in my experience is valued and respected by clients, even if they do not like what they are told. 'At least we knew where we stood with her', is a typical comment. It seems to me that genuineness and congruence are actually valued more highly than the 'niceness' which many of us fall into when we are trying hard not to be bureaucratic and distant.

It seems to me too that Rogers was right. Honesty and genuineness are valued not just for their own sake but because a person who is experienced as genuine is actually more useful and effective as a helper because their reactions, positive and negative, are experienced as real and dependable.

If you have ever been in the client position yourself, if not in relation to a social worker, then perhaps in relation to a therapist or counsellor, you will probably know how extremely important genuineness and acceptance are, and how inhibiting the slightest whiff of falseness can be – whether in the form of professional distance or faked niceness.

(Continued)

(Continued)

(2)   I cannot guess of course the areas in which you personally might find it hard to live up to
      Roger's criteria but I do suggest there will certainly be aspects of genuineness, acceptance and
      positive regard, or separateness which you will find difficult and could usefully think about. Our
      natural tendency is to put a mask over these things and to conceal them. To some extent this
      is inevitable. But part of Rogers' point is that this doesn't entirely work. Our clients are able
      to tell when we are hiding behind a mask or faking, and this radically reduces our potential
      helpfulness.

There are however aspects of social work which make it difficult to apply a Rogerian approach in full. For one thing, a significant proportion of social work clients (as I will discuss in Chapter 10) are involuntary clients, who are required to work with social work agencies whether they want to or not and whose behaviour is to varying degrees under the scrutiny of social workers acting in a 'control agent' capacity. In this context social workers are simply not in a position to offer their clients the degree of 'acceptance' that Rogers advocates. They may *really* represent a threat to their clients and they are *required* to engage in what Rogers referred to as evaluation.

Even voluntary clients cannot expect that a social worker will simply accept whatever they have to say: there are many circumstances in which a disclosure by a service user will result in a social worker being obliged to take some sort of protective action whether the service user wants it or not. Social workers need to be careful to avoid a sort of pseudo-Rogerian approach in which they offer the semblance of the kind of acceptance that Rogers prescribes, without being honest about the limitations that actually exist, or the other agendas which the social worker is working to. Karen Healy (2005: 58) found in her research with young parents that they 'were confused and often disappointed by what they understood to be offers of unconditional support and friendship which appeared to be implicit in service providers' emphasis on mutuality'. (See Chapter 11 for some further thoughts on the way that social work 'kindness' could be seen as a 'cover' for other agendas.) In addition – and this is something I will come back to later in the chapter – when assessing future risk, social workers cannot simply disregard causal and predictive factors in the past and the present.

More generally, it is also important to recognise that social workers typically play other roles than that of direct change agent. Apart from the control agent role which I have just referred to, social workers operate as 'almoners', 'care managers' and 'co-ordinators' (to use the terminology I proposed in Chapter 1). People come to social workers for assistance in resolving practical problems and not simply, or even mainly, for 'therapy' and it is important that social workers do not fall into the 'trap of thinking that forming and maintaining good relationships, sometimes called relationship building, [is] an end in itself, rather than a practice approach that provides a foundation on which to build future work' (Trevithick, 2003: 166). A simplistic application of Rogerian principles could result in social workers attempting to offer a nurturing relationship to people who are looking for no such thing. (I say a simplistic interpretation because Rogers specifically warns about encouraging dependency.)

Having said this, the basic qualities which Rogers proposes for effective helping are surely things that we would appreciate in anyone that we have to deal with. Genuineness, congruence and acceptance are qualities that I personally would welcome in a plumber or a computer repairman – and certainly in a care manager who came to assess my personal care needs. With all the caveats I have made, Rogers' emphasis on the importance of genuineness in helping relationships still seems to me to be extremely important in social work, for social workers can very easily hide behind bureaucratic systems, or become punitive, officious or simply superficial. In spite of all the limitations to the application of Rogerian ideas which I have discussed, there are plenty of situations in which a helping relationship is precisely what a social worker is being asked to provide.

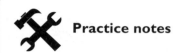 **Practice notes**

The ideas of Carl Rogers

Skill requirements

- The skill requirements of client-centred therapy seem to relate in particular to self-awareness: an ability to recognise and manage our own feelings in a helping situation so as to be able to strike a balance between, for instance, maintaining separateness while offering full attention, acceptance and positive regard.

Ethical considerations

- There do not seem to be any serious ethical pitfalls in offering a genuinely client-centred approach. However, there is a need in social work to be careful about offering what I have called a pseudo-Rogerian approach, by which I mean one in which a social worker seems to offer acceptance of a more global kind than the requirements of her job will really allow.
- The general 'effective helper' stance proposed by Rogers should be applicable to any 'helping' role and is therefore relevant to any social work role, but 'therapy' of any kind is an intrusion into privacy, which should not be entered into without a clear understanding between all concerned that this is what is happening. Healy (2005: 57) (writing about the use of psychotherapeutic ideas in social work generally) makes the point well: 'The emphasis on concepts such as empathy and mutuality can be misleading and confusing for service users in contexts where social workers bear statutory responsibilities such as in child protection, corrections and some mental health roles.'

Real-world Constraints

- Social workers are not there simply to offer helping relationships and we should not imagine that a helping relationship in itself is necessarily or usually an adequate response to a request for a service.
- The principles of being an effective helper are in principle applicable even when a social worker is operating in a 'control agent' role, but many people will understandably be reluctant to see a control agent, who may perhaps deprive them of their liberty or remove their children into care, as a confidant or a source of personal help.

Solution-focussed brief therapy

> After 15 years of doing and studying brief therapy, I have come to the conclusion that … for an intervention to successfully *fit*, it is not necessary to have detailed knowledge of the complaint. It is not even necessary even to be able to construct with any rigor how the trouble is maintained in order to prompt solution … All that is necessary is that the person involved in a troublesome situation does *something different* … . (de Shazer, 1985: 7, original emphasis)

The similarities between this quote and the one from Rogers with which I began this chapter are, I think, noticeable enough to justify my suggestion that de Shazer's SFBT can be included in a broad 'family' of ideas alongside Rogers' client-centred therapy. However SFBT is certainly *not* the same thing as client-centred therapy and is in some ways almost the opposite of it. It is, for one thing, more 'technical' by which I mean it offers a number of quite specific techniques – some might call this more *manipulative* – and is, for another, much less 'personal' in that there is much less discussion in the SFBT literature, as compared to Rogers writing, about the appropriate personal stance of the therapist.

SFBT also has close affinities with strategic family therapy, which I will mention briefly in the next chapter and with behaviourism. Formerly a professional researcher, Steve de Shazer developed his techniques through a systematic process of trying different methods and testing their outcomes. In this respect, and also in its preference for brief focussed interventions rather than lengthy professional involvement, SFBT also has something in common with Task-centred Case Work, arguably the most widely used method of intervention in social work, which I will discuss separately in the next chapter.

De Shazer's viewpoint is that most traditional forms of therapy and of helping have the effect of encouraging service users to talk and think about, their problems. (In behavioural terms, most traditional approaches to therapy *reward* problem talk with sympathy and attention and thereby *reinforce* the behaviour of 'problem talking'. De Shazer's approach reinforces solution talking.) His approach is not to dwell on the problems at all. Indeed, as the above quote shows, he claims that he can help people without even knowing the details of the problem they want help with. Instead he suggests that therapists should focus in various ways on solutions. I cannot give a full account of the approach here, but the following description of some key concepts may give a flavour of the approach.

'Exceptions'

'Exceptions' are times when the 'problem' was temporarily absent. If 'exceptions' can be identified, then the therapist asks the client to describe exactly, and in detail, not the problems but *the way things are when the problem is not present*. This has a general effect of getting the client to think of herself as someone who does not necessarily always have the problem. It has the more specific effect that, by identifying the circumstances surrounding 'exceptions', the therapist is able to give the clients therapeutic tasks to perform which are clearly already within the client's capability, because:

> the intervention just asks the client to continue to do something. This process of solution development can be summed up as helping an unrecognised difference become a difference that makes a difference. (de Shazer, 1988: 10)

If this seems obscure, the following account of the case of a child with a bed-wetting problem illustrates the point:

> A family came to therapy in an attempt to help their 10-year-old son stop wetting the bed. Every once in a while, in the previous six months, they had discovered a dry bed (an exception). However, most nights it was wet ... Mother, father and son were unable to describe any differences between wet bed nights and dry bed nights, but the six-year-old daughter pointed out that her brother was dry every Wednesday morning. (A difference had been noticed.) On Wednesday morning it was father who woke the boy while mother did it the rest of the week. After dismissing the children from the session, the therapist suggested that waking the boy should be the father's job during the two-week interval between sessions. (de Shazer, 1988: 54)

According to de Shazer, in this case the changed morning pattern resulted in the child having dry beds every day. We might speculate as to *why* this happened – did the father give the son a subtly different message in the morning to the mother, a message which he came to anticipate when he went to bed on a Tuesday night? From the point of view of solution-focussed therapy this is irelevant: it is sufficient to identify the exception and note what was different about it.

The 'miracle question' and 'scaling questions'

> *Suppose that one night, while you were asleep, there was a miracle and this problem was solved. How would you know? What would be different?* (de Shazer, 1988: 5)

The so-called 'miracle question,' on the lines of the above, is typically used in SFBT in a first session. It has the purpose of eliciting in as concrete detail as possible where the client wants to get to and it gets the client to define where he wants to get to in positive terms rather than simply in terms of the absence of the problem. It then becomes possible to ask if any part of this imagined future is already happening some of the time – and to begin to generate exceptions.

'Scaling questions', in which the client is asked to rate things on a scale of 0 to 10, are another technique that has the effect of (1) helping the client 'to get away from the idea that they are either in the problem or out of it' (Parton and O'Byrne, 2000: 105) and (2) helping the identification of exceptions or differences that can be the basis of change, even in situations where the client feels that the problem is never entirely absent. For example, if a client feels that most of the time the problem is so severe that her quality of life is 0, but is able to identify times when her quality of life was 4, then it is possible to work on the latter as an exception.

'Constructive social work'

'Constructive social work' (Parton and O'Byrne, 2000) draws heavily on the ideas of de Shazer but also forges links (as indeed de Shazer himself has done) between SFBT, other therapeutic approaches such as the narrative-based approaches of Michael White and

David Epston (1990) and a body of ideas which may loosely be categorised as 'postmodern' which originate in the field of literary and cultural criticism. This interest in postmodernist critical theory reflects that of a number of other writers about social work (see, for instance, Fook, 2002).

The important insights that these ideas offer concern the relationship of reality to language. Very roughly, some key points are the following:

- Much of what we call 'reality' (or, in some versions *all* of it) is in fact an artefact of language. To use illustrations from a social work context, words and phrases like 'depression', 'child abuse', 'mental illness', 'learning disability' – or indeed 'social work' itself – do not refer to some sort of fixed objective entity 'out there', but are socially constructed categories that, in a given social context, are treated as if they were real, but that, in another social context, might have a different meaning or no meaning at all.
- Power in society is closely related to the ability to determine what is regarded as 'true' in this way. 'Every society has its own regime of truth … [consisting of] types of discourse which it accepts and makes function as true' (Foucault, 1980: 131). These regimes of truth are used by the powerful to regulate the powerless. (In Chapter 11, I will discuss a critique of social work itself based on this idea.)
- We are all in a way the prisoners of the language that we use because of the limits it sets on what we are able to imagine and conceive of (for example, de Shazer's approach is partly based on the idea that, simply by defining themselves as 'having a problem' people become entrapped in certain patterns of behaviour.)
- Those defined as deviant in any given society are doubly prisoners in this sense, because it is the particular regime of truth which they inhabit which defines them as such and which justifies society in controlling and regulating them in various ways. (For instance, in the past male homosexuality was defined as an illness, justifying the 'treatment' of gay men by psychiatrists. Yet at other times, for example in Greece at the time of Plato, male homosexuality was regarded as entirely acceptable and normal.)
- In general, rather than looking for grand theories to explain things, we should think instead of a multiplicity of stories that people inhabit and use to make sense of their lives.

Parton and O'Byrne suggest the application of these ideas to social work to develop a new kind of practice that is not about imposing an external 'regime of truth' onto clients, which *is* in a sense what we do when we apply explanatory theories such as those discussed in the previous chapter, but about collaborating with service users in re-constructing their personal narratives in whatever ways seem helpful to them.

Applications and limitations: 'constructive' approaches

When discussing the application of particular ideas to social work, I have tried to consider both *specific* applications of particular techniques, but also more *general* applications in terms of insights which particular ideas have contributed, so to speak, to our toolkit of ways of thinking about what we do. In terms of general applications, SFBT and other 'constructive' approaches seem to me to contribute the important insight that it is not necessarily

Figure 5.1 Children made subject to care orders in England and Wales, 1992–2003

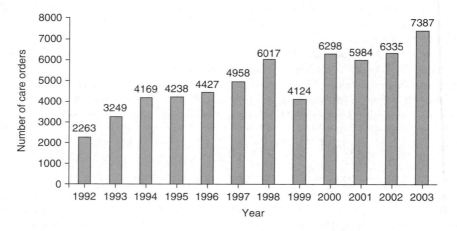

Source: Annual Judicial Statistics published by Department for Constitutional Affairs, formerly the Lord Chancellor's Department.

helpful to talk about problems. Looking at it from the perspective of these constructive approaches, I am struck by how absolutely flooded with 'problem talk' much social work practice is. A good parent – or a good teacher – wouldn't think of constantly dwelling on a child's problems and deficiencies without balancing this by noticing strengths and achievements. A good boss would not dwell constantly on the faults of her staff without noticing their strengths. But much of social work is orientated towards identifying problems and deficiencies, needs and risks, rather than identifying strengths and positives on which to build. SFBT – and the related ideas discussed by Parton and O'Byrne – offer specific techniques for redressing this balance.

These specific techniques can be used in some social work contexts, though there are limitations to their use, which I will shortly discuss. More generally, they raise difficult and uncomfortable questions about the negativity of much social work practice. Figure 5.1 shows the numbers of children made subject to care orders (that is, taken compulsorily into public care) over the period 1992–2003, showing a more than three-fold increase over an 11-year period. There may be a number of explanations for this extraordinarily rapid increase but I wonder whether one reason might be that, as Parton and O'Byrne (2000: 1) put it, 'social work has lost its way' and has lost faith in the possibility of working with parents and families to achieve positive change. Certainly, one would predict that an inability to identify and work with positives in families, coupled with a hyper-awareness of possible negatives, would result in social workers feeling that they had no choice but to remove more and more children from their families each year. Since the rate of increase shows no sign of slowing down we should perhaps begin to ask ourselves where this trend is going.

Another important challenge for conventional social work that is raised by 'constructive social work', as well as by the Rogerian client-centred philosophy discussed earlier, is the challenge to the conventional cause-and-effect model that I discussed at the beginning of the chapter. All the approaches discussed in this chapter set aside the idea of the social worker (or therapist or helper) as an expert who interprets what clients say or do in terms of some sort of scientific explanatory theory. They are all based on the premise that people construct their own meanings and stories which the social worker/therapist/helper needs to respect. The role of the professional helper is not to tell people what is wrong with them, but to help them to explore other ways of, so to speak, telling their own story, which might help them to move on from painful and unhappy situations in which they feel stuck. This is an attractive notion to social workers who are concerned to empower rather than oppress their service users.

But there are limitations to 'constructive' approaches as a social work model. Most obviously they are applicable mainly to 'direct change agent' roles and much less so to the other roles that social workers play. In fact the specific techniques offered by de Shazer and other 'constructive' are really only applicable in situations where what is going on is agreed – by social worker and service user – to be 'therapy.' Whether these or other therapeutic techniques are applicable in situations where the clients are involuntary is a difficult point. There seem to me to be real ethical as well as practical difficulties in doing therapy with people who have no choice in the matter, though it is possible to argue that a person may still choose to engage in therapeutic work even in a context where he is an involuntary social work client (De Jong and Berg [2001], for instance, propose a model for carrying out solution-focussed work with 'mandated' – that is, court-ordered – clients).

Another major limitation of all approaches that eschew cause-and-effect analysis is acknowledged by Parton and O'Byrne (2000: 67) as follows:

> However, there is a difficulty where oppression is operating or there is a serious risk of harm – then the worker has a duty to care, to state their view and to use their knowledge of such dangers and of the resources needed to deal with them.

We cannot for example, when working with a sex offender, allow ourselves to accept uncritically his view of the world, however sincerely he believes in it. We can't set aside our knowledge of the compulsive nature of such behaviour or ignore his past when thinking about what he may do in the future. If a person has committed a number of sexual offences in the past, we know it is extremely likely that he will commit more in the future: this – along with the harm that sexual offending causes – is a fact that cannot simply be abolished by changing the language we use.

A sex offender is an extreme example, but it is the case that the limited resources of social work agencies, and the demands made upon them, make it in most contexts inevitable that they prioritise their work rather rigorously and sometimes really only deal with situations where there is, as Parton and O'Byrne put it 'oppression or serious risk of harm'. In situations where social workers have to form judgements about risk in the future and about the likelihood of change they simply cannot be guided solely by the views and meanings of service users, but have to draw on ideas about how given present circumstances are related to possible outcomes in the future. In other words they have no choice but to fall back on cause-and-effect thinking, however approximate and imperfect it may be.

Practice notes

Solution-focussed and 'Constructive' approaches

Skill requirements

- Like any practice technique solution-focussed work requires not only knowledge but fluency in practice. All therapeutic approaches require that we behave in ways which in some respects differ from our normal ingrained habits of behaving in human interactions.
- In particular, since problem-focussed thinking is so ingrained in us, considerable skill is required to avoid lapsing into 'problem-talk'. This involves walking a fine line between helpfully maintaining focus and being overly directive. Service users may want to talk about problems and may be resistant to attempts to steer them away from it.

Ethical considerations

- The point just made about skills contains a value question also: to what extent should social workers prevent service users from talking about problems if they feel they need to do so?
- With any therapeutic approach, there are questions as to the ethics of working in this way with involuntary clients and, in particular, in situations where 'therapy' is not in fact what the client asked for.
- Optimism about the possibility of change is often helpful and empowering. But people are not always able to change, for a variety of reasons, and a purely solution-focussed approach may set people up to fail.
- There are often good ethical reasons why we cannot simply accept the client's own story. I have just given the example of a sex abuser (who may well tell a story about his actions being wanted by his victims, or of doing harm.)

Real-world constraints

- As already discussed, there are limits to the extent that cause-and-effect thinking can be set aside in situations where there are serious risks of harm to vulnerable people, or where people are suffering oppression at the hands of others.
- Any specifically therapeutic approach is relevant only to situations where a social worker has a mandate to work in a therapeutic capacity. I mean by this, situations where working in such a way is: (1) consistent with the social worker's brief; (2) is understood by the service user to be what is going on; and (3) agreed to by the service user.

'Postmodernist' thinking and social work theory

In view of the recent vogue for 'postmodern' ideas in social work – or at any rate in *academic* social work – I will conclude with some brief comments on this way of seeing the world. I have already indicated above that I recognise, and myself make use of, insights that originate in 'postmodern' critical theory, notably those of Foucault, but I think there are serious limitations also to this kind of theorising.

For one thing, simplistic or lazy application of these ideas can end up as a facile notion that there is no such thing as external reality and that, simply by changing the words for things, we can change the world. This can result in a kind of Orwellian 'doublespeak' in which words like 'needs-led assessment' or 'partnership' or 'empowerment' or 'anti-oppressive practice' can end up describing processes that seem almost opposite to what we imagine these words to mean.

In fact in social work we have to deal with many realities, some of them very mundane, which cannot be changed simply by giving them new names: the fact that there is only so much one can do in a given amount of time, for instance. (Perhaps social work would be less prone to taking some of the impossible tasks which are given to it if we were clearer about this.) There are also real world limits to the human capacity to change. I have already alluded to the fact that certain patterns of behaviour, such as sexual offending, are known to be extremely resistant to change. The view that early childhood experience has a lasting effect on how we view the world, discussed in the previous chapter, is surely borne out for most of us by personal experience. Indeed, there is evidence that neural pathways irreversibly laid down in our early years permanently shape the way that we deal with the world (Schore, 1999), a physiological basis for Bowlby's internal working model. This does not mean that change isn't possible or that optimism and self-belief are not important in achieving it. Change is always possible. But there *are* real-world constraints, as well as linguistic socially imposed ones, on the extent and direction of the changes that are open to us.

Without wishing to minimise the importance of ideas such as those of Foucault, I think it is wise to bear in mind that these ideas were not developed in social work, or even in a field akin to social work, but in the context of purely academic disciplines whose practitioners are not required to make decisions about how to respond to problems in the real world. When challenged about a lack of his consistency in his ideas, Foucault once replied as follows:

> What, do you imagine that I would take so much trouble and so much pleasure in writing, do you think that I would keep so persistently to my task, if I were not preparing … a labyrinth … in which I could lose myself? (Foucault, 1972: 17)

That is fine for a professional thinker, but when we think about theory for social work we are not – or, at any rate we certainly shouldn't be – in the business of constructing labyrinths to hide in. The purpose of theory in social work is to provide tools which practitioners can use to relieve suffering and to make the best possible decisions about difficult messy situations. A child is allegedly being used by an adult for sex. What should we do about it? A man believes his dead grandfather is ordering him to execute the world's evil doers. What should we do about it? A five-year-old boy finds his mother unconscious on the bedroom floor after taking an overdose. What should we do about it? Social workers have to come up with answers to these questions and live with the consequences. Critical theorists do not.

Chapter summary

The headings in this chapter were as follows:

- **Forgetting about causes:** Solving problems doesn't have to mean looking for causes and explanations.
- **Carl Rogers and client-centred therapy:** An introduction to the ideas of Carl Rogers on the nature of an effective helping relationship.
- **Rogerian principles in social work:** The application of Rogers' ideas in social work and the limits to their applicability.
- **Solution-focussed brief therapy:** The solution-focussed approach of Steve de Shazer, the idea of 'exceptions' and some of the techniques de Shazer and his colleagues have developed.
- **'Constructive social work':** Nigel Parton and Eugene O'Byrne's proposal for an approach to social work based on SFBT, 'narrative' therapies and postmodern constructionist theory.
- **Applications and limitations – constructive approaches:** The useful insights offered by the 'constructive' approaches and some limitations to the application of the techniques.
- **'Postmodernist' thinking and social work theory:** Some brief comments on postmodernist theorising in general.

The next chapter will look at change at different 'system levels', particularly in families, groups and communities.

6 Different levels

- System levels
  - Biological
  - Physical/environmental
  - Individual/psychological
  - Families and groups
  - Community
  - Societal/political
- Family systems
- Group work
- Community work
- Society as a system

In the previous two chapters I discussed various approaches to the business of bringing about, facilitating or supporting change. Although, there were many differences between them, most of these approaches were focussed primarily on change at what might be called the individual psychological level. This chapter draws attention to the fact that there are other 'system levels' at which change can occur and other ways of looking at the world than individual psychology. I will begin by saying a bit more about what I mean by 'system levels' and drawing your attention to the very different perspectives that come from looking at the world at different levels. I will then look at the concept of 'systems' and discuss ideas from family therapy, which are based on the idea of families as systems, moving on to talk about group work as an alternative to individual work and at community work. Finally, I will note that society as a whole is also a system level and raise questions as to the role that social work plays in that system.

System levels

I will use the term 'system levels' to refer to the many different levels at which it is possible in principle, in any given human situation, to look for explanations and at which it is possible, in principle, to intervene in order to bring about change. Some of these could be crudely summarised as follows.

Biological

One common way of approaching emotional and behavioural problems is by prescribing drugs that alter mood by changing the chemistry of the body. Professional intervention at this biological level is, in our society, an extremely common way of approaching a range of problems including depression (in 2001, the UK National Health Service [NHS] bill for anti-depressant drugs was £342 million [www.statistics.gov.uk]), anxiety, impotence, acute shyness and compulsive behaviours as well as the more florid psychotic conditions. The drug Ritalin is an example of an intervention at the biological level that is now very widely used to manage behaviour problems in children. By defining these problems as ADHD psychiatrists are offering an explanation for these problems at the biological level. Of course prescribing drugs is completely outside the province of social work, but it is certainly not something that social workers can ignore, for social workers do regularly encounter the following:

(1) Service users who are taking prescribed drugs of various kinds or are attempting to 'self-medicate' with over-the-counter or illegal drugs.

(2) Service users for whom going to a doctor for a prescription might be one way of dealing with their problems – and something that a social worker might or might not want to encourage. Opinions certainly vary on the extent to which it is helpful for phenomena such as anxiety or child behaviour problems to be treated as medical conditions.

(3) Cases where the use of prescribed drugs may be part of an interagency plan. For example, in the case of a client with mental health problems a social worker might be part of a team working to a plan, which includes, among other things, encouraging him to take prescribed medication and monitoring his compliance with this.

Physical/environmental

Changing a person's physical environment is another level at which intervention commonly occurs. Providing practical care or arranging for alterations to be made to a person's home are two examples. Other examples are moving an elderly person to a residential home or a child to a foster family. (Of course these moves involve profound changes in the individual's social environment as well as the purely physical one.) Social work often intervenes at the physical and environmental level. In fact one of the characteristics that distinguish social work from other caring professions is that social workers frequently take the lead (in what I called in Chapter 1 an 'executive role') in arranging such moves and changes.

Individual/psychological

Many interventions take place at the level of the person as an individual and are addressed at the person's thinking, emotions or behaviour. These have been the subject of the previous two chapters. For example CBT (as discussed in Chapter 4) is typically applied in the context of one-to-one work and addresses problems experienced by individuals.

Families and groups

We do not have to confine ourselves to working with individuals one at a time. Many of the problems which social workers are asked to address concern the relationships *between* individuals and can be addressed at that level. This applies both to families and to groups of people brought together in contexts such as residential homes. It is also possible to *create* groups with the express purpose of achieving some kind of therapeutic change for the group's members, or to work with groups of people who live together – or come together regularly – in a group care context.

Community

The idea of working to support change in whole communities is arguably a natural extension of the idea of moving away from working with individuals towards working with families and groups.

Societal/political

Many users of social work services are poor or marginalised by society in other ways. The problems that they face may in fact largely or at least in part be the *result* of poverty or marginalisation. If this is the case then arguably the most effective and genuine way of intervening would be to act at the *political* level in order to bring about structural change. Of course, no social worker has in her job description a mandate to change the laws of the land or to replace one political system with another. This level of action lies outside the scope of social work as a professional activity, though of course not outside the scope of social workers in their capacity as citizens. This can leave social work with a dilemma as to how it should respond to problems which are structural in origin.

These levels are not mutually exclusive and we can find explanations and come up with interventions at several different levels simultaneously. For example, heroin addiction could be 'explained' at the biological level (in terms of the effect of heroin on the brain), or at the individual psychological level (in terms of the vulnerability of people with certain types of family background to heroin addiction, for instance, or in terms of the patterns of reinforcement that maintain the behaviour of heroin use), or at a societal level (heroin addiction is linked to social deprivation for instance.) Different professional groups and academic disciplines might place a different emphasis on which of these different levels are most important in explaining heroin addiction and might have different ideas about the level at which it is appropriate to intervene. Doctors and nurses, not surprisingly, tend to be fonder of biological explanations and biological interventions, while social workers tend to reach for psychological or social explanations and interventions. This can lead to interprofessional disputes. (Should a child's challenging behaviour be diagnosed as ADHD, for instance, and treated as a medically defined syndrome or should it be seen as an adaptive response to particular experiences?) Even within social work there has been an ongoing debate as to the relative importance of the individual/psychological level and the societal/ political level. Those who are particularly interested in the former are likely to be more interested in direct change agent roles, those who are more interested in the latter may be more drawn to advocacy roles.

The recognition that we can't really expect to make sense of the experience of service users at a single system level has long been part of social work thinking. More recently it has become enshrined in government policy, in that it forms part of the rationale for pre-scribed assessment frameworks such as the UK governments *Framework for the Assessment of Children in Need and their Families*, which advocates an 'ecological approach':

> An understanding of a child must be located within the context of the child's family ... and of the community and cultures in which he or she is growing up. The significance of understanding the parent–child relationship has long been part of child welfare practice: less so the importance of the interface between environmental factors and a child's development. (Department of Health, 2000: 11)

However, this approach is about recognising the effect of factors at different system levels – family, community, culture – on individual children. For the remainder of this chapter I will be looking at approaches to change which do not focus on individuals but on systems of various sizes.

Family systems

The insight of family systems theory is that many human situations are more helpfully understood in terms of the interactions between individuals rather than in terms of individuals in isolation. The case example in Exercise 6.1 describes a scenario that is perhaps more likely to come up for a marriage guidance counsellor than a social worker, but it provides an illustration of my point.

Exercise 6.1

Mr Fox says that Mrs Fox never seems to want to have sex with him – and Mrs Fox confirms that is so. Mrs Fox, for her part, is upset that Mr Fox is constantly asking for sex, and doesn't seem ever to take pleasure in other kinds of physical intimacy. Mr Fox admits that, yes, any other kind of intimacy is now overshadowed for him by his anxiety about whether or not it will end in sex.

What do you think the problem is here and whose problem is it?

Comments

One could look at this as being a problem of one or the other of the individuals concerned: Mrs Fox's lack of libido, or Mr Fox's excessive libido. Or we could just see the two of them as having different and incompatible needs.

(Continued)

(Continued)

But all these interpretations assume that Mr and Mrs Fox just are as they are and ignore the way that they affect one another. Perhaps, in fact, their needs are not so very different, but they have got themselves into a vicious circle? Perhaps, Mrs Fox's loss of interest in sex results from her feeling overwhelmed by Mr Fox's demands – and if he was less demanding she would relax and feel more responsive? And at the same time, perhaps Mr Fox's preoccupation with sex is the result of his anxieties about his wife's apparent sexual rejection of him – and perhaps if he could be more sure that she was actually interested in having a sexual relationship with him then he would be able to relax a bit more, and enjoy other kinds of intimacy without always worrying about whether or not they would end in sex?

This is not to say that Mr Fox and Mrs Fox do not bring different things to their relationship as individuals. Both of them doubtless bring different feelings and ideas about intimacy to the relationship which date back to early childhood ('internal working models' to use a term from attachment theory), both of them doubtless bring different expectations and meanings that come from the different expectations of men and women in this particular society. The point is, however, that it may not be meaningful to ask whether Mr Fox or Mrs Fox is the cause of the problem here. The problem exists within the relationship between them rather than in either one of them.

Some of the things that systems perspective highlights when looking at a situation like that of Mr and Mrs Fox are the following:

- a vicious circle can develop between the members of a couple which exacerbates individual differences (not just in relation to sex but in relation to any other issue that causes problems);
- the vicious circle does not exist *in* either one of them, but can only be understood in terms of the two of them *as a system*. Neither of them 'started it'. It is a loop which encompasses them both;
- even those aspects of the problem that come into the loop from 'outside' (childhood history, societal expectations) can in themselves be seen in terms of other overlapping systems: their families of origin, their friendship group, the society in which they live, and so on.

The vicious circle – and its opposite the 'virtuous' circle – is a characteristic idea of family systems theory, which proposes that families, like other kinds of system, tend to settle into self-perpetuating loops of mutually reinforcing behaviour and attitudes. We are accustomed in everyday life to look for the ultimate causes of things (and in a human context this is often linked to the question of who is to *blame*). The insight of a systems approach is that, in human relations, 'Who started it?' or 'Who is really to blame?' is as often as meaningless a question as 'Which came first: the chicken or the egg?' In biology and in engineering where systems theory has its roots, it is very common for A to cause B *and* for B to cause A at the same time. (Or for A to cause B, B to cause C and C to cause A.) A very simple example is a thermostat, a simple switch designed to turn off a heating system when the temperature in a room rises above a certain level, and switch it on again when the room temperature falls below that level. Does the room temperature control the thermostat or does the thermostat control the room temperature? The answer if of course that both are true, and that each controls the other. A thermostat is an instance of a negative feedback loop and, since we really cannot say whether the thermostat controls the room temperature or the room temperature controls the thermostat, we can refer to the way these two things are causally linked as an example of *circular causality*. There are countless instances of this kind of mechanism not only in engineered systems but in biological ones, which need to keep themselves in equilibrium in order to survive.

Advocates of the various schools of systemic family therapy argue that many, if not most, apparently individual problems can be seen in this kind of way. Parents might identify their problem as being, for instance, that the teenaged son is behaving appallingly badly (just as Mr Fox in my example might identify the couple's problem as Mrs Fox's lack of interest in sex) but closer examination will reveal that the teenaged son's behaviour is part of a pattern of family interactions in which the entire family is implicated. Characteristically, a family crisis comes about when some major event – whether it is an unexpected event or a predictable 'life cycle' event such as a child leaving home – disrupts the functioning of the family system so that it is no longer able to maintain its equilibrium. A child leaving home, for instance, may force a husband and wife to reappraise the way they relate to one another.

I would suggest that no social worker can afford to ignore the systems dimension when thinking about families (or indeed when considering the functioning of other groups of people). Our toolkit of theoretical ideas needs to include some framework for thinking about the patterns of interaction that undoubtedly occur in groups of people. But a family systems perspective is not just an explanatory model. It is also the basis for techniques of intervention, which we can loosely group together as systemic family therapy. In some contexts, such as Child and Adolescent Mental Health services, social workers may actually work as family therapists, for all or part of the time. In other contexts, social workers may incorporate ideas and approaches drawn from systemic family therapy in their interventions with their clients.

Not surprisingly, given the focus on whole families as systems, family therapists typically like to work with families as a whole, though it is perfectly possible to apply systemic ideas to work with sub-groups of families or with individuals. There are many different approaches under the general umbrella of family therapy but a feature of all of them is that the therapist pays as much attention to *process* as to *content*. In the simple example of Mr and Mrs Fox, given earlier, the *content* of an interaction between the two of them might be what Mr Fox and Mrs Fox each think the problem is, but the *process* is the way they interact with each other, the pattern into which they characteristically fall.

Exercise 6.2

The following is an imaginary transcript of a conversation between three family members: mother (Jane), father (David) and son (Joe). What is the *content* of the conversation? What *process* can you see?

David: The reason why we are so short of money is that we are living above our means. We need to spend less time shopping. Only go to the shops when we really need to.

Jane: In other words, you are blaming me for it.

(Continued)

(Continued)

David: No, I ...
Joe: (Interrupting) Why don't you listen to what mum has to say instead of trying to blame her for everything.

[Later]
Joe: Now that I'm 15 I feel that I should be allowed to stay out as late as I want.
David: Well, I don't agree with that. I think that ...
Jane: (Interrupting) It would be nice to hear you giving some support to Joe for once instead of immediately contradicting him.
Joe: Well at least I've got *one* parent who understands what I want.
David: Well, *I* understand what you *want*. It's just that I ...
Jane: (Interrupting) You're doing it again, contradicting your son as soon as he opens his mouth.

Comments

The content of this conversation would include things like: the family has money problems, there are disagreements about what causes these money problems and there are also disagreements about coming-in times for Joe.

In terms of process, however, you might notice Joe and Jane seem to support each other against David. Both of them tend to interrupt David. When David attempts to set some boundaries as a parent, for instance, Jane does not support him but aligns herself with their son instead. Looking deeper into the family's characteristic patterns of behaviour might tell you more about the reasons for this apparent alignment of mother and son against David.

This is a very crude, brief example, but I hope it illustrates that considering the process is as important to understanding the family as looking purely at the content. If the family were to seek help with their problems then it might well be more fruitful to try and help them change the process than to be drawn into an endless discussion about coming in times or the family budget.

There are a number of different schools or styles of family therapy and two of the most well-known are:

- *Structural* family therapy centres on the idea that 'problematic family organisational structures' may make it difficult for families 'to meet the demands of lifecycle changes or unpredictable ... stresses' (Carr, 2000: 91). Structural therapists (for example, Minuchin et al., 1996) work with families on establishing or re-establishing them as functional problem-solving systems. Thus, in the example in Exercise 6.2 a therapist might suggest tasks for the family which would encourage the parents to work together as parents rather than one parent undermining the other by taking sides with the child.
- *Strategic* family therapy particularly focuses on the way that families are 'ambivalent about change, usually because family problems serve some important interpersonal function for family members' (Carr, 2000: 86). Strategic therapists (for example Madanes, 1981) aim to find ways of disrupting or unsettling long established patterns, and undermining this 'resistance' so as to create opportunities for change to occur.

In family therapy, as in other areas, it is possible to take more past-, present- or future-orientated approaches in the sense that I used these terms in Chapters 4 and 5. The solution-focussed approach, discussed in the previous chapter can be used in work with families and can be described in that context as a form of 'strategic' family therapy, insofar as it aims to help a family shift away from being stuck in patterns of behaviour centred on 'problem talk' but does not start with any preconceptions about family structure.

Many social workers will not be in positions where it is practical or appropriate to offer formal family therapy to their service users. But a systems perspective is important when thinking about people in groups of any kind.

Practice notes

Systemic Family Work

Skill requirements

- Working with families together requires an ability, not entirely unlike that required in chairing meetings, to ensure that everyone has a say and that the agenda is not dominated by one or two individuals. This is an important skill — a form of assertiveness — which is required in many different social work contexts.
- Within the context of therapeutic family work, the social worker (or therapist) is having not only to manage the session, but also to participate and also to observe the interactions of the family members. To do this alone is quite a tall order and for this reason family therapists may co-work, or make use of observers behind screens, or linked by video, who may feed back suggestions and observations to the therapist as she interacts with the family.
- Different schools or approaches in family therapy have distinctive styles: different ways of structuring family interviews, different kinds of questioning. To use these effectively and with confidence, and to still leave yourself some mental space to observe the family, requires considerable familiarity with the technique.
- All approaches involving systems theory require that: (1) we learn to think in 'circular' terms about the causes of problems rather than in 'linear' terms (in Mr and Mrs Fox's case, this means getting away from asking 'who started it' and thinking instead about the nature of the vicious circle in which they find themselves); and (2) and that we are able to pay attention to process without being distracted too much by content. This requires some practice: we are accustomed to think in linear terms and, while we may notice process, the normal rules of conversation tend to direct us not to refer to it.

(Continued)

(Continued)

Ethical considerations

- Family systems approaches raise a number of difficult issues about *power*. One of these is that, by treating families as whole systems, family therapists may overlook the power relationships within the family, including adult–child differences and gender differences. Some members of the family may feel less able to express their point of view than others and may feel more obliged to paraphrase the opinions of others.
- Another power issue is the relationship of the 'therapist' to the family. Some forms of family therapy are intimidating and perhaps mystifying for service users and the methods used – video, one-way mirrors, unseen observers, strange and unfamiliar types of questioning – may be threatening. This is also an issue with other therapeutic approaches which involve the therapist directing the content of the session and taking a position of professional distance. (See Howe [1989], or Reimers and Treacher [1995] for more on this. Masson [1990] offers a more general critique on these lines of 'therapy' in general.)
- Looking at process as well as content may be useful, but it is important not to ignore content, for 'content' is after all what the members of a family feel they want to say.
- If a social worker is to use a therapeutic approach such as this, then it is important to be clear of her mandate to do so. Are the family – or some of the family – entering into this work because they genuinely wish to do so? And are they aware what they are agreeing to and what the ground rules are?
- If the social worker also has a 'control agent' role in the case – for example, if the social worker also has a child protection function – there are real difficulties in also working in a 'family therapy' role.

Real-world constraints

- Many social workers are simply not in a position to undertake formal family therapy for resource reasons as well as for reasons to do with their primary role.

Group work

... a method of social work practice which is concerned with the recognition and use of processes which occur when three or more people work together towards a common goal. (Doel, 2000: 148)

Part of the case for systemic family work is that we may not get anywhere if we try to work with an individual while ignoring the family group of which he is part. The individual may well be unable to sustain any change unless the family itself is able to change too and so give him space to function in a different way.

This demonstrates that groups are powerful and that group pressures can be a brake on individual growth. Working with people in groups, as opposed to working with them as individuals, is really a way of harnessing that power. Among its attractions are the way that it can empower service users because the members of a group are not just recipients of 'help', but are also themselves 'helpers' for other members of the group. Indeed, advocates of the group work approach would argue that mutual support from other people grappling with the same issues is often much more effective than any amount of one-to-one professional help. It can encourage self-reliance, promote self-esteem and, by putting people in contact with each other, build informal support networks with the potential to outlast professional involvement.

Groups can also reduce the sense of isolation that, for people struggling with life challenges of many different kinds, is often one of the hardest things to cope with. Think of bereavement, coping with the demands of a disabled child, or working as a foster parent or recovering from mental illness. Finding we are not alone is, for most of us, a positive experience, and it is an experience that groupwork can provide very effectively.

Of course, groups vary a great deal, in size, in duration, in composition. Some groups have a fixed time limit; others are open-ended. Some are 'closed', in the sense that once established, they do not take in new members; others can be joined at any stage. Some are organised around a very specific agenda; others evolve their own agendas as they progress. Some have their agenda set for them by those setting up the group (for example a group run for sexual offenders in a prison); some have an agenda chosen by their members. Preston-Shoot (1987: 11) divides groups into a number of (not necessarily mutually exclusive) different types:

- *Social groups*: such as youth clubs, clubs for elderly people or people with learning disabilities, which are intended to provide opportunities for recreation and friendship.
- *Psychotherapy groups*: here the group is a therapeutic resource intended to provide the members with an experience which they can use to bring about personal change.
- *Counselling groups*: aimed at helping group members resolve specific problems. A group for people with eating problems might be an example.
- *Educational groups*: aimed at providing information or skills training. Antenatal classes would be an example, as would parenting skills groups in which specific information is offered to parents.
- *Social treatment groups*: aimed at helping group members to modify behaviours or develop new behaviours: anger management groups, for example, or groups for offenders.
- *Discussion groups*: not focussed on problem-solving but on areas of mutual interest.
- *Self-help groups*: there is an element of self-help about groupwork in general, but these are groups in which the role of a professional group leader either does not exist at all, or is purely in a supportive, advisory role. (Preston-Shoot also gives a separate category of *self-directed groups*.)
- *Social action groups*: groups set up to campaign for the purposes of achieving some form of social or political change. A neighbourhood group set up to campaign for better facilities would be an example.

What happens within a group, and the role of group leaders or facilitators, will of course vary depending on the type of group, its purpose and the way it is set up. A social group is a very different kind of entity from a social *action* group and the skills required to facilitate a self-help group may be very different from those involved in running a psychotherapeutic group. Specifically in a therapeutic kind of group (including what Preston-Shoot calls 'counselling' and 'social treatment' groups) the same distinction between *content* and *process*, that we discussed in relation to family work, becomes important (a family is, after all, a particular type of group). Awareness of the process is important in any type of group, but in groups set up with a therapeutic purpose, the process may in a sense be the *point* of the group, the source of change:

> In a successful group, process ... operates to change basic raw materials – that is the individual members – by generating a situation in which the members gradually become a functioning unit and thus gain access to resources which were not available to them before. (Douglas, 2000: 86)

Among the different processes that occur within the life of a group, Douglas (2000: 37) identifies the following:

- *Interaction.*
- *Structural processes*: including group development, establishment of roles and status of group members, the formation of sub-groups.
- *Operational processes*: including the formation of goals, decision-making and making use of resources.
- *Regulating processes*: including setting norms, standards and values, developing cohesion, acquiring influence and developing an ethos.

Effective groupwork consists of harnessing these processes in the service of whatever is the purpose of the group and in the interests of the group's individual members.

Exercise 6.3

The Greytown Children and Families social work team spend a lot of time working with young single mothers who are struggling to cope with their children's behaviour. They have always responded to this on an individual casework basis, carrying out 'assessments' of families who self-refer or are referred to them, and then offering some combination of the following services:

- Referral on to Child and Adolescent Mental Health services.
- Referral to the local Family Centre for parenting skills work.
- Family Aid visits home to work with mother on parenting skills.

What is the drawback of these responses? What might be a groupwork alternative?

Comments

The disadvantages of the responses offered (which are not untypical of those offered by social work teams in these circumstances) seem to me to be:

- *They deal with cases in isolation and offer no opportunity to struggling parents to discover that there are others in the same boat, or to build their own networks of support.*
- *The individual casework approach, even if this is not intended, can suggest a medical model in which the parent is in need of treatment and the social work team are the experts who carry out an 'assessment' (diagnosis) and prescribe an intervention (treatment).*

(Continued)

(Continued)

A groupwork response might be not to try and respond to such cases on an individual basis but to set up groups which struggling parents might be invited to join. Ideally, several types of groups would be offered to meet different needs and preferences. Some groups might serve a largely social function for isolated parents, some might be educational groups, imparting information on child development or behaviour management techniques, or counselling groups in which the participants worked together on behaviour management problems. Some groups might be helped to evolve involve into self-help groups or social action groups; working to improve facilities for parents in the area.

Groupwork is an attractive and useful alternative to individual casework in many respects, for all the reasons given earlier. But it is important to remember that 'small groups are a microcosm of the wider society: status and stereotypes will be transferred from the wider society to the group' (Phillips, 2001: 55). In other words, power imbalances will exist within a group and, since group pressures are powerful, groups have the potential to be oppressive.

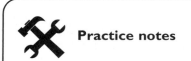 **Practice notes**

Groupwork

Skill requirements

- Ability to recognise group processes.
- Setting up groups in a way appropriate to the task in hand.
- Striking an appropriate balance as group leader/facilitator between being overly directive and failing to provide structure when needed.
- Assertiveness and ability to deal with conflict.
- Ability to deal with distress in a group context.
- Ability to deal with beginnings and endings.

Ethical considerations

- Openness and clarity about purpose are important in group work.
- Rules about acceptable communication and confidentiality need to be clear.
- A group facilitator needs to recognise his powerful position.
- Significant issues to do with power may arise in respect of group members (issues of gender, class, race, disability, sexuality, and so on) and it is necessary to be aware of and sensitive to individual vulnerability.

(Continued)

(Continued)

- In the case of groups where there is an element of compulsion about participating (for example, groups set up for offenders who may be labelled as unco-operative if they do not attend), the usual ethical issues arise about mixing therapeutic and policing roles.
- An exclusively group work response to a given problem area might be discriminatory in respect of people who do not like joining groups and prefer the individual approach.

Real-world constraints

- Although, at first sight a cost-effective alternative to individual or family work, group work involves a significant amount of additional work in terms of setting up and maintaining a group, and the associated logistics.

↗ Group care and therapeutic communities

In some contexts, social workers work with groups of service users as a matter of course, not in a formal group work context but because of the nature of the task. Such contexts include working in day centres, working in residential establishments and working with service users living in group homes. We can loosely categorise these settings together as different forms of 'group care'. Although work in this context does of course involve individual work, it is worth noting that it also involves working with groups of a very particular kind and in which the social worker has a particular sort of relationship with the service users involved:

- The social worker may be involved in delivering practical, physical care, or in supervising others who are delivering such care (feeding, bathing, taking people to the toilet, taking them to school, arranging doctor's appointments: the precise tasks will vary from one context to another).
- More than in many other contexts, social workers typically have what I called in Chapter 1 a 'responsibility holder' role: they carry responsibilities and perform tasks which might otherwise normally be carried out by close relatives.
- Social workers do not just come together with service users to carry out specific tasks, but are also informally in contact with them, sometimes for long periods. Residential social workers in a children's home, for instance may eat with residents, watch television with them, go on outings with them.
- Social workers operate as part of a team in a much more total sense than is the case for fieldworkers. They do not just share an office with other staff, but actually share the same group of service users and must pass on information and uncompleted tasks to other staff at the end of shifts.

(Continued)

(Continued)

The idea of a *therapeutic community* draws on the potential of a group living situation for a group based process of a particularly intensive kind, in which 'all members of the community, whether staff or "clients", work together on understanding and resolving whatever difficulties and conflicts may arise, whether for individuals, or for groups or for the community as a whole' (Ward, 2003: 33).

Community work

... the methods and skills used to work with people around a shared interest or concern. At the core of the methods and skills is the idea of organizing: helping people to come together to form an autonomous group. (Henderson, 2000: 72)

If it is sometimes more effective to work with groups or families than with individuals, then it seems to follow naturally that in some respects it may be better to work with communities. Community work is not a completely separate activity from group work, however, since a community work intervention typically involves the community worker attempting to encourage the development of groups. But the interest in community work lies particularly in the self-help and social action end of the group work spectrum, rather than the psychotherapeutic end. Community work is not about experts doing things for people, either individually or in groups, but about promoting the development of organised activity by the community itself either to:

- create its own resources to meet its needs (setting up a playgroup for example or a club for old people); or
- campaign to bring in resources from outside (setting up a neighbourhood pressure group, for instance, aimed at getting the local council to provide better facilities for children or old people).

In this context the community worker tries to be an enabler, a catalyst, rather than a solver of problems. But there are tensions in this role. As Popple (1994: 24) notes: 'Historically community work has developed from two distinct roots: benevolent paternalism and collective community action.' The difficulty is that community workers who are employed by the state are to a degree always outsiders, professionals, external to the community that they serve and therefore, however much they are committed to collective community action, a degree of 'benevolent paternalism' is inherent in the role.

The word 'community' is a rather vague term. It is a rather romantic notion that a whole neighbourhood does, or can, function as a single entity. A neighbourhood really consists of a series of overlapping communities – communities of interest, ethnic communities, geographical communities, extended families, workplaces – many of which will extend outside that specific neighbourhood. One of the things that a community worker needs to be clear about is *what* community she is working with (or indeed what community she is trying to help build). A community worker will typically single out for attention groups within a neighbourhood who may be losing out from mainstream services.

Practice notes

Community work

Skill requirements

- Networking skills; social confidence.
- Political skills (for example, the ability to recognise leaders, form alliances, make deals).
- Entrepreneurial skills.
- All the skills identified under 'group work'.

Ethical considerations

- All the values issues identified under 'group work' are relevant here.
- In forming alliances with local leaders, the community worker needs to bear in mind that the interests of the leaders are not necessarily the same as those they lead, and indeed the status of 'leaders' may be debatable. After all a local gangster may be a leader in his community but this does not mean he is necessarily welcomed or acknowledged as such.
- Particularly in relation to ethnic minority groups, the notion of 'community leaders' can promote a rather racist tribalised stereotype of ethnic minorities.

Real-world constraints

- Community work is unlikely to be an option for social workers other than those employed with a specific community work brief.

Society as a system

All the ways of working that I have described in this chapter share what might be called the 'systemic insight'. They recognise that the human individual does not exist in isolation but in relation to other people and that bringing about change for an individual may be inseparable from bringing about change in the social groups of which she is a part.

A logical extension of this way of thinking is to look at society as a whole as a system and to look at the interactions that take place within society itself in terms of process rather than simply content. This is basically what sociologists and anthropologists do for a living. It is also, in a sense, what I recommended in Chapter 1 when I suggested that it was important to distinguish rhetoric from underlying reality: what we are told is the purpose of some new policy is not necessarily the same thing as the social function it will actually serve.

Thinking in this way, one of the paths to follow is to ask what is the purpose that social work plays in the system that is society as a whole? Clearly in terms of *content* that purpose is to help people who are marginalised or disadvantaged, but some radical critics of social work argue that in terms of *process* what social work really does is something more like controlling those people or keeping them out of sight. (But this is something that I will discuss more fully in Chapter 11.)

There is certainly a danger that, in focussing too exclusively on any one level it is possible to overlook really important factors on other levels. Social workers might sometimes criticise health workers for focussing too much on the biological level – prescribing drugs for example to 'treat' behaviour problems the origin of which could easily be accounted for in terms of the family history or family environment – but social workers themselves may sometimes be guilty of focussing too exclusively on the individual/psychological level or on intermediate levels such as that of family systems, and failing to recognise the societal or political factors in a situation. Social workers who view their primary role as essentially therapeutic can sometimes be prone to discount the importance of factors such as poverty, poor housing and other kinds of social deprivation, or to look at requests for help with purely practical matters such as housing as being merely 'presenting problems', which the worker should try to look behind to identify underlying psychological difficulties. The traditional left-wing critique of social work points out that this type of manoeuvre, by locating 'all social work's problems in the personal sphere and in the psychological sphere' (Bailey and Brake, 1975: 19), has the effect of obscuring social injustices by in effect blaming the victim, even making the victim herself feel that her problems are the consequence of the flaws and shortcomings of her personality.

There is of course also a right-wing critique of social work (or rather of welfare provision generally), which is almost the mirror image of this: social work pays too much attention to the societal and family system levels and not *enough* to the level of the individual. By allowing people to blame their problems on other people, or on society, it undermines people's ability to take responsibility for themselves. The following extract from an interview with the former UK Prime Minister, Margaret Thatcher, in which she made the famous comment that there was 'no such thing' as society, is a statement of that point of view:

> I think we have gone through a period when too many children and people have been given to understand 'I have a problem, it is the Government's job to cope with it!' or 'I have a problem, I will go and get a grant to cope with it!' 'I am homeless, the Government must house me!' and so they are casting their problems on society and who is society? There is no such thing! There are individual men and women and there are families and no government can do anything except through people and people look to themselves first. It is our duty to look after ourselves and then also to help look after our neighbour and life is a reciprocal business and people have got the entitlements too much in mind without the obligations, because there is no such thing as an entitlement unless someone has first met an obligation. (Margaret Thatcher, interviewed by Douglas Keays, 1987)

I find it interesting that, while the right- and left-wing critiques are in some respects opposites, they both share the concern that help provided by the state may be in some way disabling to its recipients; by discouraging them from acting on their own behalf.

Chapter summary

In this chapter I have looked at working with service users from the perspective of various different levels, from the level of families and groups to the political level. The topics covered have been:

- **System levels:** Different levels – from biological to societal/political – at which we can look for explanations and plan interventions.
- **Family systems:** The idea of families as systems, the concept of circular causality, the distinction between process and content and a very brief introduction to family therapy as an approach.
- **Group work:** The use of groups as an alternative to working with individuals.
- **Community work:** Work aimed at strengthening a community's own resources.
- **Society as a system:** Society is itself a system. What role does social work play in that system, in terms of process rather than content?

The next chapter will look at task-centred casework and at crisis intervention work.

7 | Tasks and crises

In my experience, social workers, asked about how they do their job, will often refer to 'task-centred work' or 'crisis intervention'. Sometimes what social workers seem to mean by 'task-centred work' is that they do a great deal of work that involves practical tasks, as opposed to (say) work of a more therapeutic kind, so that what they are really referring to is the fact that a lot of their work seems to place them in what I described in Chapter 1 as 'executive' roles. As I've said before, I regard the executive roles as important and integral parts of social work, if not *the* most distinctive of social work's roles. However, they are not really what was originally meant by the term 'task-centred casework', which is a distinct framework for social work practice based on rather simple but persuasive ideas about what helps people to change. However, even allowing for the fact that the term is sometimes misused, I would guess that approaches related to task centred work are among the most widely used methods in social work.

Just as the term 'task centred' is sometimes used in a rather general way, so is the term 'crisis intervention'. When social workers talk about 'crisis intervention', they sometimes mean simply that they spend a lot of time having to work with people who are at the point of crisis. This is of course true of most, if not all, social workers. We might prefer to be able to intervene before things got to crisis point, or even to provide universal services that prevented the need for any social work intervention at all, but when resources are limited and have to be rationed, it is often the case that a situation has to be at or near crisis point before it is regarded as high enough priority for a social worker to become involved at all. However, though all this is so, the term 'crisis intervention' strictly refers to something rather more specific than simply intervening in a crisis. It referred to methods of intervention that drew on ideas about the psychology of people in crises.

So this chapter looks at two terms that are often used rather loosely, and considers what they meant in their original, more specific, senses. Themes linking the two are an interest in how people move forward when they are feeling overwhelmed and a belief in the value of focussed, time-limited work.

Order and chaos

Exercise 7.1

Margaret Brown is the mother of four sons aged 11, nine, seven and five. She has been bringing them up on her own since the suicide of her husband Tom two years ago. With her agreement, she has been referred to a social work agency by the head-teacher of the boys' school for help with coping with the four boys who Margaret says are completely out of her control. She says they eat when they want to, get up when they want to, come in when they want to. If she attempts to stop them from doing anything they ignore her or are abusive. They have destroyed much of the furniture in the house.

In fact the social work agency have received a number of previous referrals about this family. Neighbours have expressed concern that all four boys are out in the street until late at night and that they have been involved in minor acts of vandalism in the area. Visitors to the house have reported that the house is dirty and chaotic and that there is a strong smell of urine.

The boys have until recently been going to school regularly, but increasingly are not doing so. Their school reports that one problem for them there is that they smell of urine and are teased by other children.

Margaret says that the younger two boys still regularly wet the bed. In fact she says they regularly wet *her* bed, because the whole family typically ends up sleeping together in one bed, a habit the boys got into at the time of their father's death. Margaret, described by the referrer as 'an intelligent, thoughtful and articulate woman' who once trained as a teacher, says that when Tom was alive 'we had problems but it was nothing like this'.

Although the family has been referred with Margaret's agreement, and although the head-teacher has a great deal of sympathy for Margaret – a former member of his own profession – the referrer, and other professional agencies are increasingly worried about the emotional development and well-being of these children and consider that the status quo cannot be allowed to continue.

What are your thoughts about how things have got like this and how the members of the family might now be feeling about their situation?

(Continued)

(Continued)

Comments

Margaret herself identifies the death of her husband as the turning point for this family. 'Things seem to have fallen apart from that point' is how you might have put it. You might have thought in terms of unresolved grief or depression or suggested that for some reason the family had failed to 'move on from' their bereavement or 'work through' their grief.

If you forget about explanations and labels and simply look at how things might now feel to Margaret you might use words such as 'defeated', 'overwhelmed'. You might say that she has just 'given up'. Whatever the origins of the problem, it is not hard to see why she might feel like this now because she has so many different problems to deal with. The fact that the headteacher who made the referral considers her care of her children to be inadequate is quite likely to add to her feelings of failure and of inadequacy.

If you look at it from the point of view of the boys, you might conclude that they too have given up. They are simply distracting themselves as best they can from painful and uncomfortable feelings, without any purpose or direction in their lives.

I imagine that everyone must be familiar with the experience of having so many things to do that they 'don't know where to start'. It is quite easy in such situations to panic at the size of the task and to feel slightly paralysed; ending up doing nothing useful at all. A way that people often cope with this type of situation is to compile a list of all the things that they feel they need to do and then to prioritise – *these are the things I need to do immediately, these can be put off for a short while, these I could perhaps decide not to do at all* – and to break down the jobs into smaller, more manageable tasks. As most people probably know from personal experience, a strategy of this kind can break the log-jam because, by giving yourself permission not to think about the other nine tasks for the present, you make it possible to focus on one. It is a strategy that we are all aware of and that we advise one another to follow at difficult times: 'One thing at a time'; 'You've got to take one day at a time.'

Task-centred casework is a method of doing social work that uses this very basic principle – the principle of breaking problems down into manageable chunks which can be taken one at a time – to provide a set of tools and techniques. Mark Doel and Peter Marsh note, with some justice, that there is a noticeable tendency for writers about social work to make 'The Grand Statement (for example, "social workers should combat this or that aspect of racism/sexism etc.") unaccompanied by much in the way of practical advice' (Doel and Marsh, 1992: 7). But practical advice is precisely what task-centred casework offers.

Behind each of the sets of ideas I have discussed in the previous three chapters lies a characteristic key insight. The key insight of task-centred casework, on the face of it so straightforward as barely to constitute a theory at all, is surely that many of the clients of social work services are indeed in the position of being overwhelmed by the challenges they face that it is hard to know where to start. (Social workers in busy agencies of course often feel in the same position.) If the intervention of a social worker is not going to be in danger of *adding* to the problems of service users, by becoming yet one more thing to deal with, the social worker needs to be clear about the following:

- The intervention should have a purpose.
- That purpose should be possible to be clearly stated and there should be a shared understanding with the service user about what it is.
- Steps towards achieving that purpose need to be practical, clearly defined – in terms of goals, responsibilities and timescales – appropriately prioritised and broken down into achievable chunks.
- Except in certain clearly defined and legally mandated situations the entire plan – its purpose, the steps to be taken and the priorities – should be chosen by the client or with the client and have the client's agreement and support, not just for ethical reasons, important though they obviously are, *but because otherwise the intervention will not work.* (The exception to this principle is the type of compulsory intervention that social workers are sometimes required to take to protect vulnerable people. In the UK this would include, for instance the compulsory removal of a person to a safe place under Section 47 of the National Assistance Act, 1948 or the removal of a child who is at serious risk of harm into public care.)

To someone with no experience of social work practice these principles might seem so obviously sensible as to be almost self-evident. The reason why they are so vitally important in social work is that, in practice, a whole host of pressures are on social workers which militate against having a clear plan at all, with the result that there is a constant danger that social workers' energy will end up being wasted and dissipated in ineffective activity with no overall end in view.

Exercise 7.2

Supposing you were the social worker assigned the case of Margaret and her sons described above in Exercise 7.1. How would you feel about the case? Do you think that you might be in danger of losing your sense of clear overall purpose? If so, why?

Comments

If I was the social worker for this case I can imagine that, if I wasn't careful, I might end up feeling overwhelmed by the family's problems rather in the way that the family members themselves are. I might have difficulty 'knowing where to start' with the family's many problems. What other factors might make a social worker lose a sense of direction in this case? Margaret Brown is a thoughtful, articulate person and it might be quite easy for the social worker to fall into a sort of quasi-friendship with her, consisting of a series of interesting conversations about Margaret and her problems without any end in sight. Therapeutically inclined social workers might find themselves inclined to fall into a therapist mode in which Margaret's own history and feelings became the focus and practical problem solving is forgotten.

Alternatively, pressure from other agencies to 'do something' (which can become quite acute in situations like this) could result in a social worker feeling that it was necessary to introduce a whole range of different services to the family – bereavement counselling, parenting skills training, activities for the children, input from child psychiatric services – thus dissipating the families energies to the point where all these services effectively cancelled one another out.

It is a law of the universe (the Second Law of Thermodynamics, in fact) that order tends to disintegrate into chaos. Human life in a sense represents a constant struggle against this tendency and when we are tired, or overwhelmed by the demands on us, the struggle can seem too much, for clients and for social workers alike. The task-centred casework model provides a framework for keeping a focus and helping social workers and clients from being defeated by the scale of the problems which face us:

> The basic strategy of brief, task-centred casework rests on one central assumption: that the effectiveness and efficiency of methods normally used in casework practice can be increased considerably if they are concentrated on helping clients achieve specific and limited goals of their own choice within brief, bounded periods of service. (Reid and Epstein, 1972: 146–7)

The task-centred method

Task-centred casework is 'one of the few practice theories used within social work which originated and developed wholly within social work, rather than being an existing set of ideas imported from outside' (Payne, 1997: 49). It has in common with SFBT, discussed in Chapter 5, that it is not about offering explanations and that it emphasises brief, focussed interventions, aimed at empowering the service user to resolve their own problems within a defined period of time, rather than create dependency through long-term, unfocussed 'support' (the word 'support' is, in my experience often used by social workers to describe visiting with no clear objective or purpose, which service users may not necessarily even find supportive). Like SFBT, task-centred casework has affinities with behaviourism and, like SFBT and behavioural approaches, also claims to be evidence based, that is: based on rigorous trials of what works in practice (see, for instance, Reid, 1997).

Task-centred casework does not offer an explanatory theory, but a means of structuring the process of working towards solutions to problems with the aim of: (1) helping resolve the specific problem in question; and (2) giving the service user a positive experience of problem solving in general. This general approach, like that of SFBT, also sits well with the behaviourist view that I discussed in Chapter 4. Task-centred casework, properly done, should help to reinforce problem-solving behaviour rather than dependant behaviour.

The following are the main elements of the task-centred approach.

Exploring problems

The first stage of the process is to identify the areas that the service user is finding a problem and wants to change. The skill here is to ensure that all the problems which are important to the service user are identified, without going into too much detail on any of them: 'The intention is to get as many of the problems as possible out in the open, and in brief form, so that the range of difficulties can be seen' (Doel and Marsh, 1992: 27).

In a pure version of the task-centred model, what constitutes a problem would be defined entirely by the service user. In practice, in a variety of circumstances, there are often problems which the *social worker* needs to put on the list ('you are leaving your children on their own in the house and this isn't acceptable'). The method doesn't work if clients are forced to work on problems which are of no interest to them – Reid, (1997: 135) identifies 'the degree of client commitment or motivation to do the task' as a key predictor of success in outcome studies – but in practice there is often scope for negotiation. Clients may at least partly acknowledge that problems identified by the social worker are problems and they may be willing to work on these problems if they can see that the issues that they themselves have identified as priorities are also firmly on the agenda. What is more, for involuntary clients (often called '*mandated* clients' in the US literature), the very fact that they *are* involuntary clients is often a priority problem – so that they may be willing to work on key issues defined by the professional agencies in order to end this unwanted status. (This is really the basis of what I will define in Chapter 10 as 'protective leverage'.) Central to the task-centred model, though, is the principle that the client has the right to refuse 'help'. As Doel and Marsh (1992: 34) put it: 'if there is no agreement on problems and no acceptance of mandated problems, it cannot be said to be task-centred practice.'

Two important aspects of problem exploration using a task-centred approach are as follows. First, social workers need to avoid jumping ahead of the process by immediately identifying solutions. What is needed at the exploration stage is clarity as to the problems themselves. Second, and this is one of the most attractive features of the model, social workers need to be clear from the outset about the model itself:

> The practitioner shares assessment information and avoids hidden goals and agendas. The client's input is used in developing treatment strategies, not only to devise more effective interventions, but also to develop the client's problem-solving abilities. (Reid, 1997: 132)

Having identified the main problems, the next stage is to put those problems in some sort of priority order and to identify a small number (up to three at any one time is suggested) to be worked on first. Reid and Epstein (1972) speak of 'target problems'; Doel and Marsh (1992: 32) refer to 'lead problems':

> Some explanation is likely to be useful at this stage to point out that no problem need be lost forever, it is just a case of tackling things in order … . The workers may point out that this way of working is known to be effective, and that tackling too much at once risks not being able to achieve anything at all … . It may be useful to bear in mind that achieving a small success is likely to be much better than achieving a spectacular failure.

The written agreement

Having identified the lead problems to work on, the model now moves onto the question of what to do about it. One part of this is to agree on goals. What, in relation to this particular problem, does the client want to be different? These goals should be realistic and should be defined in terms which are clear and unambiguous and which lend themselves, as far as possible, to some sort of measurement so that social worker and client can tell what progress is being made towards meeting them. ('To do more things together as a family' is a goal, but a slightly vague one, 'To go out as a family at least once a fortnight' is more specific.) Alongside goals, a clear timescale should be agreed for the achievement of each goal. Selected problems, goals and timescales then form the basis of a written agreement between social worker and client, or clients, which provides a framework and focus for subsequent activity.

Tasks

Tasks are incremental steps towards achieving a goal and, as the name of the model suggests, they are at the core of the task-centred process. Having negotiated a written agreement the process then consists of agreeing tasks, meeting regularly to monitor progress and offering support to the service user in completing the tasks. Part of the skill required for effective task-centred work lies in ensuring that the tasks selected are doable, for setting the client up to fail with impossible tasks would be counterproductive. Another part of the skill lies in the way that the client is supported during the process.

This is not to say that *all* tasks need necessarily be the responsibility of the client. Tasks can be taken on by the social worker as well – and this is usually appropriate. But if the social worker takes on all the tasks the work ceases to be task-centred casework and becomes something more akin to care management. In a case such as that of Margaret and her sons in Exercise 7.1 this would not be appropriate for at least two reasons. First, it would deprive them of the experience of resolving things for themselves and very likely confirm their sense of helplessness. Second (and more fundamentally), it would simply be ineffective, since the kinds of problem that exist in this case – the children wet the bed, they stay out late at night, they do not do what their mother asks – are to do with the behaviour of Margaret and the boys. Services and support can be provided but, however, much one feels for their plight, it is quite literally impossible for the home situation to change unless she and they are willing to do some things differently from what they are doing now. Whatever tasks the social worker takes on, and services he provides, these can only support Margaret and the boys themselves in making changes. They cannot make the changes for her. I emphasise this point because it is something that it is easy to get confused about. It can feel 'unfair' to expect people in desperate situations to make changes themselves. But there is often no alternative. What the task-centred model offers is a means of making this unavoidable fact less daunting.

The task centred model is eclectic with regard to the support offered. Having no particular explanatory model of its own, it is perfectly possible, for instance, to offer Rogerian counselling or psychodynamic therapy as an adjunct to a task-centred piece of work. Equally it would be perfectly consistent with the model for the social worker to switch to a 'care management' role and provide services such as activities for the children as part of the work. But at the core of the approach is the idea of helping to focus the client's own problem-solving abilities in a way that will maximise the chances of success:

> Once a task is agreed on, the caseworker's techniques are concentrated almost exclusively on helping the client carry it out. It is assumed that this focusing of activity is one key to the relative success of brief, time-limited therapies. Not only is a maximum of caseworker effort brought to bear upon a narrow sector of the client's life-space, but the client's efforts are concentrated there as well. (Reid and Epstein, 1972: 147)

Termination of involvement

Central to the task-centred approach is the need for *clarity* and *transparency* about what is happening. I mentioned earlier the universal tendency of things to degenerate from order into confusion, and it is certainly true that social work can very easily lose focus to a point where both the social worker and the client cease to be clear about where they are heading and what they are trying to achieve. Task-centred work involves being explicit about the method used and about things such as goals, tasks and timescales. It also involves being completely clear about the *mandate* (that is: the basis for the social worker being involved at all), which I will discuss shortly. Finally, and very importantly, it involves being clear when social work involvement ends. The ending should not come as a surprise to the client because the timescale for the work should have been agreed at the outset and, if extensions have been found to be necessary, these too should have been discussed, agreed and placed on the shared record of the process. But when the end is reached the task-centred model proposes that it should be formally marked by a review of the process. Here the client is given an opportunity to comment and place on record what they have found helpful or unhelpful about the work, how successful it has been and what they have taken from it.

Clarity about mandate

As I have already noted, the task-centred model can only be used to address problems which clients themselves are motivated to do something about. This position can be easily parodied, as in the old joke about how many social workers it takes to change a light bulb (answer: 'One, but the light bulb has got to *really want* to change'), but in fact it ought to be obvious that trying to work with people on problems that they have no interest in tackling is normally both a waste of time and unethical – and often actually counter-productive. A failure to grasp this can result in social workers drifting into casework relationships where there is no clear understanding with the service user as to the purpose of their involvement. One of the key insights at the heart of task-centred casework is a recognition of the futility of much of this sort of unfocused visiting, which social workers nevertheless still often undertake, either to allay their own anxieties or the anxieties of other professionals who are often keen for a social worker to be involved in cases even if there is no clear purpose.

However, as I have already noted, a task-centred approach is applicable in work with involuntary service users when there is at least some genuine agreement with the service user about the nature of at least some of the problems to be addressed and at least some willingness to work on agreed problems. Chris Trotter (2004: 80), writing about involuntary clients, concludes:

> In our study we anticipated that clients would do better if their workers talked to them about a range of problems. We also anticipated that the clients would do better if they defined the problems rather than the worker. This was clearly the case.

I will come back to these matters in Chapter 10, which explores the particular issues involved in working in a 'control agent' role. Sufficient to say for the moment that if there is *no* agreement at all on the problems to be addressed, then task-centred work, along with other kinds of 'direct change agent' work, cannot take place. People really cannot either usefully or ethically be 'sentenced to help' (Bottoms and McWilliams, 1979, as cited by Doel and Marsh, 1992: 34). If a client is not interested in working with a social worker, and if the client or someone else is placed at risk of serious harm as a result, then (depending on the context and her precise legal responsibilities) the social worker may have to resort to taking protective action in a 'control agent' capacity. Otherwise the social worker should consider closing the case. Much social work time is wasted in my experience by not being clear about the need to make this basic choice, so that social work 'involvement' continues in cases where there is *neither* a legal mandate for protective intervention, *nor* a mandate from the service users themselves.

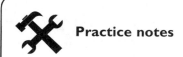 **Practice notes**

Task-centred casework

Skill requirements

- To apply the task-centred model, like other models, requires not only knowledge of the model in principle, but fluency in practice. The general principles are exceptionally easy to understand and to explain to others, but considerable skill is involved in negotiating a workable agreement with realistic goals and tasks, and in supporting service users during the process of carrying out tasks.
- Most aspects of the process require skills in listening and communicating clearly.
- An ability to convey confidence in the service user and in the method is likely to be crucial to success.

Ethical considerations

- I have already quoted the very important point, made by the originators of task-centred casework themselves, that the client should have the right to refuse the social worker's help. A strength of a task-centred approach is that it allows the social worker to be clear with the service user about the nature of the help that is on offer.
- However, just giving the service user this right is not necessarily enough, because of the power difference between social worker and service user (for example, a service user might be reluctant to actually exercise the right to refuse help if she felt that this might adversely affect her relationship with the social worker). We should be very wary about the nature of 'agreements' (or 'contracts') drawn up between social workers and service users in situations – such as child protection cases – where the social worker is there is a 'protective' role, exercising, or potentially exercising, statutory powers. In law a contract is not valid if one of the parties was under duress – and we should remember this principle in social work.

(Continued)

(Continued)

- Agreements in writing are also distrusted by many people – particularly those with limited literacy skills – and may make people feel pinned-down or trapped unless they are very confident that nothing is in there that they have not understood or agreed to.
- An approach that essentially supports the service user in sorting through and then working to resolve her own problems is, in many ways, empowering. It avoids setting the worker up as expert or the service user as victim or passive recipient. The process is also exceptionally transparent. 'The openness of the model allows the client and others the opportunity of challenging the work undertaken' (Doel and Marsh, 1992: 4).
- On the other hand, 'task-centred practice might be criticized for focusing on the individual case ... and thus locating the problem with the individual' (Doel and Marsh 1992: 97), even if the problem is caused by factors external to the individual (for example racial harassment). Having said this, though, there is no reason in principle why advocacy and self-advocacy, should not be chosen as tasks: in which case the task-centred process would simply be about supporting the client in getting what she is entitled to, and would not in any way mean locating the problem itself with her.

Real-world constraints

- This model is probably easier than many to use in the real-world context of limited time and constant pressure put on social workers to take on new cases and close existing ones as quickly as possible. It isn't appropriate where there is no agreement between client and social worker as to the problems to be worked on. It isn't appropriate when the client is not capable of sustained rational thought. It may not be appropriate where the social worker has a very narrow brief of assessing eligibility for material help and services: for example, the parent of a disabled child has contacted the social worker's agency to request some assistance with day care and has no interest in any form of casework help.

Equilibrium and crisis

I commented earlier on the tendency for order to disintegrate into chaos and the word crisis is often used to describe times when the established order of our lives seems to have disintegrated or to be in danger of doing so. 'A time of intense difficulty or danger,' is the first definition given by the *NODE* (2001). We think of public events like the Cuban missile crisis of the 1960s, when the balance of power of the cold war seemed likely to disintegrate into all-out nuclear war, or personal events such as being made redundant, or the break-up of a marriage or a sudden bereavement – times during which people often feel that 'their world is falling apart' and that the whole purpose and meaning of their life is under threat. Gerald Caplan referred to a crisis as 'something that is, for a time, insurmountable by the use of customary methods of problem solving.' This results in a 'period of disorganization ...., a period of upset, during which many abortive attempts at a solution are made' (Caplan, 1961, cited by Kanel, 2003: 1). A crisis is an event which stops us from being able to maintain equilibrium in the ways that we have been maintaining it up to now. Losing your job, for instance, makes it impossible to carry on with the same daily routine, to rely on the same monthly budget or to see yourself – and be seen by others – in the same way as before. The old ways of dealing with life, the old sources of security, simply don't work anymore. This can be profoundly disturbing.

So crises are threats to our equilibrium, to our established way of seeing the world. All kinds of events can be 'crises' in this sense, not just disasters but even events that seem positive, such as unexpectedly becoming a millionaire. Lottery winners often say things like 'it won't change my life' but of course it will, and statements of this kind can be seen as last-ditch attempts to stave off the threat posed by change and to hang onto equilibrium, not unlike the way that recently bereaved people for a short time are simply unable to take on board the reality of what has happened. Normal life events – the onset of adolescence, the birth of a child, retirement – can all be crises in this sense and can, for some people, be profoundly disturbing and disorientating.

However, the word crisis also has a rather different meaning. The word derives from the Greek *krisis* which means 'decision' and the *NODE* gives as a second definition 'a time when a difficult or important decision must be made'. A crisis is a 'crunch time': not simply a disaster but also potentially an opportunity for change. A crisis event destroys the old equilibrium but makes possible the development of new ones, which might otherwise never have surfaced. Being made redundant, for example, is for most people, a very distressing event. It can precipitate further catastrophic events, which in turn become crises: mental health breakdowns, marriage break-ups, even suicide. But for many people too it opens up new opportunities, which might otherwise never have been taken. When a caterpillar goes into a chrysalis its body disintegrates completely but, if all goes well, the new body of a moth or butterfly is able to form as a result of this disintegration. Even bereavement can be an occasion for growth.

We tend to react initially to any serious threat to our equilibrium by attempting to stave it off. If the threat is unavoidable, we may resort to various psychological defences ('it won't change my life', 'I refuse to accept that this is true'). If *these* fail we may become angry, disorientated or depressed. But if we are able to begin to accept what has happened – to stop hanging onto the old equilibrium – and instead begin to construct a new way of dealing with the world, then we may in due course arrive at a new equilibrium. I imagine that most people will know this is the case from personal experience of one kind or another.

⬀ Post-traumatic stress disorder

It is characteristic of our response to any crisis event that we cannot take it all in at once and cannot simply move forward without going through a stage of renegotiation and adjustment. Post-traumatic stress disorder (PTSD) is perhaps a very extreme instance of

(Continued)

(Continued)

this pattern. First described in relation to soldiers traumatised by their experiences in the front-line in the First World War (when it was known as 'shell-shock') PTSD occurs when people have been exposed to exceptionally frightening and horrific events. Its characteristics include recurrent recollections of the event which intrude into everyday life, recurrent dreams about the event and 'flashback' phenomena in which the event itself seems to be recurring. They also include intense psychological distress and actual physiological reaction (for example sweating and trembling) to situations that remind the sufferer of the traumatic event, avoidance of these situations and a general reduction of the sufferer's ability to focus on other aspects of life. It may be encountered by social workers in connection with people who have suffered rape, abuse or violent attacks, and people who have been involved in accidents and disasters (see Kanel, 2003: 202–39).

Crises and social work

Crises are central to social work for several reasons. First, it is typically a crisis of some sort that precipitates the involvement in the first place of social workers in the lives of their service users. Hospital social workers, for instance, are typically dealing with people whose everyday lives have been disrupted by illness. Social workers with the elderly first meet their clients at the point when they are no longer being able to manage their own day-to-day lives without outside help – for many people a hugely difficult point to have reached and a hugely difficult point to *admit* to having reached. Many people require long-term input from social work services after the point of crisis is passed but most social work involvement begins with a crisis of some kind, even if not necessarily a very catastrophic one. As I noted at the beginning of this chapter, this is exacerbated by the rationing systems that social work agencies typically have to put in place because of limitations on their time and resources. Sometimes a crisis has to become acute before a person is able to reach the eligibility criterion for a service.

Second, and this is something not so often discussed either in the literature on social work or the literature on crises, social workers are not uncommonly in the business of *deliberately precipitating* crises in people's lives. To give an example: precipitating a crisis (albeit, perhaps, a comparatively small one) is what, in essence, a youth justice worker is doing when she tells a young offender that if he does not co-operate with the terms of the supervision order by showing up to appointments with her, she will have to take his case back to court. She is creating a situation in which the existing equilibrium (of carrying on without bothering to come to appointments) can no longer be maintained and in which a decision of some kind must be made. I will come back to these kinds of scenario in Chapter 10 when I discuss what I call 'protective leverage'.

Third, even if a social worker has no intention of deliberately precipitating a crisis in the way I have just discussed, social work intervention in people's lives can, in itself, represent a crisis event. Social workers themselves may not always be aware of this. A social worker carrying out a child protection investigation may not ever know what kind of devastation this can leave behind in a family, even in cases where the investigation concludes that there is no risk to a child – in fact such situations may be the ones in which a family may feel most alone as it is left to pick up the pieces. A series of studies commissioned in the UK by the Department of Health (1995: 43) in the mid-1990s all confirmed 'the sense of shock, fear and anger' felt by families in the aftermath of child protection investigations, though many families were able too to identify positive consequences.

Crisis intervention

Crisis intervention is not a single model in the way that task-centred casework is a single model, but rather a group of models for short-term work with people at points of acute crisis, drawing on psychodynamic, systems theory and other branches of psychology, which focus on the known particular psychological characteristics of people in such situations. They are about 'helping people in crisis recognise and correct temporary affective, behavioral and cognitive distortions brought about by traumatic events' (James and Gilliland, 2005: 8), as illustrated by the following example:

> A student fails one algebra test and concludes that he or she can never pass algebra, therefore cannot become an engineer (as the parents are perceived to expect/demand). The student progresses to a feeling of helplessness, then to hopelessness, and then contemplates suicide. (2005: 8)

The distortion in this case lies in what, to an outside observer, seems the vastly inflated importance that the student is attaching to this single event. The aim of crisis intervention is to help the student to recognise that her perceptions and feelings about this are temporary ones, and that decisions should not be made on the basis of these alone. The example is also a reminder that what may seem like a relatively small event to one person may seem to be a catastrophe to another. In social work, we are apt to become inured to the significance of events that we witness all the time, and are therefore in danger of overlooking the effect that they have on others. The admission of an old person to a residential home, for instance, is a routine event for a social worker working with the elderly. But for an individual elderly person, for whom this may represent the end of 60 years of living as an independent adult, it may be an event of devastating importance. (Old people in this situation are sometimes wrongly assumed to be suffering from some form of dementia, because they seem confused and out of touch with their surroundings, when in fact this is simply the initial defensive response to the crisis).

Of course, many crises are precipitated by events which, even to an outside observer, do indeed seem catastrophic, but even in these situations, it is possible to move on from the feelings of paralysis, helplessness and despair that typically follow on from initial reactions of denial and disbelief. What the example of the student demonstrates is that without help some people may fail to make the necessary transition and emerge from the immobile state which is characteristic and normal in the immediate aftermath of a crisis event.

As I have said, there are a number of different models of crisis intervention. James and Gilliland (2005: 21–2) offer a 'six-step model', Kanel (2003: 29–59) describe a three-part 'ABC model'. I will not attempt to describe these models in detail here, partly because it seems to me that the response that is appropriate does depend on the scale and type of crisis involved, and that some of these models may be overly 'medical' and mechanistic. But among the essential components of crisis intervention are:

- It is important to establish a relationship with the person in crisis and provide her with space in which it is possible to describe what has occurred and express what she is feeling, bearing in mind that people in these situations may need to repeat this process many times and cannot be hurried through. Moving forward does not entail the suppression of painful feelings but rather a recognition of them.
- Understanding the effect of an event requires not only clarity about the actual facts of the event that occurred, but about the meaning of that event to the individual (as the example of the student above illustrates).
- People in acute crisis situations do not process information in the way they would otherwise. Things may need to be gone over many times.
- People in acute crisis situations typically feel paralysed. Their normal repertoire of responses is inadequate to deal with the new situation with which they are now faced, and they feel helpless. Part of the process of crisis intervention is helping bring people to a point where they begin to make choices again about how they are going to cope in the new situation in which they find themselves.
- At the same time (and here the task-centred approach becomes relevant) people in crisis need to be reassured that the process will take time, that moving on is a matter of taking small incremental steps and that it is not necessary to do everything at once. But, if a person is to move on, it is necessary to begin to do something:

  In the realm of crisis, *not to choose is a choice*, and this choice usually turns out to be negative and destructive. *Choosing to do something* at least contains the seeds of growth. (James and Gilliland, 2005: 4, Original emphasis)

- States of crisis do not last forever, and people are more receptive to help and to suggestions during the crisis state than they are at a later time:

  A crisis is by its nature a time-limited event in that a person cannot tolerate the extreme tension and psychological disequilibrium of the state for more than a few weeks … . Whether a person emerges stronger or weaker from a crisis is not based so much on previous character make-up, although this factor is relevant, as on the kind of help he or she receives during the actual crisis. (Kanel, 2003: 3)

Crisis intervention does not offer a single technique that can be taken up and applied by social workers, though it does offer a number of alternative intervention models. The important insight that it does offer, in my opinion, relates to the idea of crisis itself. I have suggested already that social workers are often insufficiently aware of the degree to which those they work with are in crisis and of the way that this will affect their functioning.

Exercise 7.3

Returning to the case of Margaret Brown and her sons, discussed in Exercise 7.1 and subsequently, do you see any useful application of the idea of crisis intervention to this scenario?

Comments

The obvious crisis point in this family was the loss of Tom, the father of the family, in a particularly distressing way two years ago. It would appear on the information available that this family did not find a way of coping successfully following this appalling crisis and may never have emerged from the feelings of paralysis and helplessness that followed it. With the benefit of hindsight, one might think that some intervention at the time of Tom's death might possibly have helped to prevent things from getting to this state.

However, the family have reached another kind of crisis with Margaret's own acknowledgement that she is not coping as a parent. A new crisis does provide opportunities to revisit issues from previous crises which have not been dealt with.

You might argue that this kind of work may need to be done with Margaret and/or the boys alongside, or prior to, more practicial tasks if the family are really going to be able to move on.

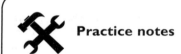 **Practice notes**

Crisis intervention

Skill requirements

- Working with people in a crisis requires the qualities of an 'effective helper', discussed in Chapter 5. It is necessary to convey empathy without being overwhelmed by the other person's distress; not necessarily an easy thing to do.
- To apply a specific crisis intervention approach requires not only knowledge of the model in principle but fluency in practice.

Ethical considerations

- Because someone is having a crisis does not necessarily mean they want professional help of a 'therapeutic' kind. Crises are a normal part of life – indeed a necessary part of life – and people usually prefer to deal with them with the help of family and friends. There is a danger of over-professionalising such things and making them the province of 'experts'. It would be wrong to assume that everyone who is experiencing a crisis or suffered a traumatic event necessarily needs professional help. And some people who *do* turn to professional agencies do so purely for practical help and do not want to be 'therapised'.

(Continued)

(Continued)

- The emphasis in crisis intervention theory on the crisis state as a window of opportunity, while intuitively convincing, raises serious issues about client vulnerability and professional power. Noting that 'a crisis worker can gain significant leverage at this time because of greater client vulnerability' Kristi Karel (2003: 4) acknowledges that 'It would be easy for an unscrupulous worker to take advantage of a client at a time of crisis'.

Real-world constraints

- Social work intervention following crises is not a theory or an aspiration but an existing fact. However, it is not always possible or appropriate for social workers to undertake crisis intervention work in a therapeutic sense. Apart from resource constraints which may prevent this, there is also the perennial issue about the way in which social work's different roles can clash with one another. For instance, from the point of view of a service user, the person who has just admitted you to an old people's home may not be the best person to work with you on the personal crisis that this has created; the person who is writing a report on you for a court may not be the person that you would wish to entrust with your feelings of loss, grief and fear.

Chapter summary

The headings dealt with in this chapter were as follows:

- **Order and chaos:** The tendency of things to disintegrate into chaos and disorder and how this applies both in the lives of people with whom social workers work and in social work itself.
- **The task-centred method:** An outline of the essential components of task-centred casework.
- **Clarity about mandate:** The importance in social work of being clear of the basis for your involvement with any given service user.
- **Equilibrium and crisis:** Crisis as an event that disrupts the equilibrium of life and which cannot be dealt with by a person's normal repertoire of responses.
- **Crises and social work:** Social workers normally deal with people in crisis and also often themselves bring about crises, sometimes deliberately, sometimes inadvertently.
- **Crisis intervention:** Brief outline of the principles of crisis intervention.

In the next chapter, which begins Part III, I will look at various approaches to advocacy and at the idea of empowerment.

Part III

IDEAS ABOUT ROLES

Introduction

Part II looked at a range of ideas about change and explored their relevance to social work practice. In this part of the book I am going to come at the question of theory and practice in social work from a somewhat different angle. The starting point of the following three chapters will be different roles that social workers play. Instead of discussing particular 'theories', I will be inviting the reader to think about some of the issues involved in performing these roles. Using the terminology I proposed in the first chapter: Chapter 8 will look at 'advocacy' roles, Chapter 9 will look at the 'control agent' role and Chapter 10 will look at roles which particularly involve working with other people, particularly the 'care manager', 'co-ordinator' and 'responsibility holder' roles.

8 Advocacy and empowerment

- Defining advocacy
- Rights
- Unheard voices
- Indirect advocacy
- Advocacy and other roles
- Advocacy, power and empowerment

  - Power-sensitive practice
  - Recognising the need for advocacy
  - Involving service users

- Limits to empowerment

Part II looked at various approaches towards the business of helping people bring about change in their own lives. But people who seek the help of social workers are not necessarily looking to change the way that they lead their lives. Often the change they seek is in the world around them, which is failing to provide them with what they need or what they are entitled to. This chapter is, in essence, about helping people to bring about change in the world around them.

'Advocacy' describes a role, or set of roles, which social workers and others can take on, involving either speaking up for people or supporting people in speaking up for themselves. 'Empowerment' is a more general term, describing not a particular role but an approach or stance that fits well with the advocacy role, but could be applied in other ways. Both concepts are attractive alternatives for those who suspect that the more traditional 'therapeutic' strand in social work often 'blames the victim' by making external problems – problems caused by social exclusion of one kind or another – look like problems of individual psychological functioning. (If a person with a disability is depressed because he cannot get a job, we *could* see the problem as being his depression. Conversely, we could see the problem as the fact that no one will give him a job.) Advocacy, the role and empowerment, the idea, are not about examining why people are as they are, or about helping them to change the way they live, but about supporting them in getting things to which they are, or should be, entitled.

Defining advocacy

In modern English the word 'advocacy' seems to have both a broad general meaning and a rather more specific meaning. The more general meaning is something on the lines of 'Public support for or recommendation of a particular cause or policy' (*NODE*, 2001). The more specific meaning refers specifically to *one person speaking on behalf of another or others*. 'The function of an advocate; speaking on behalf of' is the definition of 'advocacy' given by the *Shorter Oxford English Dictionary* (*SOED*, 5th edition, 2002). This dictionary's definition of 'advocate' includes 'a person whose profession is to plead cases in courts of law' (a lawyer) and 'a person who pleads, intercedes or speaks for another'.

The word 'advocacy' has a similar range of meanings when it is used in social work. Definitions of the word produced by writers about social work typically include both the meaning of supporting a cause and the meaning of representing an individual or group:

> *Social work advocacy is the exclusive and mutual representation of a client(s) or a cause in a forum, attempting to systematically influence decision making in an unjust or unresponsive system(s).* (Schneider and Lester, 2001: 65)

Considering this definition, one begins to see just how central the advocacy role is to social work. Social workers in most specialisms are engaged in a daily basis in attempting to influence the decision-making of 'unjust or unresponsive systems', on behalf of their service users. They try to persuade other agencies, or their own agency, to provide services, they negotiate with benefits agencies to provide new benefits or to resolve problems with existing benefits on their clients' behalf, they negotiate with housing agencies, they support their clients when they are being interviewed by the police or immigration authorities, they try to represent the views and/or interests of their clients in court reports. Other professionals also engage in advocacy, and there are some professions (such as the law) for which advocacy is the primary task. But social workers tend to be the ones in any multi-professional group who take on tasks that involve negotiation around practical problems such as money or housing, and are therefore particularly likely to be involved in advocacy work.

There is some disagreement, though, in the social work literature however about whether all of this activity can strictly be described as advocacy. David and Toby Brandon (2001: 20, original emphasis.) believe that an essential core of advocacy 'lies in *the accomplishment of tasks defined by the client*'. They are making the important distinction between a social worker acting *at a client's request* and a social worker acting in what she perceives as being *in a client's best interests*, with only the former counting in their terms as real advocacy. On this definition, writing at a service user's request to support her application for a housing transfer *is* advocacy but arguing in a court report that a child should be removed from her abusive parents is not advocacy, unless the child herself has requested it and even though you may be convinced that this is necessary for the child's safety and well-being and may feel that you are (in the broader sense of the word) advocating for the best interests of the child.

In the English and Welsh legal system, an independent social worker called a *children's guardian* is appointed by a court when there are proceedings of this kind, with the rationale that there needs to be someone who is solely there to represent the child's interests, as well as the social worker who is representing the child protection agency, which has (in most cases) brought the case to court. The guardian might *seem* to be more straightforwardly an advocate for the child than the social worker from the child protection agency, but even the guardian is not obliged to simply represent the child's views, and may make her own different proposals if she feels this is in the child's best interests, so neither social worker is practising advocacy in the Brandon and Brandon sense, though both are legally required to make the interests of the child paramount in their thinking. If the child is a small baby, it is of course impossible for a social worker to be an advocate for the child in this narrow sense.

I don't think David and Toby Brandon would disagree that there are at least some situations in which a social worker may need to go against the wishes of a client and speak out for a course of action which she believes is in the client's best interests. I think their concern would be that, if this too is defined as *advocacy*, it weakens the distinctiveness of advocacy as an essentially service user-led process and allows advocacy to become yet another way in which professionals impose their own views about what is best for people. Brandon and Brandon are particularly concerned to protect the idea of advocacy as an *alternative* to approaches in which the professional is assumed to know, *better than the client himself*, what the client really needs, as well as being an alternative to 'treatment' models (that is, broadly what I have called 'direct change agent' work) in which it is assumed that the client's own functioning is the thing that needs to change.

Most writers on advocacy seem to take a similar view but there are variations. Neil Bateman (2000: 48), for instance, believes that 'acting in the client's best interests may ... mean that the advocate has to steer the client away from a particular course of action'. Freddolino et al. (2004) offer a four-part classification of advocacy which includes *best interests advocacy*, in which the social worker 'identifies the needs of the recipient [that is, service user] and advocates for their fulfilment independent of the recipient' and *client-centred advocacy*, in which the social worker 'identifies the needs of the recipient that will be met and involves the recipient in the advocacy process to address these needs' (Freddolino et al., 2004: 126). Neither of these would be regarded by the Brandons as genuine advocacy, though Freddolino et al.'s other two categories *enabling advocacy* and *consumer-controlled advocacy* would seem to correspond to the Brandon's *representing clients directly* and *supporting advocacy indirectly*, which I will discuss presently.

There are certainly many situations in which a social worker cannot simply act on a service user's wishes, but perhaps it is better, rather than trying to stretch the definition of advocacy to include these situations, to simply acknowledge that social workers have to combine advocacy with other roles (a subject I will come back to shortly) and to retain the word advocacy only for those situations where the social worker is acting on the service

Table 8.1   Social work advocacy involvement

Representing clients directly ['direct advocacy']

Micro: advocate for a client trying to access social security benefits; writing to a housing office making a case for a housing transfer.

Macro: whistleblowing about deficiencies in whole services [...]; lobbying or collectively advocating for improved welfare rights, better facilities for immigrants, changes in social legislation.

Supporting advocacy indirectly ['indirect advocacy']

Micro: supporting self-advocacy, backing up a client complaining about services: working with a self-advocacy group; advocacy component in care planning – basing the plan more on what the client wants than on some notion of 'needs'.

Macro: helping neighbourhood groups to articulate deficiencies in the collection of rubbish and repair to damage done by vandals. [*Note: this is essentially community work, as briefly discussed in Chapter 6.*]

Source: Brandon and Brandon (2001: 64), my additions in square brackets.

user's own wishes? In Chapter 1, when I discussed social work roles, I suggested the term 'responsibility holder' to describe the role played by social workers when they act to protect the best interests of people – small babies would be a particularly clear case in point – who are not thought to be capable of making decisions completely by themselves.

I have already mentioned the distinction that Brandon and Brandon make between 'representing clients directly' (advocacy in the sense so far discussed) and 'supporting advocacy indirectly', which means supporting clients in being advocates for themselves (see Table 8.1 above, which also includes their distinction between advocacy at the 'micro' and 'macro' levels). I adopted this distinction in Chapter 1 when I subdivided advocacy roles into 'direct' and 'indirect' advocacy.

Rights

Assessments carried out by social workers acting in other roles, for example, in a 'care manager' role, tend to turn on the concepts of *need* and *risk*: a social worker, along with the service user, identifies needs and risks in the current situation and attempts to meet the needs and minimise the risks. In advocacy work an equivalent position is occupied by the concept of *rights*. Rights, as Neil Bateman puts it, 'are the fulcrum upon which advocacy balances' (Bateman, 2000: 40). Rights are not a completely different thing from needs and risks, for by and large they are legal guarantees that people can have certain needs met and be protected against various risks. (Consider the right to free healthcare in the UK, or the right to protection against injury at work enshrined in health and safety legislation.) But herein lies the distinction: needs and risks are defined either by the individual concerned themselves or by professionals exercising their judgement or expertise, but rights are defined in law.

A needs- or risks-based process arguably steers us towards a kind of medical model in which we are trying to find out 'what is wrong with people', while a rights-based process arguably avoids this, since the issue isn't what is wrong with someone, but what they are entitled to under the law.

Unheard voices

Exercise 8.1

Some years ago, when I was a social worker in a fieldwork team, I had for a time the respon-sibility of running an outposted call-in office where, on a Thursday morning, members of the public could come without an appointment to seek help or advice on problems. On one occasion a woman came in who was having a problem with her benefits. I forget what the problem was but I remember that, while the woman was sitting with me, I telephoned the benefits agency to see if I could resolve it. After a short conversation with me, the benefits officer agreed to sort the problem out. Feeling rather pleased with myself, I turned back to the woman, expecting her also to be pleased – and perhaps impressed with my skills as an advocate. Instead the woman was quite angry:

   'You didn't tell them anything that I hadn't already told them,' she said, 'so how come they agree to sort it out when it's you that speaks to them, but not when it's me?'

   What do you think was the answer to her question?

Comments

Of course I don't know what the answer to her question was in this particular case. It is possible that I was better at making a case than she was (though as I recall this was a perfectly articulate person, quite capable of making her own points.) It is possible that I was more diplomatic in the way I went about it. (If the woman had been very aggressive, for instance, or accused the benefits agency of incompetence, it's possible that the benefits officer might have been less inclined to find a way round the problem.) If she had been black, or disabled, I might have wondered whether the fact that I am white and not disabled had made the difference. Perhaps the fact that I am a man made the difference, or the fact that I speak with what to British ears is a recognisably middle-class accent?

   However, in this situation I think it likely that the difference was due to the fact that I represented a professional agency and she was, like most people the benefits agency deals with all day, a benefits claimant. My professional status, and perhaps simply the fact that I was a bit different to the bulk of this agency's callers, was enough to tip the balance in favour of the benefits officer listening to me and carrying out the small steps that were necessary to resolving the problem.

What the situation in Exercise 8.1 illustrates is that we only *need* advocacy because some people find it harder than others to get themselves heard. There is no good reason why the benefits officer should respond differently to facts about a benefits claimant when pre-sented by a social worker to how he would respond to the same facts when presented by the claimant herself, but he did. The fact that this sort of thing is common is the reason why

Schneider and Lester's definition cited above referred to advocacy influencing decision making in 'an unjust or unresponsive system'.

The point of the story is not to criticise the benefits system in particular. I have no doubt that social workers themselves do the same kind of thing in many circumstances. (Imagine you are presented with the same set of facts and the same demand for a service by (1) a member of the general public and (2) by a consultant psychiatrist. Can you be entirely sure that you would respond in exactly the same way in either case?) Everyone is selective about who they listen to and who they don't and we are all liable to influenced by a whole range of factors from the clarity, presentational skills and demeanour of the speaker, to their physical appearance, their gender, their accent and their ethnic background. Most of us find it easier to hear the views of people who are 'like us' in some way, than the views of those who seem very different from us.

Probably most of us have at some time also had the experience of not being listened to, but the fact is that some groups of people face this experience far more often than others, particularly those who are marginalised in some way by society, such as disabled people, immigrants or homeless people, or those seen as not fully capable of knowing what is in their own best interests, such as children, old people with dementia, people who have mental health problems and learning disabilities. The problem is compounded when people have specific communication problems such as poor grasp of the English language, inability to read and write, or (as is the case for instance with many people with cerebral palsy) actual difficulty with speaking in a way that other people can comprehend.

The great appeal of advocacy as an approach is that it is about redressing the balance and helping voices to be heard which otherwise would have gone unheard.

Indirect advocacy

I suppose one of the reasons why the woman in Exercise 8.1 was angry was that she had been made aware of the fact that she was (at least in respect of this particular problem with the benefits agency) one of the people who doesn't get listened to and that I (in this context and on this occasion) was one of the people who do. While I had helped her with her benefit problem, I hadn't helped with this 'not-being-listened-to' problem at all. I had used my (relative) power in this situation to assist her with a specific problem arising from her (relative) powerlessness, but I had not assisted her in gaining more power.

What I am calling indirect advocacy (and Brandon and Brandon call 'supporting advocacy indirectly') might be described as an approach that addressed not just the immediate problem but also the more general 'not-being-listened-to' problem. I suppose (if she had wanted this) I could have invited the woman in Exercise 8.1 to make the telephone call herself from my office, advised her how to go about it and given her some feedback on her performance. Actually, I'm not sure such an approach would have been very welcome in her case – it might have made her feel even more belittled and patronised – but it would seem entirely appropriate with people whose difficulty may simply be that they lack the skills and experience to advocate effectively on their own behalf: young people leaving the public care system, for instance, or people with disabilities moving from some form of institutional care to their own accommodation.

Although a lack of skills or experience on their part may be one reason why some people don't get listened to, it is far from being the only reason. For many people the problem lies in assumptions and prejudices about the groups they are perceived to belong to. In these cases, indirect advocacy would not consist of helping people acquire skills (offering help with skills that people already have is, of course, not only patronising and belittling, but entirely pointless) but of supporting them in collectively building a stronger voice that is less easy for those in authority to ignore. This kind of indirect advocacy might include: putting people in touch with self-advocacy support groups, helping people to form self-advocacy groups, and offering support and facilities to self-advocacy groups. Community work, as discussed in Chapter 6, is typically a form of indirect advocacy.

Advocacy and other roles

In characteristically robust fashion, Brandon and Brandon (2001: 49) describe the role conflicts involved for a social worker in one fairly typical-sounding social work case as 'beyond the wit of a committee compromising the Buddha, Christ and Mohammed'. All social work involves some advocacy, but the extent to which a social worker can actually be an unreserved advocate for her service users varies greatly according to context. On the one hand there are some voluntary agencies whose main function is advocacy on behalf of service users. On the other, in a state social work agency a social worker has a number of other roles and responsibilities which may conflict with the practice of advocacy:

- *Control agent* roles involve social workers in some circumstances in overruling the wishes of service users. Social workers acting as control agents cannot simply implement the wishes of service users. Service users may also be reluctant to discuss their views and wishes with social workers who may be recording what they say as evidence.
- *Responsibility holder* roles require social workers to discharge parental- or familial-type responsibilities for clients. While good parents are in many respects the best of all advocates for their children, they are not advocates in the pure 'Brandon and Brandon' sense, because they do not necessarily implement their children's wishes in every respect if this would go against their children's long-term interests.
- *Almoner* and *care manager* roles involve social workers in making decisions about the distribution of their agency's resources. It is impossible to be a wholehearted advocate for one client while simultaneously attempting to manage the distribution of resources in a way that will be fair to all clients, as Andrew Maynard and I (2005: 96–7) have discussed elsewhere. We also noted that even advocating wholeheartedly for a single client can have unintended negative consequences for that client if it involves emphasising that client's level of need and thereby 'labelling' him.
- *Direct change agent* roles (such as the role of therapist or counsellor) may require that a client's way of doing things is challenged or questioned. This doesn't sit well with the position of an advocate acting on a client's instructions. Supporters of advocacy, such as David Brandon, tend to argue for advocacy as an *alternative* to direct change roles. Crudely, direct change agent work can be characterised as locating and addressing problems *within* a person, while advocacy work can be characterised as locating and addressing problems *outside* the person, a distinction analogous to the distinction between the medical and social models of disability or mental illness.
- *Conflicts of interest* may occur when a social worker is working with a family and not an individual, her ability to act as an advocate for one member of the family may be limited by her responsibilities

to other family members. A social worker for the elderly, for instance, has responsibilities towards both elderly people and their carers.

- *Duties and obligations towards her employer* inevitably compromise social workers' ability to serve as an advocate for a client who may be disputing a decision made by that agency because, as David Brandon (1991: 118) bluntly put it, 'The alleged oppressor pays their salaries'. These duties and obligations may also get in the way of advocating for a client in dispute with another agency with which the social work agency is closely linked through inter-agency working arrangements, something which is increasingly common, as I will discuss in the next chapter.

The fact that there are constraints and limitations on the capacity of social workers to act as advocates for their clients does not mean that they cannot do so at all. As I have already noted advocacy is a mainstream social work role and one of the characteristics of the profession. But being aware of the limits of one's capacity to act as an advocate is important and is one of the benefits of thinking about what advocacy really means. Social workers who recognise that their other roles prevent them from acting as an advocate for a particular service user are then in a position to refer the client on to independent advocacy services, such as parents groups which support parents on the receiving end of child protection investigations. And recognition of the limits to its capacity to truly advocate for its service users, allows an agency to consider ways of building opportunities for self-advocacy into the structure of the agency itself, for example by having committees of service users, or service users involved in running the agency and/or in appointing its staff. Formal complaints procedures too can provide a mechanism that makes it possible for the voices of service users to be heard when they are unhappy with the service they are receiving.

Advocacy, power and empowerment

Exercise 8.2

Referring back once more to the example in Exercise 8.1, put yourself into the position of the woman who has had to ask for someone else to advocate on her behalf in order to resolve a benefits problems. Suppose that she has repeatedly had this experience, or experiences like it. What effect might this have on her?

Suppose the woman had a learning disability, say, or was a gypsy. What difference would that make?

Comments

I have already said that, while the benefits problem was resolved in this case, the 'not-being-listened-to' problem was not resolved at all. Indeed one of the effects of experiences of this kind would be to highlight for the woman the fact that she cannot get people to listen to her in her own right. This in turn might have a number of different effects, depending on the woman's personality and her past experiences. She might very well (and with justice) feel angry and unfairly treated. She might simply

(Continued)

> *(Continued)*
>
> *become resigned to the fact that 'they don't listen to people like me'. If she was a gypsy she might put this down to widespread negative stereotypes about gypsies and travellers among the rest of the population. Many people might come to the conclusion that it was their own fault in some way: 'I'm no good at explaining things,' 'I'm a nuisance to people.' A person with learning disabilities might well have received and internalised a lot of messages to this effect.*
>
> *The general point, though, is that these experiences are likely to make people aware of being powerless. Some might react to this by fighting in order to get more power, others might feel that they simply had to accept it, others again might conclude that they deserved it.*

What I have called a 'not-being-listened-to' problem is really the problem of powerlessness. Powerful people get listened to; their needs, wishes and views are taken seriously. Powerless people do not get listened to; their needs, wishes and views are not taken seriously and their existence is often only seriously considered when it affects the powerful in some way. For instance, public debate about mental illness often seems to focus more on the possible problems posed by people with mental health problems to the rest of the population as on the needs of people with mental health problems themselves.

Direct advocacy can address particular problems caused by lack of power – in direct advocacy, the advocate effectively *lends* her power to the person she is advocating for – but does not address the underlying problem of powerlessness, except in so far as it may encourage people to recognise that they have rights and that they are entitled to be heard. Indirect advocacy, in its many forms, does attempt to address the problem of powerlessness more directly by trying to help or encourage or support people in taking power for themselves through *self-advocacy*. The term 'empowerment' – one of those words so widely used in social work discourse that it is in danger of losing its meaning – refers simply to this process of people taking power for themselves. Robert Adams (2003: 8) defines it as:

> the means by which individuals, groups and/or communities become able to take control of their circumstances and achieve their own goals, thereby being able to work towards helping themselves and others to maximise the quality of their lives.

One of the dilemmas that social workers face is that 'help' can itself be *dis*empowering. As Brandon and Brandon (2001: 21) put it:

> Social services are traditionally disempowering. Staff behave in ways that clientalise the individuals under their care. They no longer remain authentic citizens after entry to the day centres, old people's homes, psychiatric hospitals.

But this process of 'clientalisation' doesn't just occur in institutions. A student of mine recently described to me a child protection case conference attended by two very young and very nervous parents and a dozen older professionals. When the young man attempted to advocate on behalf of himself and his partner, two of the professionals looked at one another and smirked, almost as if the very attempt to offer a different view to that of the professionals was laughable. There are countless examples like this of the ways in which social workers, their agencies and their professional collaborators can belittle and disempower the users of their services. Even the routine process of conducting a full assessment of needs when a member of the public requests a service, useful though it in some ways is, is in a way disempowering. It is a kind of throwback to the high days of therapeutic social work in the 1970s, mentioned earlier, when the 'presenting problems' offered by clients tended to be seen as mere symptoms of underlying problems, which the clients themselves might not be aware of. (If you went into a shop to buy a television set, how would you feel if the shop assistant insisted on carrying out a full assessment of your needs to see if a television set was what you *really* needed?)

Empowerment, in a social work context, means working in a way that is aimed at increasing people's sense of power and control over their own lives, rather than diminishing it. It is not a single method or technique and, perhaps partly because of this lack of specificity, it is a word (like 'partnership') which can easily be used in rather a cosmetic and superficial way to give a warm glow to a social worker, to include in the publicity literature of a social work agency, or to provide a social work student with a named 'theory' to include in an essay or a placement report. Just as the word 'partnership' is often misused in social work to describe work in which the client is in *no* sense an equal partner, so the word 'empowerment' can unfortunately be used to put an acceptable face on practice which in truth is anything but empowering. 'Empowerment', as Brandon and Brandon (2001: 20) observe, can 'become a method used to reconcile people to being powerless. Our systems are extremely seductive and manipulative.'

It seems to me that we are bad at calling things by their true names in social work and are prone to try and cover up things that we find uncomfortable with anodyne language. Sometimes it *is* appropriate for social workers to exercise power to control situations and overrule the wishes of clients or carers – I discuss this further in Chapter 10 – but when we do this we should not pretend we are working in partnership with people or empowering them, for this simply debases the words and ideas themselves, making them harder to use even in situations where they are or should be applicable. But there are many ways in which the idea of empowerment can genuinely be applied to social work practice, some of which are the following:

Power-sensitive practice

By this I mean simply practice that which is sensitive to the existence of power differences between social worker and service user and find ways, not to pretend that the power differences do not exist, but to prevent the service user from being intimidated and silenced by them. For example, I mentioned earlier two young parents in the intimidating and disrespectful environment of a case conference. Sensitivity to their position might mean planning the meeting to ensure that they had a proper hearing, or allowing them to bring an independent advocate or supporter. Transparency – of the process, of the options at any given stage, of matters such as recording and confidentiality and of mechanisms for appeal and complaint – is important. People feel powerless when they feel they have no control or don't know what is going on. At their worst, social work agencies are opaque, arbitrary bureaucracies which communicate in incomprehensible jargon, keep people waiting for weeks and months for a service, and make decisions behind closed doors without revealing the criteria they use, not unlike the nightmarish bureaucracies invoked in the novels of Franz Kafka.

↗ Consciousness-raising

Implicit, and often explicit, in the discourse of empowerment is the idea of consciousness-raising. The purpose of empowerment is to enable people who perceive themselves as having no power to take power. Society has disempowered groups of people by teaching them to locate their difficulties within themselves, as personal deficiencies, rather than locating them externally to themselves, as structural injustices. Paulo Friere's (1986) *Pedagogy of the Oppressed* is widely quoted in the empowerment literature and, as the title of the book indicates, Friere saw the work of empowerment as being pedagogical (that is: educational) in character. It involves people who are oppressed *'learning to perceive* social, political, and economic contradictions' (1986: 66, my emphasis). People who have been oppressed or abused do indeed often locate their difficulties quite erroneously inside themselves, and it makes sense that part of the process of empowerment is correcting these misapprehensions and enabling people to get a more realistic view of the world than the one that has been given to them by their own oppressors or abusers. (I recall working with a child who had been sexually abused by a group of adults at the age of about six, but who was still convinced that the abuse had been somehow his fault: one of the aims of working with this boy was to teach him that it was not.) Empowerment means not only that the worker should be, in my terms, 'power-sensitive', but that the client should also be helped to be power-sensitive, aware of the pervasive and distorting role of power in shaping the way we see the world.

However, there is a paradox here, in that any such work must start with the assumption that the person doing the work knows the truth about the world better than the person who is being worked with. Is this so different from the psychodynamically minded social worker who is convinced that he understands his clients *real* needs better than the client himself? This paradox sits at the heart of the whole notion of empowerment as a professional activity.

Recognising the need for advocacy

Introducing independent direct advocates to service users when necessary is a basic element of power-sensitive practice. Indirect advocacy as discussed earlier in this chapter – supporting service users, individually or in groups, to effectively advocate for themselves – is perhaps one of the purest forms of empowerment work, since its whole aim is to increase people's power in their dealings with the rest of the world.

Involving service users

Busy social workers sometimes grumble that their job would be fine if it wasn't for the clients. There always seems to be plenty to do apart from actually dealing with service users – meetings to attend, forms to fill in, files to write up – so that it really *is* quite possible to lose sight of the fact that all this activity is supposed to be for the benefit of service users. In fact, of course, no service *is* just there for its clients. Social work services are there also to meet the needs of those who work in them, those who manage them, those who fund them and set them up. The problem is that these other stakeholders tend to be a lot more powerful than the service's own clients. This can result in a service which is inclined to ignore the views of the very people it is actually mandated to serve.

One way of off-setting this and ensuring that service users remain at centre stage is to involve service users in shaping the service itself. Braye (2000) identified four levels at which this can occur:

(1) Individual service users, or prospective service users, being involved in their own service.
(2) Involvement of groups of service users in planning services.
(3) Developing independent user-led services (that is, non-statutory organisations which are actually run by service users.)
(4) Involvement of service users in research.

It is desirable that service users should be involved at all these levels not only because it is consistent with the idea of empowerment but also because it is likely to result in a more efficient service.

↗ Producer capture

The idea of empowerment as *consciousness-raising* comes from the political left. The idea that it is important for users of a public service to have control over it is an idea also strongly associated with the political right.

A general criticism of public services from the perspective of classical free-market economics is that they do not have to compete to attract customers. Or at any rate, no incentive exists that is comparable to the incentives that exist in the market place, the market mechanism being the so-called 'hidden hand' which, according to the 18th-century free-market economist Adam Smith (1996: first published 1776), channels people's basically selfish interests into serving the common good.

In the view of classical economics people basically act in their own self-interest. The argument goes that in the absence of the incentive provided by the market place to maximise the quality and efficiency of the service – for service users cannot 'take their custom elsewhere' – the staff in public service organisations will develop other priorities. They may for example be more interested in promoting their own prestige, or in having as

(Continued)

(Continued)

quiet and as stress-free life as possible, or in doing the jobs that happen to interest them, rather than the ones which may most need doing. Public services are effectively *captured* by their producers. Producers then shape the service to meet their own needs – schools are run for the benefit of teachers rather than pupils, hospitals for their staff rather than their patients – effectively disempowering the users of those services. Attempts to introduce market mechanisms and consumer choice into public services by a succession of British governments over the past 25 years, have been intended to address this problem of producer capture.

Social workers have a tendency to align themselves with the leftward end of the political spectrum and may be inclined to dismiss theoretical ideas that originate on the right, but I suggest that we should be open to ideas wherever they come from. I find the idea of 'producer capture' a useful one.

I have already alluded in this chapter to a time during the 1960s and 1970s when workers influenced by psychodynamic ideas would often operate on the assumption that 'client's own definitions of their personal problems' could not be relied upon and that 'the more profound and relevant reasons for their difficult situations and relationships lay outside the direct knowledge of the distressed individual and within the competence of the professional' (Brandon and Brandon, 2001: 63). Given that the role of 'therapist' has a rather more prestigious and glamorous ring to it for many social workers than that of 'care manager', and given that many find therapy more personally interesting and rewarding, perhaps the fact that clients were 'receiving treatment when they were asking for representation' (2001: 63) was in part an instance of producer capture?

Limits to empowerment

Since involving users in the delivery of their own services would seem to be beneficial for service users and in most circumstances likely to be more efficient than not involving them, why is there not more of it? Of course there are many answers to this. For one thing most people are reluctant to give up power – we should be careful not to rule out the possibility that this may apply to our own virtuous selves and not just to 'other people'. But there are also sometimes genuine limits to the practicability of user participation. These have to do, first, with *capacity* (some people – children or people with profound learning disabilities, for example – may not be able to make judgements about their own long-term best interests) and, second, with *conflicting interests*. As Sarah Banks (2001: 38) says, 'in the interests of justice, it may not always be morally right to prioritise the user's rights at the expense of those of others'.

Perhaps the most difficult situations are those in which there are several different parties who all have some call on social work services, but whose interests are not identical and whose capacity and/or power is markedly different. Here it is easy to fall into a pattern of bending over backwards to meet the needs of one party and forgetting about the needs of the other. When working with the families of children of disabilities, for instance, this might result in trying to understand and meet the needs of the parents while forgetting that the children (who may be more difficult to communicate with) do not necessarily have the same needs as their parents.

Practice notes

Advocacy and empowerment

Skill requirements

- Genuinely *representing* service users and allowing service users to make their own decisions requires an ability to operate without the security that is conferred by the traditional 'expert' role of the professional. Paradoxically, this may require a higher level of skill and confidence – and a more genuine expertise – than working in more traditional ways.
- One reason that some groups of service users tend not to be adequately involved in the delivery of their own services is that they are harder to communicate with: I think, for example, of small children, people with learning difficulties and people with motor impairments which make speech difficult. Specific communication skills may therefore be important.

Ethical considerations

- The needs and rights of people other than the primary service user, for whom social workers may also have responsibilities, may conflict with the service user's own needs.
- Issues of capacity (ability to make informed decisions) need to be considered.

Real-world constraints

- Sometimes the rhetoric of service user participation fails to acknowledge the huge differences in capacity that exist among the members of a group to which society happens to assign a single label. When we speak about learning disabled people, for instance, we are talking about a group in which are included people with an IQ of 70, who are able to read, write, go to work and parent children – people who clearly can and should be involved in the design of services intended to meet their needs – but it includes also people who lack the intellectual capacity to develop language or to meet even their own most basic needs.
- Involving service users in the delivery of their own services can seldom be just a matter of delivering whatever the user asks for, but engaging in a kind of negotiation in which other factors need to be taken into account, including possible competing claims (as discussed above) and limitations to what the agency can deliver (for reasons to do with resources or to do with its mandate.) This applies not only to social work service users but to all users of public services.
- The reality though is that some people get more of what they want or need than others, and this is where advocacy and the idea of empowerment are valuable in the real world.

Chapter summary

The following are the headings that have been covered in this chapter:

- **Defining advocacy:** Different ways of defining advocacy. Direct and indirect advocacy.
- **Rights:** The idea of rights as central to advocacy, occupying a similar position to 'needs' and 'risks' in other areas of social work.
- **Unheard voices:** 'Not-being-listened-to' as the fundamental problem which creates the need for advocacy.
- **Indirect advocacy:** Supporting service users in advocating for themselves.
- **Advocacy and other roles:** The way that advocacy as a role can clash with other social work roles and make wholehearted advocacy difficult.
- **Advocacy, power and empowerment:** The relationship of advocacy to empowerment. Empowerment as an alternative paradigm to 'treatment'.
- **Limits to empowerment:** Competing claims which limit the degree to which empowerment can be adopted as the sole principle of practice.

The next chapter looks at the various social work roles that involve collaboration with people other than service users themselves.

9 | Working with others

- Working with carers
- Working with other professionals and agencies

  - Status differences
  - Different priorities arising from different responsibilities
  - Different perceptions arising from different value bases or theoretical assumptions
  - Disagreements about respective responsibilities
  - Differences as to primary client

- The downside
- The co-ordinator role
- The care manager role

  - Needs-led assessment
  - Thinking about resources
  - Direct payments

- The responsibility holder role

It goes without saying that social work involves working with others. For social workers in what I have called a 'service development' role, these 'others' may not actually include the users of the service, but in most cases the central 'other' with whom social workers are involved is the user or recipient of the service. At the centre of social work, you might say, is a working relationship with a person, or group of people, who have either identified themselves, or been identified by others, as having some kind of problem. The same is true of activities like therapy and counselling and it is presumably for this reason that the body of 'theory' referred to in social work texts (including this one) tends to draw heavily on ideas that come from various branches of therapeutic work.

But as I have emphasised more than once in this book, social work is actually a very *different* kind of job to that of a therapist or counsellor, because social workers undertake a whole range of different roles, which may not even include a therapist/counsellor role, or may include other roles that sit very uneasily with this one. In the last chapter, for instance, I discussed the distinct role of 'advocate'. In the next chapter I will look at the 'control agent' role. This chapter will look at issues that arise, to varying degrees in all of what I have called 'executive' roles, which, to recap, I divided up in Chapter 1 as follows:

- Almoner
- Care manager
- Responsibility holder
- Control agent
- Co-ordinator
- Service developer

All of these roles involve the social worker in working with people other than simply the service user in a variety of different ways. Figure 9.1, for instance, represents the working relationships of a social worker working with an elderly woman, Mrs Brown.

In this case the social worker has responsibilities to assess, and try to meet, the needs of two people whose interests may not be the same: Mrs Brown and Mrs Brown's main carer, her daughter. The social worker has commissioned the services of two provider agencies, one providing day centre care, one providing care assistants to support Mrs Brown at home. (The social worker has arranged for her agency to enter into a contract with these agencies under which they are paid to provide a specified service.) The social worker also needs to liase with other professionals involved in supporting Mrs Brown, in this case the GP and the community nurse. The community nurse is also providing care for Mrs Brown, so her input will need to be co-ordinated with that of the other service providers and with the daughter. It is these characteristic webs of relationships with people other than the recipient of the service herself that will be the subject of the rest of this chapter.

Working with carers

In a rather poor attempt at a definition of social work in Chapter 1, I described a social worker as a '*Professional with special responsibility for people who are in some way vulnerable, excluded or disadvantaged in society*'. But in fact most of the work of caring for and supporting such people is done not by professionals at all but by unpaid carers. These carers, of whom the majority are female, include the spouses and partners of elderly people and people with health problems or disabilities, the parents of adults and children with health problems or disabilities, and the adult children of elderly people and people with health problems or disabilities. They also include a substantial number of children still of school age – 'young carers' – who provide care for parents who have disabilities or health problems. (The Office of National Statistics in 1996 estimated that there were between 19,000 and 51,000

Figure 9.1   Working with Mrs Brown

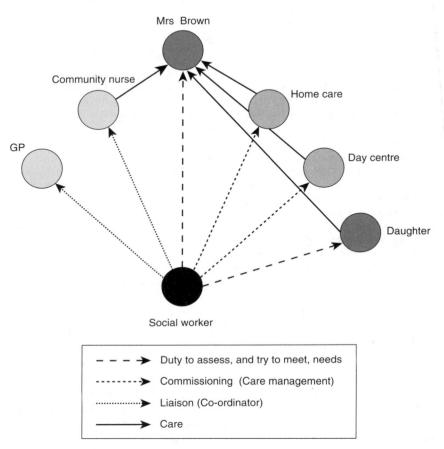

young carers in the UK [ONS, 1996]). In England and Wales, *The Carers (Recognition and Services) Act* represented an acknowledgement that all these carers are people with needs in their own right, though significantly it gave carers the right to have their needs *assessed*, but not necessarily the right to have their needs *met*.

One difficulty in assessing the needs of carers is that, for a whole range of different reasons, carers' needs do not necessarily marry up with the needs of the primary service user. The assessing social worker therefore has to attempt to balance these needs and achieve some kind of compromise, bearing in mind that ultimately the carer may need some support if she or he is going to be able to continue to *be* an adequate carer. The same issues arise incidentally when working with non-disabled children and their parents, who, while not carers in the sense of the Carers Recognition Act, are of course carers in the wider sense of the word.

The following exercise considers a case where both primary service user and main carer are elderly people.

Exercise 9.1

Mrs Rotherham is 92. She is physically very frail and moves about her house only with great difficulty, using a Zimmer frame. She requires help with getting in and out of bed, getting to the toilet and bathing and she needs all her meals prepared. Since she can easily get stuck or fall over, she also requires regular checking during the day. However, she is mentally extremely alert and has always been a woman of sharp intelligence.

Mrs Rotherham's main carer is her widowed daughter, Mrs Lucy Down, now aged 64, who has let out her own house and moved back in with her mother to care for her.

Mrs Down has contacted social services to request help. She says that she is exhausted by the demands of caring for her mother and needs a holiday. Could respite care be arranged for Mrs Rotherham for a two-week period while she takes a break? Mrs Down's GP has also written in support of this request, saying that Mrs Down is not in good health herself. She has a weak heart and is prone to depression, for which she is currently receiving treatment. The GP suggests that if she does not have a break, Mrs Down will become ill and will no longer be able to offer care to her mother.

A social worker visits Mrs Rotherham and Mrs Down.

'Lucy will have to do as she thinks fit,' says Mrs Rotherham flatly, 'but I am not going into a home and that is final.'

'How about if I arranged for care for Mrs Rotherham at home?' asks the social worker. He says he thinks he could arrange for care assistants to get Mrs Rotherham in and out of bed and see to her bathing and toileting needs – and also arrange for meals to be delivered – though this would mean that Mrs Rotherham would have to be on her own in between the care assistant's visits.

Mrs Rotherham makes it quite clear that she would be very unhappy with such an arrangement but she does not absolutely veto it. However, Mrs Down says, if that is all that can be offered, she will have to abandon the idea of a holiday, because it would be no rest for her at all if she was worrying all the time about her mother, who might fall and hurt herself during the times of day in between the care assistant's visits.

How would you deal with this situation if you were the social worker?

Comments

The fact is that both Mrs Rotherham and Mrs Down are adults who are capable of making their own decisions. This is a relationship which has existed for 64 years and the social worker cannot reasonably expect to transform it. Mrs Rotherham and Mrs Down have different needs, but their needs are also to some extent interlocking (for example, it is actually in Mrs Rotherham's own interests that her daughter gets a break.) The social worker cannot force services on Mrs Rotherham, nor can he insist that Mrs Down takes a break if her own sense of guilt does not allow her to do so. But perhaps it would be possible to engage in a dialogue that might help to move things on. Perhaps, Mrs Rotherham might be persuaded to be more supportive to her daughter's need for a break (and to desist from using 'emotional blackmail' to stop her going)? Perhaps Mrs Down might be persuaded that she needs a holiday and that, if Mrs Rotherham prefers to stay at home rather than go into residential care, then that is Mrs Rotherham's own choice?

Practice notes

Working with carers

Skill requirements

- The same kinds of skills are involved as those involved in working directly with primary service users.
- There is an added complication in that, the interests of carers are very rarely identical with those of primary clients, and there is a need to be very clear about your respective responsibilities to each.

Ethical considerations

- Who are you responsible for?
- How should your priorities be determined? Does your agency's brief make this clear? Or does your agency have responsibilities both for primary service users and carers?
- If the latter is the case, how do you prioritise their needs when they are not compatible? How do you avoid just going for the line of least resistance?
- Is your commitment to the carer in danger of obscuring the needs of the primary service user?
- On the other hand, are you in danger of effectively exploiting the carer's goodwill by failing to provide alternative care services?

Real-world constraints

- Resource constraints often make it difficult to provide services for carers at the level that they would wish.

Working with other professionals and agencies

Among the goals set in the UK by the *National Service Framework for Mental Health* was the following:

> *Ensure that education and training emphasise team, inter-disciplinary and inter-agency working.* All education and training should be evidence-based, and should stress the value of team, inter-disciplinary and inter-agency working. Service users and carers should be involved in planning, providing and evaluating education and training. (Department of Health, 1999c: 109, original emphasis)

Government and non-government publications are full of exhortations to members of the caring professions to work more closely together, not only in mental health but in children and families work (Department of Health, 1999a) and all the other main areas in which social workers operate. There has been a trend for some time in the UK towards setting up multi-disciplinary teams in which social workers operate alongside professionals with other backgrounds (Youth Offending Teams are an example), and there are now increasing moves towards amalgamation of services. See for example the moves to amalgamate education and children's social work services and create 'Children's Trusts' that originated in the green paper, *Every Child Matters* (Department for Education and Skills, 2003) and in the *Children Act, 2004*. Behind these kinds of proposals is an assumption that lack of understanding between different professions or different agencies causes problems that result in an inferior service being delivered.

Certainly problems are created for service users when services are fragmented between several different agencies, one of which is that 'each agency defines the needs of clients in terms of the services the agencies are mandated to provide, rather than what the client requires to resolve effectively the problem being experienced'. (Adkins et al., 1999: 1). The other kinds of problem that typically occur between different agencies and/or different professions are misunderstandings and communication problems. These can arise for a number of different reasons, including the following.

Status differences

Some professions have a higher status in society than others. The medical profession, for instance, is widely seen as having a higher status than social workers. This may lead to difficulties in working together as genuinely equal collaborators. In several child abuse inquiries, social workers have been criticised for taking medical opinion on trust, notably the Cleveland Inquiry (Butler-Sloss, 1987) and more recently the inquiry into the death of Victoria Climbié. In the Cleveland case, social workers were criticised for accepting on trust that there was medical evidence that children *had* been abused. In the Climbié case social workers were criticised for uncritically accepting a medical opinion that said that apparent non-accidental injuries were in fact scabies scars (Laming, 2003: 97).

The issue is not unique to child protection work and problems can arise, among other areas, in hospital social work and in the mental health field. In England and Wales, for instance, Approved Social Workers under the Mental Health Act, 1983, are placed in the position of deciding whether or not to act on the recommendation of psychiatrists that a person needs to be compulsorily detained in a mental hospital.

Different priorities arising from different responsibilities

Different agencies have different jobs to do and limited resources to do these jobs. These can result in one agency having very different priorities to another in any given situation and this in turn can result in frustration and mutual mistrust. For example, in the UK, the preoccupation of the NHS with moving patients out of hospital beds as quickly as possible can seem cold and heartless to a social worker whose client would benefit from being able to take the process much more gently. However, the social worker may not have to think, as the hospital staff do, of acutely ill new patients coming in who urgently need beds.

Schoolteachers likewise often express frustration about the fact that social services are often unable to follow up on their referrals about children who are causing them concern, and it may seem to those teachers that the social services department is a 'heartless bureaucracy' that simply does not care. But the teachers cannot be aware of all the other demands on the time of the social services department, which are forcing it to prioritise calls on its time. In the same way, social workers sometimes get frustrated with schools who exclude children from the classroom or demand that they move elsewhere. To a social worker, knowing all the problems that these children may be facing in their lives, *this* can seem very heartless, but of course the social worker does not have to think about the other children in a class whose learning may be disrupted by a pupil who is behaving badly.

Different perceptions arising from different value bases or theoretical assumptions

Another potential source of misunderstanding and friction lies in the fact that their different training will lead professionals from different backgrounds to focus on different aspects of a problem. Doctors and nurses, for instance, may be inclined to look for explanations of emotional or behavioural problems at the level of biochemistry and may be inclined to try to deal with it at that level using drugs (that is, they incline to the 'medical model'). Social workers, in contrast, may be more inclined to look for explanations in terms of the social context and a person's individual life experience within it (that is, they incline to a 'social model').

These kinds of differences can be very positive: they can result in a 'creative tension' in which each professional group is forced to examine its own assumptions. But they can also result in conflict and stalemate.

Disagreements about respective responsibilities

Another source of tension between professionals, or between agencies, occurs when there are arguments about who is responsible for what. For example, there can be disagreements between local authorities and the NHS about whether a given problem is 'social' (and therefore the responsibility of social services) or 'medical' (and therefore the responsibility of health). It is perhaps these kinds of problems in particular that combined teams or inter-agency trusts are intended to avoid. Flexibility and willingness to compromise do tend to result when people know each other personally and work together on a day-to-day basis, although these kinds of difficulties are not unknown even in multi-agency/inter-professional teams.

Differences as to primary client

It is often the case that different agencies focus on a different primary client. In a family case where the parents have learning disabilities, for instance, the learning disability agencies will see the parents as their primary clients, but a child and family social worker will see the children as their primary clients. Since each member of the family has different needs, it can be very useful for each to have their own advocate, so to speak, within the professional system. But it can also lead to conflict if there is not a constructive dialogue between the professionals involved – this in the end can work against the interest of all family members. There are many other situations where different agencies or professionals may have a different primary focus. The following exercise deals with a case where an elderly man is living with a son who has profound physical and learning disabilities.

Exercise 9.2

Harry Thompson is a widower aged 80 living with his son James, who is 58, in the house into which Harry and his wife first moved when they married, a year before James was born. James has limited mobility as a result of cerebral palsy and also has a profound learning disability. Although he can make sounds to express his emotions, he has never acquired any sort of language. He requires help with feeding, toileting, dressing. He has a regular daily routine, which he seems to be comfortable with. His pleasures in life include watching television, food, playing in the bath and the company of the family cat, Jessie. Harry is himself in fairly good health for his age, but he is getting very weary of the business of providing physical care for James and is finding it increasingly difficult, even though he is devoted to his son and would not settle for any arrangement in which James was going to be unhappy.

Harry's GP insists that, at 80, Harry should be entitled to retire not only from work, but from the daily grind of meeting all James' personal needs. He says that Harry's health will start to suffer if he is made to carry on and that it would be better to get 'something sorted out for James' now, while there is time to make proper arrangements. What the GP has in mind is that James should be cared for in a residential establishment. He thinks that additional help in the home will be insufficient and in any case will be intrusive and worrying and will not give Harry the rest he needs and deserves.

The GP refers the case to the local Adults with Learning Disability Team and a social worker is allocated to the case. However, the social worker takes a very different line to the one that the GP was expecting. The social worker insists that James is her primary client and points out that, since James cannot speak for himself, it is particularly important that his own needs are properly taken into account. She points out that this is every bit as much James's home as Harry's (James has lived there all his life) and that, if the GP is concerned about the effects on Harry of continuing to care for James, she, as James' social worker, is very much more worried about the effects on James of moving him at 58, from the home in which he feels secure and comfortable to a new and, to him, alien, environment for which he cannot be prepared in advance and about which he cannot be consulted.

What are your thoughts about the way forward here?

Comments

Here we have a situation where the GP very definitely sees his responsibility as being to protect the interests of his patient, Harry. What is right for James seems, for the GP, to be a secondary consideration. Conversely, the social worker sees her brief as being to look after the interests of James. What is good about this situation is that both father and son have a strong supporter in the professional system.

(Continued)

(Continued)

(Situations like this can arise in which one party really has no-one to speak up for them and in such situations it may be particularly important to arrange for that person to have an advocate of their own.)

There is potential for deadlock in a situation like this. It could end up with the social worker and the GP at loggerheads, each one accusing the other of being callous and uncaring about the needs of the person each one sees as their primary concern. But this should not be necessary if they work to avoid taking up unnecessarily polarised positions. For one thing there is a good deal of common ground between Harry's and James' needs. On the one hand Harry is devoted to James and will not be happy unless James is properly cared for – so there is no question of being able to meet Harry's needs while disregarding James'. On the other hand, there is clearly a limit to what Harry can offer (he will not live forever after all), so it is not in James' interest to act as if the present arrangements can go on indefinitely.

It is therefore a question of reaching a solution, which meets Harry's need to step down the amount of care he offers to James while at the same time meeting James' need for continuity and routine. You may have had other ideas but one imaginative solution I have actually seen used in a similar situation to this was as follows.

Harry (or his equivalent) was provided with alternative accommodation of his own nearby, leaving James in his familiar environment. Twenty-four-hour care for James was funded using his benefit entitlements and community care funds that otherwise might have been spent on providing him with a costly residential bed. Night cover was provided by specially recruited live-in carers in exchange for free accommodation. Harry visited daily and continued to provide a part of James' care, but at a very much lower level.

The downside

As we have seen, good communication between professions and agencies is generally seen as a 'good thing'. Thus in the UK, the government Green Paper *Every Child Matters* aimed to avoid children 'slipping through the safety net' by:

improving information sharing between agencies to ensure all local authorities have a list of children in their area, the services each child has had contact with, and the contact details of the relevant professionals who work with them. The Government will remove the legislative barriers to better information sharing, and the technical barriers to electronic information sharing through developing a single unique identity number, and common data standards on the recording of information. (Department for Education and Skills, 2003: 8, original emphasis)

In the wake of a terrible tragedy, such as the death of Victoria Climbié, which could have been avoided if there had been better communication between agencies, it is hard to argue against the idea that information sharing is a good thing. But there is another side to it.

Exercise 9.3

Imagine that you went to see a counsellor or therapist for help with personal problems or difficult life decisions (some readers of this workbook will doubtless have done so at some point and will not need to imagine it). Imagine that, in the course of the sessions with the counsellor you discussed very personal matters, such as your intimate relationships, your sexuality, your doubts about your own abilities (as a parent, as a worker, as a partner), your use of alcohol or drugs, your mental health, your negative and positive feelings about other people in your life, secrets which, for one reason or another, you had not been able to share with those around you.

How would you then feel if your counsellor then wrote all this down and passed it on to your GP, a teacher in your children's school, a local police officer? Or how would you feel if your counsellor was to phone round these and other agencies (probation, social services, drug and alcohol services) to see what other information they had about you? How would you feel if all this information were combined into a common record to which all these agencies had access?

How would you feel if you yourself did not have full access to the information that these agencies were passing between themselves?

Comments

I think it probably safe to say that you would feel pretty uncomfortable about the counsellor behaving in this way. If she had not told you in advance she was going to do this, you would probably be very angry. Conversely, if she did tell you in advance, then that would substantially alter your views on what you would be prepared to discuss with this person – and whether you wanted to get involved with them at all.

Of course, as I began this session by saying, the job of a social worker is not the same thing as that of a counsellor or therapist. Nevertheless, a social worker's job does often entail winning the trust of clients and communicating with them about very personal matters.

One thing that makes the question even more sensitive in relation to social work is that the information being circulated may have a major effect on a service user's life (decisions about where they can live, for example, or whether or not they are able to parent their own children may be based on it!) If we ourselves did not have access to information about us that was being used to inform decisions of this kind, this would seem very unjust indeed.

Service users do feel uncomfortable about the information-sharing that goes on between professionals. This is particularly so if they feel that the information in circulation is inaccurate or only tells one side of the story (and the fact is that professionals will tend to note deficits and problems more than they note strengths, because it is the deficits and problems that cause their involvement in the first place.) Adkins et al. (1999: 227) note that collaboration among agencies is not necessarily seen as desirable by service users:

Clients have a number of concerns that mitigate their support of interagency collaboration:

- their sense of control of their own lives is eroded by increased violations of privacy;
- their understanding of what they have committed to in seeking services is uncertain;
- a perception of exclusion emerges – 'I want to be at that meeting if they are talking about me' …

Leslie Margolin, in a particularly savage critique of social work which I will discuss further in Chapter 11, makes a number of telling points about the way in which the gathering of information, and the sharing of information between agencies, increases the power of those agencies at the expense of the client:

Because the client knows nothing of the social worker's birth, family of origin and work history, yet the social worker possesses an intimate awareness of these details in reference to the client, one party is anonymous to the degree that the other is individualized, exposed. (Margolin, 1997: 38)

The following quotation refers to systems for sharing information between agencies as they emerged in the USA in the latter part of the 19th century, but it remains entirely relevant today:

Because each social worker's point of view was coordinated with that of other accredited officials, power was automatized and disindividualized. The social worker never faced any given family as an individual, nor even as the representative of a single organization; she became instead the stand-in for an entire class of people …

[So] when social workers visited the client's home, they were accompanied by many people. But only the social worker knew the identities of these uninvited guests. And only the social worker knew the uses to which these guests were put … (Margolin, 1997: 39)

Margolin is not the first to observe how disempowering it could feel for clients to know that information sharing was going on and he cites a social work textbook, published in 1935, that recommends *deceiving* clients as a way round this problem:

It is often best for interviewees not to know that an interviewer is in communication with outside sources of information as they might gain the feeling that he may be rendered prejudiced by someone else who did not quite understand them: they often feel their past is trailing behind them wherever they go. (Young, 1935: 194, cited in Margolin, 1997: 38)

This kind of deceit, I have to say, is still regularly practised. On numerous occasions I have encountered professionals of one kind or another passing on information with the request that the service user not be told that this has happened. The reason typically given is that 'it will damage my working relationship' with the service user, who will feel that trust is being betrayed. (So it is necessary to deceive someone in order to maintain their trust.)

Nowadays, of course, the technology exists to store and share information to a quite unprecedented degree. At time of writing the possibility of a national database of children is under discussion, which would allow all agencies access to basic information and would allow 'practitioners to flag on the system early warnings when they have a concern about a child which in itself may not be a trigger or meet the usual thresholds for intervention' (Department for Education and Skills, 2003: 53). I suggest that in our thinking about such developments, we should not make the uncritical assumption that working together and sharing information are necessarily 'good things.'

Practice notes

Working with other professions and agencies

Skill requirements

- Assertiveness is an important skill in working with other professionals. As a social worker you have a distinct job to do and a distinct perspective to represent and it may be necessary to insist on this in the face of pressure to fall in with the agendas of other professionals or other agencies.
- Listening skills are equally important, since no profession has the monopoly on 'truth' and no agency is in a position to see the whole picture, untarnished by its own particular local agendas.
- Networking skills are important: a matter of developing and maintaining good relationships with other professionals and workers in other agencies, and not just 'using' these other workers when a specific need arises.

Ethical considerations

- Part of effective inter-professional/inter-agency work is to do with clarity about what particular values your own agency and/or your own profession is there to promote and defend.
- Equally, it is important to apply 'respect for persons' to those who work in other professions and/or for other agencies and not to fall back into a complacent view that 'our' profession (or 'our' agency) is necessarily right and the others wrong.
- Clarity about boundaries around privacy and confidentiality are crucial in inter-agency work. You need to be clear what kinds of information you will share with other agencies and what you will not – both your clients and the other agencies need to understand what your boundaries are.
- Lying to people to maintain their trust is surely indefensible. It is not acceptable to pretend to offer confidentiality when you are not in fact doing so.
- Close co-operation and information sharing between agencies increases their collective power and may therefore increase the feeling of powerlessness of service users. This needs to be carefully considered in discussion of moves towards increased co-operation and information sharing. Professional people have an ethical obligation to participate in such debates and not merely to accept new developments uncritically.

(Continued)

(Continued)

Real-world constraints

- Although you will encounter a great deal of aspirational talk about the desirability of breaking down the barriers between professionals, the fact remains that different professionals have different jobs to do and different resources to do these jobs with. For instance, the fact that school teachers find it hard to get social workers to follow up on all their concerns is frustrating for school teachers and may make them feel discontented with social workers as a profession. But better communication between social workers and teachers will not alter the fact that both social workers and teachers only work so many hours a week and have to prioritise the different calls on their time. What good communication can do, is make different groups more understanding of the constraints that others work under.
- A more general point that was perhaps highlighted in the discussion on information-sharing is that, in the real world, initiatives that from one point of view appear to be a 'good thing' may from another point of view create new problems. In social work – as in politics and in many other areas of life – we are seldom able to simply apply one principle. More often we are attempting to strike a balance between opposing principles.

The co-ordinator role

I am going to conclude this chapter by touching briefly on some of the distinctive 'executive' roles that are sometimes played by social workers within multi-agency systems. The first of these roles is the one that in Chapter 1 I called the 'co-ordinator' role. In this role a social worker is not placed in charge of other professionals but is expected to co-ordinate their efforts by taking overall responsibility for ensuring that plans are discussed and agreed and by acting as a focal point for information sharing. This kind of role is taken on, to varying degrees, by social workers in most contexts. In residential establishments, for instance, it is common for a key worker system to operate in which one residential worker takes the lead in co-ordinating work in respect of a particular resident.

The professional who takes on this kind of role does not *necessarily* have to be a social worker. The Care Programme Approach introduced by the UK Government for mental health services (Department of Health, 1999b), includes a role originally called 'key worker' and then called 'care co-ordinator', but this role ma[...]ial workers but also by community psychiatric nurse[...]

Another co-ordinator role – one that i[...] by social workers in the UK – is that of '[...] ments set out in *Working Together* (Depart[...]

The key worker is responsible for making sure [...]veloped into a more detailed inter-agency plan. S/he sho[...] child and family, securing contributions from Core Group members and others as necessary. The key worker is also responsible for acting as lead worker for the inter-agency work with the child and the family. S/he should co-ordinate the contribution of family members and other agencies to planning the actions which need to be taken, putting the child protection plan into effect, and reviewing progress against the objectives set out in the plan. [The term 'Core Group' refers to family members, foster-parents if applicable, and those professionals who will be in direct contact with the family.]

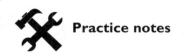 **Practice notes**

The co-ordinator role

Skill requirements, ethical considerations and real-world constraints

I do not wish to add much to the skills and values listed under 'working with other professions and agencies', except to say that:

(1)   As I have just noted, the co-ordinator role often requires that the social worker takes on a leadership role – yet does so in a context where she has no formal management responsibility for those she is expected to lead.
(2)   To key work adequately, particularly in a context such as child protection, where the professional system is engaged in managing significant risks, requires organisational skills: an ability to develop and maintain systems to ensure that you are kept adequately informed and that you adequately inform others.

The care manager role

The term 'care management' came into general use in the UK following the implementation of the NHS and Community Care Act, 1990. The term had been in use for some time in the USA. Social workers (along with other social services staff) had for many years been in the business of assessing the needs of adult service users and negotiating various combinations of residential, day care and homecare services to meet those needs. What was different after the Act was that:

(1)   The duties of social services departments in this respect were very considerably expanded. (Public funding for care in private residential homes, previously part of the benefits system, was transferred to local authorities; see Lewis and Glennerster [1996].)
(2)   A 'mixed economy of care' was introduced. In this new arrangement many of the actual providers of care services – whether residential, day care or homecare – were not part of social services departments but were private companies or voluntary agencies.

(3)   As a result of this change, the social worker's task was no longer to link service users up to services run by her own agency, but to assemble a package of care services *purchased* by her agency from a variety of *providers*, many of whom would be external to the social worker's own agency.

Social workers have always been involved in commissioning or recruiting help from a variety of sources but the NHS and Community Care Act extended and formalised this care management role, so that social workers became a kind of broker, using a budget agreed with her own agency to put a care plan into practice by purchasing (or 'commissioning') a package of services.

↗ A note on terminology

I warned in Chapter 1 about the different ways in which words are used. I should note here that those who undertake a care management role under the NHS and Community Care Act are commonly referred to as 'care co-ordinators', which is of course a different use of the word 'co-ordinator' from that in this book where I make a distinction between 'co-ordinator' and 'care manager roles'.

Needs-led assessment

One of the principles that is supposed to underlie assessment in this new environment was the idea of *needs-led assessment*, as opposed to a service-led approach. The principle of a needs-led approach is that, when carrying out an assessment, the assessor should set aside any thoughts about what services were actually available in order to focus as clearly as possible on needs as opposed to services.

To illustrate the difference, consider the example in Exercise 9.2. If a social worker had taken a purely *service*-led approach, she would have considered the services that actually existed at the time and defined James' needs in those terms. Thus, if the services provided by her agency consisted of residential care or day care, she might have defined James as being in need of residential care, or in need of day care. In fact, *no one* is specifically 'in need of residential care', though many people have high personal care needs which, in some cases, can be best met in a residential context. James had high personal care needs and also a need for continuity and familiar surroundings. The personalised solution which I described involved, in effect, creating a new service for James designed around his needs. This would simply not have been possible if he had been simply labelled a 'residential care case' or a 'day care case.'

I should perhaps add, though, that when the concept of needs-led assessment was introduced during the implementation of the NHS and Community Care Act, what was not so often acknowledged was that the Act was actually intended to provide a mechanism for rationing resources, and to control expenditure in an area where government spending was running out of control. In this context, not surprisingly, the meaning of the term 'needs-led assessment' has become worn down by use, because in reality assessments are dictated not simply by client's needs but also by the need to limit the services that are provided. Nowadays the term 'needs-led assessment' often seems to mean nothing more than a form on which needs are recorded. However, the *principle* of a needs-led assessment remains a sound one.

Thinking about resources

For better or worse a social worker acting as a purchaser or commissioner of services has to be much more aware of how *much things cost* than a social worker operating in the more traditional system, where she is merely requesting services from her own or other agencies. On the plus side, this encourages social workers to make best use of the limited financial resources that are available in any agency. If you know that service X will cost £500 a week, you might be more inclined to find creative alternatives to service X than if you had no idea that it was so expensive. (If you end up as a result, finding an alternative that is cheaper but just as good or better, then you have freed up resources that can be used to meet needs that otherwise might not have been met.) Conversely, it is hard to be 'needs-led' when you are also having to think about costs and staying within budget.

Direct payments

One consideration that should always be borne in mind when thinking about care management is whether a service user actually needs a care manager at all. After all, most of us in our private lives are able to purchase the various goods and services that we feel we need without requiring the services of someone to do it for us. Direct payments are a way in which care management can simply be handed over the service user. In the UK, under the Community Care (Direct Payments) Act, 1996, local authority social service departments can make cash payments to service users. 'Instead of arranging the services it has assessed the person as needing' (Department of Health, 1996: 4), the agency provides service users with the resources to make whatever arrangements they think fit:

> Day-to-day control of the money and care package passes to the person who has the strongest incentive to ensure that it is spent properly on the necessary services and who is best placed to judge how to match available resources to needs. (Department of Health, 1996: 3)

Of course the system is open to abuse, for example by relatives or others who might put vulnerable service users under pressure to hand over money, so service users need to be adequately safeguarded against exploitation. And for some service users, having to make their own care arrangements is either beyond their capacity or simply a burden which they do not feel up to carrying, but for many service users this is an attractive option.

Practice notes

Care management

Skill requirements

- Apart from the skills listed under 'working with other professions and agencies', care management (as its name suggests) involves management skills, including skills in budgeting, leadership skills and an ability to oversee and (if necessary) challenge the work of others.

Ethical considerations

- Pure care management involves relatively little contact with clients and a relatively large amount of dealing with systems and administrative arrangements. In this context the challenge to your values is to carry on looking at the task as a *human* one and the service user as a unique human being, rather than as a logistical problem.
- A social worker acting as a care manager needs to think carefully about her respective responsibilities to her service user and to the agency as a whole, and to the relationship between her care manager role and any advocacy role which she believes she ought to be carrying out. She cannot be a whole-hearted advocate for her client's needs, if she is required (as is commonly the case) to also take on an 'almoner' role in which the needs of one service user are weighed up against the needs of others.
- In any given situation, it is worth thinking about whether service users *need* a care manager. Would it be better for direct payments to be made to the service user who could then manage his or her own care?

Real-world constraints

- Care management as a method of delivering services works best in the context where there are a range of different services available to be commissioned and where the care manager has sufficient purchasing power to 'shop around' for the best combination of services for each service user. In practice the range of options can be limited and the funding restricted.

The responsibility holder role

The care manager role as I have described it is most prevalent in the UK in the area of services for elderly people and adults with physical disability. In child and family social work in the UK, there is less of a 'mixed economy' of care and less emphasis on a model in which those who come up with a care plan are in an actual purchasing relationship with those who provide the services. Nevertheless, in this area of work too, there is an increasing tendency to separate out the 'assessment' function from the service provider function. The term 'care manager' is less widely used, but the social worker's task is often to assess needs and to propose a care plan to meet these needs. The actual implementation of the care plan may be largely, or even entirely, down to others (family centres, family support workers, and so on) who deliver the direct work to the service user, while social workers are left with a supervising and co-ordinating function.

In the case of children in public care, social workers carry a rather unique level of responsibility in that, on behalf of their agencies, they are required to discharge the responsibilities of a parent. They are therefore typically combining elements of a care management role with what I have called the 'responsibility holder' role, a combination of roles which really is unique to social work. Here, as with a real parent, social workers have to make judgements as to the capacity of children to make their own decisions about their needs, and have to consider the lifelong needs of children as well as their immediate ones: their needs for a secure family base and a sense of identity, for instance. A common mistake that is made is to take a purely short-term care management approach in such cases, by ensuring that children's immediate needs are met while failing to lay foundations for their future. 'Drift' in care (first publicised by Rowe and Lambert, 1973) is the result, and can have devastating effects for children who are effectively denied the possibility of a family where they put down roots and have the experience of loving and being loved.

The role of responsibility holder in this context is made more complex by the fact that in most cases parental responsibility must be shared to varying degrees both with the actual natural parents of the child and with carers who discharge parental responsibility on a day-to-day basis without having overall control.

Chapter summary

This chapter has explored some of the characteristic ways in which social workers work with others. The topics covered have been:

- **Working with carers:** The importance of carers, and the issues involved in thinking about their distinct needs.
- **Working with other professionals and agencies:** The advantages, difficulties and possible disadvantages in inter-professional working.
- **The downside:** The ways in which inter-agency/inter-professional working may be disempowering for service users – the difficulties that arise in inter-professional working when it comes to confidentiality and privacy.
- **The co-ordinator role:** The social work role in which social worker co-ordinates but does not control the work of others.
- **The care manager role:** The social work role in which a social worker purchases and oversees services from other sources.
- **The responsibility holder role:** A brief note on the particular position of social workers planning for children for whom their agency has some parental responsibility.

In the next chapter I will consider the issues raised by a role played by social workers which sets social work apart from many other professions: the 'control agent' role.

10 | Coercive powers

- Varieties of power

  - Legitimate power
  - Expert power
  - Reward power
  - Referent power
  - Coercive power

- Statutory powers in social work

  - Elderly people and people with disabilities
  - Mental health
  - Children and families
  - Youth justice

- 'Control' and social work
- Towards a model of the control agent role
- Working with involuntary clients

  - Accurate role clarification
  - Reinforcing and modelling 'pro-social' values
  - Collaborative problem-solving

One of the aspects of social work that distinguishes it quite sharply from many of the other 'caring professions' is what I called in Chapter 1 its 'control agent' role. In several different areas of work, social workers are given – or can obtain through the courts – legal powers that can be used to *compel* people to do things. In this respect, however uncomfortable the comparison may make some of us feel, social work has more in common with occupations such as the police force or the prison service than it does with counselling or psychotherapy.

Power is not necessarily a bad thing and the use of statutory power is not necessarily oppressive. For example, if social workers had applied for a court order under the Children Act, 1989, to remove Victoria Climbié (see Laming, 2003) from her aunt Kouao before she was fatally injured, that would not have been an oppressive act. On the contrary, it would have liberated Victoria from a particularly appalling form of adult oppression against which, as a child, she was powerless to protect herself. But power can be abused and it is insidious in its effects both on those who wield it (there is surely some truth in the saying 'all power corrupts') and on those who are on the receiving end. Statutory power can also, even with the very best intentions, be used incompetently and ineffectively, or in ways that make things worse rather than better.

Varieties of power

This chapter is about the use of statutory, coercive powers. But it is worth noting at the outset that formal, statutory powers are only one of the varieties of power which social workers and others use. French and Raven (1959, see Raven, 1993, for developments and refinements of this model) proposed that social power could be categorised into five varieties:

Legitimate power

Power gained through rules and official roles. In a university context, an example would be the powers given to lecturers to mark the work of students. In the case of marking, various checks and balances are built into the system (second markers, external assessors and so on) to try to ensure that this power is exercised appropriately. A social work example might be the power exercised by a social worker in a team for elderly people who carries out needs assessments in order to come to a judgement about the level and type of need of a given service user. These assessments largely determine the way that resources are allocated. This power could be abused by a social worker overstating the case for service users she happens to like, or understating the case for service users she dislikes.

Expert power

This is power gained through being recognised having particular knowledge or skills. It is worth noting that this kind of power is to do with perception: a person can obtain expert power simply by being *perceived* to possess particular knowledge or skills, even if objectively she does not. (Other kinds of power too rely as much on the perceptions of others as on the objective realities.) In many contexts, the opinion of social workers as to the degree of risk that exists in a given situation will be influential in determining what action is taken. For example: at a child protection conference a social worker's firmly stated view may well prevail and determine the outcome. This power could be abused if the social worker over-stated her own level of expertise and gave the impression that, for example, what amounted to an informed guess, had the status of a fact. Other professions too are often guilty of this. Myers (1994: 24) noted the tendency of professional experts to make over-dogmatic

statements such as 'Children do not lie about sexual abuse', when in fact we can never completely rule out the possibility that in some circumstances children do lie, just as we can never completely rule out the possibility that a carer may be an abuser. By claiming more expertise than we really have, we undermine the legitimacy of what others have to say, particularly service users, who may be unfairly silenced as a result.

Reward power

Power gained through the ability to give rewards. One way in which social workers may get into a position of possessing reward power is when they are their clients' only access point to services. But there are many ways in which social workers can reward service users, one of which is simply by giving sympathy and attention to people who are desperately in need of them. In an investigation into allegations of Satanic abuse, the anthropologist, Jean la Fontaine (1998) went as far as to suggest that the desire to please their questioners (social workers, police officers and so on) might actually lead some vulnerable and needy people to invent stories to conform to what they thought the questioners wanted to hear: 'When the listener is eager to hear more, gratitude for support may impel the young person ... to find ever more dramatic memories to recount' (1998: 154).

Referent power

This is the power a person derives from the admiration and respect of others. It may derive from personal qualities on the one hand, and from social status or prestige on the other. Some social workers have a great deal of personal authority or charisma, which can be used constructively, but can also be abused. In terms of prestige and status: we may not think social work is a very high status profession compared to some, but it may seem high status to some of the people that social workers deal with. Social workers may seem to many service users to be better educated, more able and more affluent than themselves. In British society we learn to identify other people's social class from signs such as accent and dress, and on that basis, many social workers will seem to belong to a 'higher' class than many service users. Those who see themselves at the bottom of the pile can become very resigned to and accepting of being ordered around by those of higher status and it is often extremely easy for social workers, perhaps inadvertently, to exploit this, thus further confirming feelings of powerlessness on the part of service users.

Coercive power

This is the power gained through the ability to punish or to use physical force to bring about a certain outcome and it is social work's possession of coercive powers that is the main subject of this chapter. 'But surely social work isn't about using physical force or punishment?', would be an understandable objection at this point. We need to be clear therefore that, while social workers may not *themselves* use force or punishments, they do exercise legal powers that rely on the ability of the state to use force and/or punishment to make these powers a reality. For example, when a British social worker signs an application for a person to be detained in hospital under the Mental Health Act, 1983, the police will enforce this if the person refuses to co-operate. When social workers obtain court orders to allow them to remove children from their parents, and the parents refuse to comply, the police will be called on as a final resort and will if necessary use physical force. Sometimes police officers force doors and physically restrain adults to ensure that a court order on a child can be carried out. Pieces of paper such as court orders or Mental Health Act applications do not *in themselves* make anyone do anything. Their power comes from the fact that force can be enlisted to put them into effect.

Statutory powers in social work

The following is a brief summary of some of the main legal powers of compulsion that are exercised by social workers in the UK as they stand at time of writing. (Social workers in other countries also exercise such powers, though these differ from one country to another.) All of these powers are instances of coercive powers in that in each case physical force and/or punishment can be enlisted in the case of non-compliance. In fact in most cases physical force is not necessary, but this is because people are aware that it can, if necessary be called upon. In much the same way, if a person demands that we do something and we know he has a gun in his pocket, then we will tend to meet his demands, even if he doesn't actually produce the gun.

Elderly people and people with disabilities

Under a very old piece of legislation – Section 47 of the National Assistance Act, 1948 – local authority social services departments can and do still apply to a magistrates' court for an order authorising them to remove a person 'in need of care and attention' from their home and to take them to a hospital, residential home or some other 'suitable place' if:

- the person is 'suffering from grave chronic disease or being aged, infirm or physically incapacitated, is living in insanitary conditions', and
- 'is unable to devote to themselves, and is not receiving from other persons, proper care and attention', and
- the person's removal from home is necessary, 'either in their own interests or for preventing injury to the health of, or serious nuisance to, other persons', and
- the Community Physician has supplied evidence in writing to the local authority to this effect.

Seven days notice needs to be given to the person concerned or to someone who is 'in charge of' that person. If the court is satisfied by the evidence presented it can make an order lasting up to three months under Section 47(4), which can be further renewed by the court for a further three months. In an emergency an order can also be obtained from a single magistrate without giving the person concerned any prior notice, provided that the community physician and another doctor are willing to state that it is 'in the interest of that person to remove him without delay', under Section 1(1) of the National Assistance (Amendment) Act, 1951. An emergency order of this kind can last up to three weeks.

Mental health

In England and Wales, the Mental Health Act, 1983, places social workers in a unique position of authority which is not matched in any other social work specialism. Social workers 'approved' under the Act are the professional group who are entrusted with the ultimate decision as to whether people should be detained, and even given treatment, against their will, and they are empowered to make these decisions without reference to the courts. Section 2 of the Act makes provision for a 'patient' to be admitted and detained for assessment on the grounds that:

(1) he is suffering from mental disorder of a nature or degree which warrants the detention of the patient in a hospital for assessment (or for assessment followed by medical treatment) for at least a limited period; and
(2) he ought to be so detained in the interests of his own health and safety or with a view to the protection of other persons.

A person can be detained under this section for 28 days if an application is made by an approved social worker, on the recommendation of two medical practitioners.

Detention for treatment – permitting not only compulsory detention but compulsory treatment – under Section 3 of the Act can likewise be made by an approved social worker on the recommendation of two medical practitioners on the grounds that:

(1) the patient 'is suffering from mental illness, severe mental impairment, psychopathic disorder or mental impairment and his mental disorder is of a nature or degree which makes it appropriate for him to receive medical treatment in a hospital; and
(2) in the case of a psychopathic disorder or mental impairment, such treatment is likely to alleviate or prevent a deterioration of his condition; and
(3) it is necessary for the health or safety of the patient or for the protection of other persons that he should receive such treatment and it cannot be provided unless he is detained under this section.'

There is also provision for an emergency application to be made under Section 4, on the recommendation of one medical practitioner, under which a 'patient' can be detained for 72 hours.

Children and families

The statutory powers exercised by children and family social workers are certainly the manifestation of the control agent role which is most widely known to the British public at large and it is the one that rouses the strongest and most ambivalent passions. Unlike mental health social workers, though, child and families social workers never exercise these powers on their own account. They have to request courts to make orders which will allow them to remove children from their parents or to obtain access to them. It is with courts, not social workers, that the decision ultimately rests.

Section 47 of the Children Act, 1989 sets out a local authority's duties when it receives information about a child within its area who may be suffering, or likely to suffer, 'significant harm':

• It should make sufficient enquiries to allow it to determine what action needs to be taken to protect the child.
• It should arrange for the child to be seen, unless sufficient information can be obtained without doing so.

- If denied access to a child, or refused information about the child's whereabouts, it should apply for a court order. This might be an emergency protection order (Sections 44–46), a child assessment order (Section 43), a care order or a supervision order (Section 31).
- More generally it should decide whether it is in the interests of the child whether to initiate court proceedings.

But even if the case is not taken to court, the multi-disciplinary arrangements under *Working Together* (Department of Health, 1999a), create an environment – Case Conferences, Core Groups, Strategy Meetings – in which parental behaviour is placed under scrutiny. Parents are expected to comply with the Child Protection Plans put in place by the multi-agency system and, while such plans do not in themselves have statutory force, failure to comply places parents at risk of being taken to court in the ways described above. While this is a *multi-agency* system, only two agencies can take on the role of 'key worker' (an instance of what I called in Chapter 1 a 'co-ordinator' role) and only these two agencies have the job of taking cases (if necessary) to court. Both of these agencies are social work agencies, namely local authority social service departments and the NSPCC (the National Society for the Prevention of Cruelty to Children.)

Youth justice

The Crime and Disorder Act, 1998 required local authorities across England and Wales to set up Youth Offending Teams (YOTs): inter-disciplinary and multi-agency teams which can include social services staff alongside representatives from the police, the probation service, the health service, education, drugs and alcohol services, and housing officers. Each local YOT has a manager with overall responsibility for co-ordinating youth justice service work in his or her area (see Youth Justice Board [www.youth-justice-board.gov.uk]).

Social workers in YOTs are directly involved in administering the criminal justice system. They are involved in writing reports for use by courts when deciding how to deal with convicted young offenders. They are also involved in administering a number of the sentences that a court can make, including the following:

- *Supervision Orders* (not to be confused with Supervision Orders under the Children Act, 1989), which requires the offender to meet regularly with a YOT worker and participate in activities set by the YOT. Supervision orders may also have various 'specified activities' attached to them in which the offender is required to participate.
- *Action Plan Orders* described in the Youth Justice Board website as 'an intensive, community-based programme lasting 3 months ... specifically tailored to the risks and needs of the young person. It can include repairing the harm done to the victim of the offence or the community, education and training, attending an Attendance Centre or a variety of other programmes to address a young person's offending behaviour.'
- *Referral Orders*, under which the offender is required to attend a Youth Offender Panel made up of a YOT worker and two volunteers from the local community. The Panel, in conjunction with the young person, their parents or carers and (where appropriate) the victim, agree a contract lasting 3–12 months. This may include, among other things, a requirement to attend programmes

intended to address the offending behaviour or a requirement to repair the harm done by their offence.

- *Reparation Orders* that require the offender to make restitution for the harm caused by their offence either directly to the victim, which, if both parties agree to it, can involve victim–offender mediation, or indirectly to the community generally.

Among the duties of a YOT worker overseeing a young offender under orders of these kinds is the duty to ensure that the young person participates as required. In the event that a young person fails to comply with an order, then the YOT worker will take the case back to court for being in breach of the order – a step which could result in the young person being given a custodial sentence or other forms of punishment.

'Control' and social work

I find that social work texts – even government guidance – are sometimes rather coy about the use of coercive powers in social work. It *is* generally recognised that social work has both a 'care' and a 'control' function, but a notion seems to linger in our minds that 'control' is necessarily oppressive (and therefore bad) while 'care' is necessarily good, and that 'control' is therefore best swept away under the carpet and out of sight. Actually 'care' can be oppressive in its effects and 'control' can be not only liberating but life-saving. (During an acute schizophrenic episode, a man comes to believe that he is receiving radio messages from God that he should kill his family. Is it oppressive to use coercive powers to protect his family – and the man himself – from his dangerous, and temporary, delusions?) But our feeling that 'control' isn't *really* what social workers ought to be doing seems to me to lead to a lack of guidance on how to appropriately use it. Books on social work theory are typically full of ideas derived from therapy and counselling which are primarily applicable to work with voluntary clients, yet some social workers work mainly or even exclusively with involuntary clients. And, while everyone acknowledges that sometimes it is necessary to use coercive powers, there is surprisingly little theory on how to do so:

> There is no relationship between the frequency with which practitioners see mandated [i.e. involuntary] clients and the number of articles and books devoted to discussing practice with them. This is not surprising because the field's practice procedures have been developed assuming that practitioners work with voluntary clients. (De Jong and Berg, 2001: 361)

Actually, it *is* surprising in many ways that this is the case when one considers what a central position 'statutory work' (as it is commonly called in Britain) actually occupies in social work as it is actually practised. In the UK a very significant proportion of social work in the children and families field takes place with cases where children are either already subject to care or supervision orders, or with cases where parents know that social workers would go to court and apply for such orders if they did not comply with protection plans. Indeed, I would guess that *most* of the time put in by social workers in this field is spent on such cases. De Jong and Berg (2001: 361), who are based in the USA, likewise suggest that 'the majority of clients seen by social workers in public agencies are mandated, or at least to some degree involuntary'. One can argue about whether coercive powers are used too readily or not readily enough, and there are periodic pendulum swings in public policy and social work practice in this regard, but they *are* used and social work is the profession primarily charged with the task of using them. Perhaps we ought to give some consideration as to what they are supposed to achieve and how. The following are a few thoughts, drawing on the concept of 'crisis' which I discussed in Chapter 7.

Towards a model of the control agent role

Coercive powers are used in social work in two *ways* and for two kinds of *purpose*. The ways in which they can be used are *explicit* and *implicit*. Explicit use of coercive powers occurs when a social worker actually obtains a court order or, in the case of the Mental Health Act, completes an application for a patient to be detained, or, in a youth justice context, takes a young offender back to court for non-compliance. Implicit use of coercive powers occurs when a social worker does not actually carry out any of these explicit steps, but is able to secure the compliance of a service user as a result of the fact that the service user knows that the social worker can invoke these powers if necessary. I think that we are inclined to greatly underestimate the extent of our implicit powers. Social workers sometimes exercise implicit coercive powers without even realising it, imagining that they are working in a voluntary partnership with service users when in fact service users are complying with their wishes out of fear of the consequences of not doing so. For instance, in the UK, social workers in the children and families field have to operate in a context where perhaps the single most widely known fact about social workers is that they can remove children from their families.

The kinds of *purpose* for which coercive powers can be used, I will call *direct protection* and *protective leverage*. By *direct protection*, I mean actual physical separation of people thought to be at risk from other people or situations thought to pose a risk to them: the removal of a child from a family, the removal of a mentally ill person from the community. By *protective leverage*, I am referring to the ways in which coercive powers are used to encourage people to bring about changes in their lives, in order to reduce the risks that they pose to themselves or to others. Thus, in England and Wales, a Supervision Order under the Crime and Disorder Act, 1998, backed with the possibility of other measures in the event of non-compliance, may be used as protective leverage to get a young person to meet with a professional on a regular basis and discuss his offending behaviour.

Often social workers hope that steps taken to confer direct protection will also provide protective leverage. For instance a child is removed from a neglectful lone mother under a court order. The primary purpose of this would be to protect him from the risks he was facing at home, but it may also be hoped that removing him from home will demonstrate to his mother that she cannot continue to act as she has been acting and that, if she wants her son to return to her care, she will need to look at what she is doing wrong and work to make things better. In other cases, social workers hope that protective leverage will be provided by putting service users on notice that formal protective measures are being considered. For instance a man with mental health problems is persuaded to agree to go into

Figure 10.1   Coercive powers in social work

		Purpose used for	
		Direct protection	**Protective leverage**
Ways used	**Explicit**	Use of court orders or other statutory powers to either physically move a vulnerable person from an environment where he is at risk, or to physically move a person thought to pose risks to others.	Use of court orders or other statutory powers by a social worker to require co-operation in a protection plan or other plan of action intended to bring about change.
	Implicit	Without using court orders or other statutory powers, but by using the service user's knowledge that such powers are available, a social worker either physically moves a vulnerable person from an environment where he is at risk, or physically moves a person thought to pose risks to others.	Without using court orders or other statutory powers, but by using the service user's knowledge that such powers are available, a social worker obtains co-operation in a protection plan or other plan of action intended to bring about change.

hospital on a voluntary basis. One of the reasons he agrees to this is that he has been informed that an application to detain him compulsorily may well otherwise occur.

Please note that I am *not* saying here that protective measures should be used merely as a threat. This would be an abuse of power. However, in situations that are close to the threshold where protective measures will need to be taken, it is generally appropriate to warn those concerned of this fact, and it is perfectly reasonable to encourage people to act in ways that will remove the necessity of carrying out those protective measures. (I say it is *generally* appropriate to give advance warning because there are some situations in which advance warning cannot be given without placing people at risk.) Likewise, in a situation where protective measures have actually been taken, it is in most cases good practice to use this as a starting point for working towards a state of affairs in which protective measures can be lifted, as in my example of the neglectful mother. Figure 10.1 sets out the various possibilities.

In this book I have argued that there is always an underlying theory behind any intervention, and that we ought to be clear about – be able to describe – what that theory is. So what is the theory behind the use of coercive powers? How are they supposed to work and why?

In cases where coercive powers are used (explicitly or implicitly) for the purpose of direct protection, the theory is pretty obvious: when a situation is dangerous we can reduce the danger by removing from it either the endangered or the dangerous person. What must be borne in mind, though, is that short-term direct protection is in most cases only the beginning of the story. A person may be detained in a mental hospital as a short-term measure, but that still leaves us with the job of putting together a plan for rehabilitation. A child may be removed from an abusive or neglectful carer, but that still leaves us with the much more challenging task of providing that child with a secure future, either by resolving problems at home so they can return, or in some cases by preparing the child for a new family. (In the last chapter I mentioned the problem of 'drift' which occurs for children who are kept in public care without any clear plan being implemented for their long-term future. One reason that drift occurs is that we sometimes mistakenly assume that providing direct protection is all that we need to think about.)

When it comes to the use of coercive powers for *protective leverage*, however, the picture becomes a little more complicated. What kind of protective leverage do coercive powers actually confer?

Exercise 10.1

David and Eve have been worrying neighbours, extended family members and professional agencies for some time with their care of their children Harry, aged seven, and Fran, six. Over the last term, the children have been absent for over 10 per cent of school days and have been late into school almost every day – sometimes over an hour late. At school they are often observed to be very hungry and Fran has twice been caught stealing from other children's lunch boxes. Their clothing is often dirty and/or put on incorrectly (for example with the buttons not aligned properly). They seem very tired and isolated among their peer group. The school has attempted to talk to David and Eve about this, but they never respond to letters.

Professionals visiting the family home have found it very difficult to gain access. David and Eve don't respond to appointment letters and are seldom in when professionals call at prearranged times. When a social worker did manage to see Eve recently, after three unsuccessful attempts, she found that the house was in a very chaotic and dirty state. There were large piles of dirty clothes on the floor, unwashed crockery on most surfaces and there was an overpowering smell of urine. Eve seemed to have just got out of bed, although it was two in the afternoon, and the curtains were still drawn. The social worker asked to see the children's beds and found that they had no sheets, only blankets on bare mattresses.

Neighbours report that there are frequent adult visitors to the house throughout the evening and through to the early hours of the morning. David and Eve both have convictions for drug offences. There is some evidence to suggest that they are dealing in drugs. Professionals surmise (1) that they are preoccupied with a drug-based lifestyle and have little space left to attend to their children's needs, (2) that they usually don't get up early enough in the morning to give their children breakfast or help them to get ready for school.

Eventually the children's names are placed on the child protection register on the grounds of neglect and it is made clear to the parents that they need to comply with a protection plan or legal advice will be sought about the possibility of initiating care proceedings. The protection plan includes elements like: David and Eve should keep appointments with professionals, ensure the children are properly prepared for school and have properly made up beds to sleep in and so on. David and Eve both state that they love their children and do not want them to be taken into public care.

Here is a situation where coercive power is being used to try and get some protective leverage. How might this affect David and Eve and what protective leverage will it actually give?

(Continued)

(Continued)

Comments

You will probably agree that most parents would be very severely shaken by the possibility that their children might be removed from them and would be prepared to do a great deal to prevent this from occurring. The protective leverage here would therefore seem to be considerable. But what can it achieve?

One possibility you may have thought about is that this will 'bring Eve and David to their senses', force them to realise how bad things have become and provide them with the necessary push towards sorting out their lives and providing a better home for their children. This is the most optimistic view, but it can happen. In a sense the agency intervention becomes a 'crisis' for the family, in the positive sense that it becomes a turning point (see Chapter 7 for more on crises.)

Another possibility is that they will not examine their own part in this at all, but will deal with this simply as an external threat to be managed by making small gestures towards compliance with the requirements being made upon them: you could call this superficial or feigned compliance. But, to be optimistic again, superficial compliance can sometimes be a starting point for deeper change.

A third possibility is that it will have no effect at all. This, however, may in itself provide some protective leverage of a kind in that it can be seen as diagnostic. It is possible to argue that, if these parents cannot do anything about their parenting even when they have been made aware that they could lose their children if they don't, then this tells us something quite negative about their commitment to their children. This could be used as evidence by a social work agency seeking a legal mandate to make alternative plans for the children.

But we should also acknowledge the possibility that the use of coercive powers in situations like this can have negative consequences on the protective leverage of social workers as well as positive ones. It may make it harder for David and Eve to trust the professional agencies. It may make it harder for them to be honest with the professional agencies about (for instance) the extent of their drug use. It may even make them more reluctant, rather than less so, to let professionals into their home.

Given the fact that David and Eve were not working with professional agencies in any case, this last point may seem somewhat academic in this particular situation, but there is one more negative aspect to consider: the effect of a social work intervention actually has ripples that spread far wider than the particular case in question. The more social workers use coercive powers, the more the use of coercive powers will be associated with social work in the public mind, and this will cast a shadow not only over a particular case, but over the work of social workers in general. Overuse of coercive powers may reduce our overall ability to work in a co-operative way.

I hope Exercise 10.1 demonstrates that the possession of coercive power does confer protective leverage. In Chapter 7, I suggested that the way this works is by precipitating a *crisis* in the life of the client, a moment at which simply maintaining the existing equilibrium is no longer a viable option and in which change of some kind simply cannot be avoided. However, like many of the other methods used by social workers and like other kinds of crisis in people's lives, this kind of deliberately engineered crisis is unpredictable in its effects. The possible effects of the application of coercive power to obtain protective leverage in a given situation could be summarised as follows:

- Deep change: The crisis created is fully worked through by the service user, resulting in durable internalised change. (Service users sometimes say, 'It was a wake up call' or 'It was the kick up the backside I needed'.)
- Surface change: A crisis of some kind is precipitated, but it results in purely superficial or feigned compliance with the power-holder. (But surface change can *become* deep change.)
- No change: In spite of a service user being made aware of the consequences of non-compliance, compliance does not occur. This is often interpreted as diagnostic of lack of motivation or ability to change. In a case where a child has been taken into public care, for instance, non-compliance may be used by social workers as evidence to obtain the authority to make alternative long-term care plans for children. However, we should be aware that denial and refusal to face the necessity for change are known to be common psychological manoeuvres in the face of crises of any kind, and should be wary of assuming that failure to change necessary demonstrates indifference.
- Negative change: The use of coercive powers actually inhibits effective work, making those on the receiving end less, not more, willing to co-operate with social workers. (Here the crisis has indeed brought about change, but not in the hoped-for direction.)
- Wider negative change: The use of coercive powers in particular cases affects negatively not only current service users but potential service users' perceptions of the agency. The fact that social workers are known to 'take children into care', for instance, affects the relationships that all parents have with social workers, and not just those parents whose own children have been taken into care, or parents where this has actually been discussed.

Having noted it, I will leave aside the issue of *wider negative change*. It is an important question, but it is really more a matter for policy-makers than for social workers making decisions in specific situations.

In the context of decision-making about individual cases, a social worker would seek to minimise the use of coercive powers. (Although, as I have noted, it may be impossible to eliminate the effect of *implicit* coercive power and social workers may simply have to recognise and allow for its existence.) However, assuming that other approaches have been tried and that coercive powers are deemed to be necessary to obtain protective leverage, a social worker will naturally want to use those powers in a way that will result, if possible, in *deep change* and that will not, as far as possible, result in *negative change*. There is often a danger, for instance, that the use of protective leverage may achieve no more than a resentful compliance with superficial aspects of a protection plan while actually reducing a client's willingness to really work together with a social worker. (The client may feel he has no choice but to let the social worker into the house, but may be more determined than ever not to talk to the social worker about anything of any significance.)

In the event that *no change* is the result, this can be seen as diagnostic but the social worker will need to be as confident as possible that this really is diagnostic of an inability or unwillingness to change, and does not simply indicate that the wrong approach has been used.

Practice notes

Using coercive powers

Skill requirements

- The use of statutory powers requires a good understanding of the relevant law and an ability to present yourself effectively in the formal context of courts and tribunals.
- It is necessary to feel comfortable operating in a position of authority.
- Clear thinking is needed to reach a decision on whether the use of coercive powers is justified and for what purpose.
- It requires skills in working with involuntary clients which I will discuss separately below.

Ethical considerations

- Coercive powers should only be used when it can be justified in terms of a duty of care towards someone who would otherwise be vulnerable.
- Honesty and self-awareness are important. There are many reasons why we might be tempted to reach for statutory powers when they really are not needed. There are also many reasons why we might be tempted *not* to use these powers even when they really do need to be used to protect someone. Honesty allows us to separate out our legitimate motives from the ones that are really not legitimate in a professional context.
- One thing that we need to be aware of in particular is the possibility that we may be inappropriately influenced – one way or another – in our decisions about the use of statutory powers by factors such as the ethnicity of the service user. Thompson (2001) notes that research suggests that professionals are more ready to use 'control' in relation to black people than they are in relation to white people. On the other hand the Climbié report (Laming, 2003) discussed the possibility that the professional failure to intervene may have been partly the result of fears of seeming racist, given that Victoria and her aunt were of African (Ivorian) origin.

Real-world constraints

- The use of coercive powers is of course not a theoretical idea but an event that actually occurs in social work in the real world. The constraints that the real world does impose however are on what can be achieved by the use of such powers. To give a single instance. It may be possible to obtain a court order to remove a child from an abusive or neglectful situation with a view to finding an alternative family for that child. But to successfully place that child in a new family is dependant on a number of factors that may be outside of your control, such as the availability of placements, the child's ability to form new attachments. Realism requires that social workers take recourse to extreme measures of this kind (1) only when the current circumstances really justify it, but also (2) only when there is a reasonable certainty of being able to secure a better outcome as a result. In England and Wales, this principle is enshrined in Section 1(5) of the Children Act, 1989, which states that a court should not make any kind of order on a child 'unless it considers that doing so would be better for the child than making no order at all'.

Working with involuntary service users

As far as possible in a situation in which coercive powers are being used, a social worker needs to work in a way that maximises the possibility of deep change and minimises negative change. Given the sometimes enormous long-term consequences of interventions of this kind for those involved, it is important to be certain that powers have been used in a way that is as far as possible constructive. This means developing a way of working that is appropriate to the realities of the situation. In particular, we need to recognise that working in this context is very different to working with people in an entirely voluntary context, and raises some quite distinct practical and ethical questions:

- Service users are aware of your role and of the fact that what they tell you about themselves may influence the decisions you make in that role.
- Service users may not have chosen to work with you and may be only doing so because they are required to do so by law or because they know they have to do so in order to avoid some undesirable outcome.
- There are serious ethical issues about attempting to do 'therapy' with someone who is not a voluntary client. There are also issues of an entirely pragmatic kind about the *usefulness* of attempting to do so, given that no form of counselling or therapy can get far without the active participation of the client. Suggestions such as those of De Jong and Berg (2001) about how to get round these problems may be useful but they tend to relate to the scenario of a therapist working with someone who has been sent to them by a court. The situation is rather different when a social worker whose own agency took the case to court attempts to work in a therapeutic way.

When thinking about any aspect of social work it is always a useful exercise to try and put yourself into the position of a service user and consider what you would find helpful and unhelpful. The following exercise invites you to do this here.

Exercise 10.2

Imagine either:

(1) That you are a parent (perhaps you will not need to imagine that part) and that someone has reported you to a social services department, alleging that you are seriously mistreating your children (you may imagine that the allegation is true or false – whichever you prefer). You are being visited by a social worker as a result.

Or:

(2) That you are boy or girl of 15 who has got into a peer group where theft and vandalism are considered normal behaviour. You have been arrested, charged and convicted for a series of offences and are now under a Supervision Order, which requires you to meet with a youth justice officer (in this case a social worker) and work on your offending behaviour.

What would you want from the social worker? What would help you to feel that you could work constructively with the social worker? What would make this more difficult?

(Continued)

(Continued)

Comments

You may have thought of other things, but among the things I would certainly find helpful would be:

- *For the social worker to be absolutely clear and frank about the ground rules. What will happen to the information I give her? What is at stake? What can I expect from her? What will be the consequences if I don't co-operate? What kinds of help can I expect?*
- *Within these ground rules I would want the social worker to treat me respectfully as a human being, by listening to my point of view and taking it seriously.*
- *I would find it helpful to be clear about the purpose of each session with the social worker and to be able to feel confident that the social worker knew what she was doing and that the social worker was being open about what she was doing and did not have a hidden agenda.*
- *I might not like it, but it would be helpful to me if the social worker were able to challenge me (when I was being evasive, for instance, or unduly negative), but this would have to be done carefully, so that it did not feel like a put-down.*
- *I would get on better with the social worker if she seemed comfortable with her authority, but at the same time able to convey some humanity and warmth.*

What I would find unhelpful would be:

- *If the social worker adopted an officious, distant bureaucratic tone or tried to lay claim to expertise which I thought was questionable. I would not be in a very receptive mood for working with the social worker if, secretly, I was thinking she was a pompous windbag.*
- *On the other hand, I would find it equally off-putting if the social worker was overly familiar and tried to come over as a friend. For example, I would not like it if the social worker started calling me by my first name without asking me what I wanted to be called.*
- *If the social worker did not listen to me.*
- *If the social worker did not challenge me at all, even when I was being difficult or evasive. (I might at one level be relieved, but in fact I would find it unhelpful. It would suggest to me that the social worker was only 'going through the motions'.)*
- *If the social worker was overbearing and threatening.*
- *If the social worker tried to pretend that her control agent role did not exist, or did not explain it to me properly.*
- *If the social worker did not do what she said she would do (for example if she failed to keep appointments) or did not stick to her own ground rules. For example, if she passed on information to another agency without consulting me, having told me originally that she would let me know in advance if she felt it was necessary to pass something on to another agency.*
- *If the social worker attempted to win my favour by conveying to me that she was 'on my side against the system'. For example, a youth justice worker might convey to an offender that she herself actually thought his offending was quite acceptable, but she needed to go through the motions in order to 'get the system off his back'. I would find this very confusing.*

In Chapter 4, I referred to Chris Trotter's (1999) book on working with involuntary clients because of its use of behaviourist principles. As it is one of a very small number of books which are purely focussed on the issues involved in working with involuntary service users,

I will come back to it here (you could also look at Rooney, 1992). When working with involuntary clients, Trotter points out, social workers have 'two roles, a legalistic, or surveillance, role and a helping, therapeutic or problem-solving role' (Trotter, 1999: 3). Drawing on outcome research studies he suggests three keys in particular to successful work when attempting to combine these two very different roles.

Accurate role clarification

> Outcomes are improved for involuntary clients when workers focus on helping them to understand the role of the worker and the role of the client in the direct practice process. This involves ongoing discussions about issues such as authority and how it might be used, the dual role of the worker ..., the aims and purposes of the intervention from both client and worker perspectives, as well as issues relating to confidentiality. In short, clarifying role is about the question: 'what are we here for?' (Trotter, 1999: 17–18)

One point that he particularly emphasises is the need to be clear about 'what is negotiable and what is not' (Trotter, 1999: 50).

Trotter's explanation speaks for itself but I would just note that it is surprisingly easy to get this wrong. When one has been doing a job for some time it is easy to forget that what is obvious to you is not necessarily obvious to the service user. It is also easy to stop asking *yourself* the question as to what it is you are doing and what it is you are trying to achieve. If you are not clear yourself what you are doing, you will certainly not be able to reassure the service user that your intervention is purposeful.

Reinforcing and modelling 'pro-social' values

By the slightly odd term 'pro-social values', Trotter means values which are socially desirable (avoiding criminality, non-violent interaction, caring for children, responsibility, self-reliance and so on) and which social workers in various capacities are charged with trying to promote. According to Trotter, the pro-social approach

> involves workers identifying with and being clear about the values they wish to promote and purposefully encouraging those values through the use of praise and other rewards. It also involves appropriate modelling of the values the worker seeks to promote, and challenging anti-social or pro-criminal expressions and actions. (Trotter, 1999: 19)

Trotter acknowledges some might see this approach as 'manipulative' and that some social workers might also have qualms about imposing certain values on service users. However, we should be clear that an assumption that certain values are desirable are really part of what a social worker signs up to when she joins an agency that works with involuntary service users. We should also notice that these values – taken broadly – are generally fairly uncontroversial: a YOT worker needs to subscribe to the belief that it is a good thing to steer young people away from criminality; a child protection worker needs to subscribe to the view that child abuse (as it is currently understood) is something to be avoided. What *would* be more questionable would be the use of such techniques to promote more narrow notions of pro-social values (for example, to impose middle-class values on working-class service users.)

One attractive feature of the pro-social approach as defined by Trotter is that it does not need to focus only on deficits, but is about building on and encouraging strengths.

Collaborative problem-solving

Here Trotter draws on the task-centred approach which I discussed in Chapter 7. He suggests that better outcomes are associated with approaches based on 'modest, achievable goals which are the client's rather than the worker's (or at least collaboratively developed), and identifying strategies with the client to achieve the goals' (Trotter, 1999: 21).

Of course, in work with involuntary clients, it is not always possible to allow the client to set all the goals ('A sex offender, for example, might not view his offending behaviour as a problem and his goal might be to avoid detection in the future' Trotter, [1999: 22]). Nevertheless, although some goals may be non-negotiable from the social worker's point of view, there is almost always scope for other goals to be placed on the agenda by the service user.

What Trotter's work does not emphasise so much is that this kind of work is difficult on an emotional level. It is challenging for most of us to work with people who have reason to feel angry with us, who may be inclined to find fault with what we are doing, and who might prefer to have nothing to do with us at all. And it is not easy to give people messages that they are likely to find distressing such as, 'Even though I know you don't want to go, I have decided to apply for you to be detained in a mental hospital'.

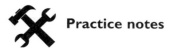 **Practice notes**

Working with involuntary clients

Skill requirements

- Clear thinking is very important when attempting to carry out two or more quite distinct roles in the same context. As we have seen, the ability to *convey* clarity to service users is important.
- The use of statutory powers can provoke strong reactions (naturally enough, since they involve imposing restrictions on other people). Therefore an ability to cope with anger and hostility is important.
- Assertiveness is important. You need to be able to give difficult messages and stick to them.
- Along with the above skills, you need the ability to convey warmth and respect, even in situations where you are also giving hard messages and, very possibly, facing an angry or distressed reaction.
- An ability to reflect and to make use of the reflective process of supervision is very important in an area of work where errors are easy to make because of the issues at stake and the strong feelings involved, but where errors can be very costly in human terms to all concerned.

(Continued)

(Continued)

Ethical considerations

- I have already mentioned the importance of clarity in this area. It is particularly important to be clear about your professional values and what they mean in this context. Lack of clarity about your role, or discomfort about your role, can lead to messages to service users being confused, contradictory or dishonest.
- Clarity about the need to show respect to service users is important in situations where conflict can occur, since a normal response in conditions of conflict is to view the 'other side' negatively.
- There is – obviously – a huge power imbalance in this kind of situation. The potential for abuse, misuse or overuse of power is enormous.

Real-world constraints

- Working with involuntary clients is not a 'theory' but a fact: it does in fact occur in most areas of social work and in some areas is the dominant mode of working. The real world constraints that exist relate more to the limits of what can be achieved in this way. We need to be aware that the protective leverage conferred by statutory powers is a blunt instrument in many respects and that the power it confers is more limited than it might at first sight appear. No legal mandate confers on us the ability to change people at will.

Chapter summary

This chapter has considered the particular issues involved when social workers – in a variety of different contexts – are expected to use legal powers to control others. The topics discussed have been:

- **Varieties of power:** The different kinds of power that social workers can exercise.
- **Statutory powers in social work:** Coercive powers given to social workers in the UK by the law.
- **'Control' and social work:** The 'control' aspect of social work, and how it seems to be relatively under-discussed in social work texts.
- **Towards a theory of the control agent role:** What is the use of coercive powers supposed to achieve and how? The *explicit* and *implicit* use of coercive power. The use of power for '*direct protection*' and for '*protective leverage*'.
- **Working with involuntary clients:** What is different about working with involuntary clients and what is required: *accurate role clarification, reinforcing and modelling pro-social values* and *collaborative problem-solving*.

In the next chapter, which is called 'Rhetoric and Reality' and begins the last and final part of this book, I will consider some of the more negative aspects of social work, which include the negative aspects of social work's 'control' function.

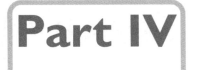

Part IV   IT'S ALL VERY WELL IN THEORY

Introduction

The theme that connects the two chapters in this final part of the book is that it is important to challenge our own assumptions. Chapter 11 acknowledges a gulf between social work as it is in theory and social work as it is in practice and considers the reasons for this. It also discusses negative public perceptions of social workers and considers what truth they contain. Chapter 12 invites you to consider what knowledge, theory and expertise mean in the context of an activity like social work that operates in an area where there is so much uncertainty and so little that we can be completely certain about. It discusses the importance of self-awareness and the need for social workers to constantly re-appraise their practice and the assumptions on which that practice is based.

11 Rhetoric and reality

- Theory and practice
  - Sweetening
  - Decoupling
  - Wishlisting
- Policy, fantasy and 'symbolic reassurance'
- Other agendas
- Negative stereotypes
- Under the cover of kindness
- Finding a balance

I now want to acknowledge that there can be quite a gulf between what is written and said about social work and what social work is like in practice, whether for those practising it or those on the receiving end of its ministrations. In other words, there is a gap between theory and practice (using the word 'theory' in a broad sense), which social work students often notice when they go out into placements or start work on qualifying. It seems important to discuss that gap in a book about theory in social work.

My intention in this chapter is to offer some thoughts about the nature of this gap and to promote a certain scepticism about models of social work that are offered to you by others, whether they are government policy makers or social work academics such as myself, while at the same time encouraging you to be cautious about your own assumptions. I hope it will provide you with a few rudimentary tools that may help you to appraise theories and ideas which are offered to you, and to make distinctions between those ideas which may be helpful to you and your clients and those which may actually make things more difficult.

Theory and practice

Exercise 11.1

Can you think of examples, from your own experience, of ways in which social work as it is taught or presented in books and government publications differs from social work as it is actually practiced?

Comments

You may well have your own particular examples but the following is a random selection of ways in which it seems to me that theory and practice often seem to differ:

- *Although social work books emphasise the importance of theory, social work practitioners frequently – in fact probably normally – do not apply specific theoretical models in their day-to-day work.*
- *Books and teaching about social work tend to identify social work with social justice and with support for those in society who are the most powerless and excluded. However, social workers are widely distrusted and even sometimes feared because of their powers to intervene in family life.*
- *The goals and techniques which are proposed for social work in social work books often seem out of kilter with what is actually practicable or achievable in the context in which social workers actually work. The books sometimes seem to be writing about a completely different job.*
- *Government guidance for social workers also often seems to set goals and expectations which are not proportionate to the resources that are actually made available and may not even be consistent with what is humanly possible.*

There are actually a number of different things going on here; some positive, some negative. To begin with the positives, it is important to acknowledge that a gap between theory and reality is in one sense inevitable because reality is inevitably more complicated than any theory, just as a landscape is always more complicated than the maps which are made of it. I will not discuss this point much further here because it will be the subject of the next and final chapter. I will just note in passing that the fact that a map is always simpler than the landscape it depicts doesn't mean that maps aren't useful. Indeed, the way they simplify things is partly what *makes* them useful. (Think of the simplified schematic maps we use to navigate the London Underground, the Paris Metro or the New York Subway.)

It is also right to acknowledge that it is perfectly appropriate to have *aspirations* which go beyond the way things actually are, or even beyond what is actually practicable in a given moment. In fact the development and maintenance of good practice in social work *requires* that we don't just write and talk about the way social work is done now, but about the ways in which it should or could be done. A gap between aspiration and existing reality is valuable in social work as it is in life generally. Without it, changes for the better would never occur.

What is *not* helpful though are disjunctures between social work talk and social work reality which are *not* acknowledged or openly recognised because these constitute a pretence that things are different from how they really are. We need to be careful not to collude in such a pretence, while the real situation remains undiscussed, like a family secret. These disjunctures can take various forms, including what I will call *sweetening, decoupling* and *wishlisting*. I will explain what I mean by these terms shortly, but they all refer to ways in which words, ideas and theories serve, neither to provide a schematic map of reality nor to offer goals to aim for, *but to obscure how things really are*. They are therefore obstacles to real progress, though they are used to create an illusion that progress has occurred.

Sweetening

By sweetening I mean the use of words and ideas which give the impression that things are other than they are, or even the *opposite* of what they really are, as in George Orwell's (1993, first published in 1948) famous novel *1984* in which the government department responsible for rationing was called the Ministry of Plenty and the department responsible for waging war was called the Ministry of Peace.

For sweetening to work, the word or idea that is used as a sweetener has, like 'plenty' or 'peace', to be in itself something good and desirable. In social work words such as *empowerment* or *anti-oppressive practice* can easily be used as sweeteners for practices which in fact are anything but empowering or anti-oppressive. Likewise, I have often heard the word *partnership* used to describe working relationships with clients in which all the power is on the social work side and in which the client may only be co-operating because he knows that otherwise he will be taken to court. (In fact I have heard social workers say that the *reason* they took a parent to court was because the parent 'was not prepared to work in partnership'.) The point I am making here (to recap on discussion in the previous chapter) is not that it is necessarily wrong for social workers to use coercive powers, for sometimes this is appropriate and necessary, but that it is wrong and unhelpful to conceal that this is what is happening through the misuse of words like 'partnership'. This devalues the word itself and gets in the way of rational discussion about the rights and wrongs of particular courses of action. Genuine partnership is harder to achieve when we no longer have a distinct word for it.

Here is another example. The concept of the 'needs-led assessment' is in itself a useful idea which I discussed previously in Chapter 9 (see page 146). But a case could be made for saying that the concept was used as a sweetener in the UK in the 1990s, when large-scale reforms of the provision of social care services for elderly and disabled people were brought in by the NHS and Community Care Act, 1990. Public rhetoric and training courses for social workers and other staff required to implement the changes presented these as an exciting new development in practice, which would expand choices for service users by moving from service-led to needs-led assessment.

What was not made explicit was that one of the main drivers for these reforms was the need to control public expenditure on residential and nursing home care. Under a loophole in social security regulations made in 1980, people in residential and nursing homes could obtain financial help from the social security system with the charges of residential and nursing homes if they did not have the capacity to pay, and it became possible for people to dispose of their assets and then claim state assistance with the full cost of residential or nursing home care without going through any sort of assessment of their care needs. As a result, social security expenditure on residential and nursing home care rose from around £10 million in 1979, to £2000 million by 1991. A main aim of the community care reforms was to make social services departments responsible for *rationing* public funding for residential and nursing homecare. Reforms billed as an exciting expansion of choice for service users were driven largely by 'the need to stop the haemorrhage in the social security budget' (Lewis and Glennerster, 1996: 8) and therefore actually to set severe limits on the ability of service users to choose an option that had previously been open to them. In true Orwellian style, less choice was presented as more choice.

Nowadays social workers often use the phrase 'needs-led assessment' to refer to a form on which a client's needs are recorded. The essential distinction between being needs-led and service-led seems often to be lost. This I suggest is a direct result of the misuse of the needs-led concept to describe a process which was not really led by client needs.

Decoupling

I am suggesting the word 'decoupling' to describe a situation that occurs when theory or talk or writing becomes disconnected from the external reality to which it is supposed to relate, with the result that theory or talk becomes an end in itself. Theorising, words and intellectual games are seductive to many of us. Human beings take pleasure in creating patterns and order and it can be very easy, either when theorising or when developing policy, to be so carried away by this pleasure as to lose sight either of the practical purpose that the theory or policy was intended to serve or of the practical constraints which any concrete action would need to take into account. What is more, theorising, drawing up policies on paper and coining new words are basically *easier* activities than bringing about change in the external world, so that manipulating words, ideas and symbols can readily become a comforting *alternative* to action: 'A dramatic symbolic life among abstractions ... becomes a substitute gratification for the pleasure of remolding the concrete environment' (Edelman, 1985: 9).

I would gently suggest that some of the more arcane discussions on theory and social work that can be found in the academic literature do occasionally fall into this category. The use of bold radical rhetoric, unmatched by bold radical action, or an excessive preoccupation with changing the *words* for things may perhaps also sometimes serve the purpose of making us *feel* we are doing something about the injustices of the world, and thereby excusing us from *actually* doing anything. The following was my response to a suggestion by Hawkins et al. (2001) that the absence of 'social justice terminology' in the everyday language of social workers indicated a need 'to examine our current language, to consciously use social justice terminology where appropriate, or to coin new "socially just" terms to suit our purposes' (Hawkins et al., 2001: 11):

> With due respect to these authors, the approach they suggest seems to me to be an example of a mistake that we in social work far too often make: believing that we can change things simply by changing the words we use. In my experience such an approach results either in the new words falling rapidly into disuse or in their being used in a way that is incongruent with – even opposite to – their ostensible meaning ('needs-led assessment', for instance, being used to

describe a system for rationing services.) There is surely too much of this kind of Orwellian incongruence between language and reality in social work, yet it is something that a simplistic 'postmodern' insistence on the primacy of language is likely to encourage. (Beckett, 2003: 637–8)

In other words, once language and reality become decoupled, language serves not to change reality but to conceal it. Even ostensibly radical ideas become simply sweeteners, and therefore obstacles to real change. My suggestion is that social workers, presented with ideas and words and policies, should always ask the question: does this relate in a useful way to the decisions I have to make in practice?

Wishlisting

Another form of social work discourse that can be found both in academic texts and in policy documents takes the form of lists of problems that social workers should do something about. Sometimes such lists are useful – see my comments on aspiration earlier – in that they set goals and standards. However, in many situations it is actually relatively easy to identify problems. The part that social workers need help with is *how* to address them and with what resources. A list which simply dumps social problems on social workers to deal with, without providing any practical guidance, and without identifying where the time is going to come from or where the necessary skills are going to be acquired, is actually of very little use. It may make my point if I parody wishlists of this kind as follows:

Example of a wishlist

Social workers should:

- *Abolish war and institute a new era of world peace*
- *Eliminate poverty and racism*
- *Defeat sin and evil*
- *Foreswear lewd and impure thoughts*
- *Create a society in which there is justice for everyone*
- *Reverse global warming*

Of course wishlists that you will actually encounter are never quite as blatantly impractical as this. But you *will* find in social work texts examples of what Mark Doel and Peter Marsh (1992: 7) call Grand Statements which, as they say, are often 'unaccompanied by much in the way of practical advice'. These wishlists can also be found in government publications and in documents such as the recommendations of child abuse enquiries. An example of the latter which I often cite is the recommendation of the Victoria Climbié enquiry that social services departments should not devise 'ways of limiting access to services' (Laming, 2003: 11). Since any public service with a limited budget and a limited amount of staff time has no choice but to limit access to services, such a recommendation is really of no more practical use than a recommendation that social workers should abolish war and institute a new era of world peace.

What is insidious about these wishlists is that they are really a special case of decoupling in the sense that I used the word earlier. Those who compile them may feel – and sincerely believe – that they are doing something useful about a problem, but in truth they are really exempting themselves from addressing that problem by passing everything that is difficult about it onto others.

Policy, fantasy and 'symbolic reassurance'

Why are there sometimes disjunctures of these kinds between social work language and social work reality? One reason is that the policies which social workers are required to implement are the product of a *political* process. Politicians, agency managers and policy-makers of all sorts, being human, naturally enough want their policies to reflect well on them and to please those on whom they depend for jobs and for advancement. For this reason policy initiatives tend to be presented as radical, new and entirely positive when they may in fact constitute little more than new names for old ideas. Usually too they serve functions which are different from their stated one, such as acting as a 'sweetener', as in the case of the NHS and Community Care Act, 1990 discussed earlier, where talk about increasing service user choices belied an underlying agenda which was about *closing off* of certain choices.

It is important too to remember that politics is about 'horse-trading'. Policy initiatives emerge as a result of power struggles between different interest groups with different agendas. Nigel Parton (1991: 176–90) gives a vivid account of such a process when he describes the lobbying and counter-lobbying by various interest groups that led to the incorporation of the 'Child Assessment Order' in the Children Act, 1989.

Actually the Child Assessment Order is hardly ever used but its inclusion in the Act may well have felt like a victory to those, such as the NSPCC, who lobbied in support of it. It is a curious fact about human nature that we can often be reassured by purely symbolic gestures that make little or no difference in any practical sense, with the result that, as Murray Edelman (1985: 41) puts it 'myth and symbolic reassurance become key elements in the governmental process'. Hence sweetening, decoupling and wishlisting as discussed earlier. Policies that are presented as means of solving particular problems do not necessarily in fact do so. Nevertheless they often serve to reassure us that 'something is being done'. Following a well-publicised child abuse tragedy, for example, there is typically a public enquiry which makes a long series of recommendations as to action to prevent such a thing happening again. This helps to reassure the public that these dreadful events are not simply being tolerated, whether or not the recommendations are actually workable and whether or not they would actually improve things.

The difficulty for state-employed social workers who, like other public servants, are required to implement new policies, is that policies intended to provide symbolic reassurance may not in fact be practicable and may not in fact help them to do their job. Suzanne Regan (2001) made this point in an article on the *Framework for the Assessment of Children in Need and their Families* (Department of Health, 2000), which at time of writing remains the UK government's blueprint for assessments of families carried out by social workers in England and Wales:

> New social policy reforms are like branded products in that they embody elements of fantasy and simulation. [The *Framework*] presents social work agencies with yet another simulated model which prescribes structures of action in an idealised world and not in the grim complicated reality of the real world. (Regan, 2001: 36)

Murray Edelman's insight was that people are often *more* attached to reassuring symbols – sweeteners in my terms – than to the realities which they supposedly represent:

> The laws may be repealed in effect by administrative policy, budgetary starvation, or other little publicised means; but the laws as symbols must stand because they satisfy interests that are very strong indeed. (Edelman, 1985: 37)

Bridget McKeigue and I (McKeigue and Beckett, 2004) have shown that, years after the implementation of the 1989 Children Act in England and Wales, commentators frequently referred to its provisions as an achievement, even when those provisions had had no tangible effect and even when things had actually been getting worse rather than better since the Act came into effect. 'However difficult the decisions that have to be made [in court proceedings concerning children], it is of paramount importance that no undue delays occur, since they may drastically reduce the options for a child', wrote Carol Sheldrick, (1998: 263) quite correctly, in 1998. She then added: 'Fortunately the Children Act 1989 recognizes this and imposes the duty of no undue delays on courts, lawyers and professionals' (1998: 263). The existence of the no delay principle in Section 1 of the Act was clearly providing her with some 'symbolic reassurance', but the fact was that when she wrote this, the average length of care proceedings had been steadily increasing every year since the Act came into effect.

Other agendas

But it is not in the political and policy-making arenas that these dynamics exist. Social work academics such as myself, for instance, also have our own agendas – and agendas set for us – which influence the way we teach and write about social work and may result in us generating talk and writing about social work which is not entirely consistent with reality. We may, for instance, be tempted to make things seem more difficult than they need to be, or to make unrealistic claims as to the role of social work in society, in our desire to prove that ours is a 'real' academic subject, worthy to be taught in universities alongside physics or history or philosophy and perhaps too out of a need to generate articles and books to meet the quotas expected of us by our employers and to progress our own academic careers.

↗ References

If you are a social work student you might like to think about the way that your teachers, myself included, insist on your providing references in your written work. There are a number of perfectly good reasons for this. It is a way of encouraging you to broaden your thinking. But you might argue that it is a way in which we social work academics consolidate our own position of authority and preserve our status as custodians of social work theory: something has to be written down in an academic text for it to 'count'.

(Continued)

(Continued)

Since becoming an academic myself I have written articles and books, such as this one, which you could, if you wished, cite in your written work and duly receive credit as a result from your markers for having referred to 'literature' or 'theory' (always assuming, of course, that you correctly reference your quotations). However, it sometimes occurs to me that, had I had the same thoughts when I was a student myself or when I was in practice, they could not have been cited in this way.

I am reminded of Michel Foucault's ideas about the relationship of power with the ability to define what constitutes the truth and is defined as real. (Foucault, 1980)

You might argue too that, the longer we are in academic life, the more likely it is that purely academic agendas will predominate over agendas to do with the practical problems of social work. Academic social work always runs the risk of becoming decoupled from social work itself. 'Social work', as an academic subject, runs the risk of becoming an increasingly abstract concept: an interesting focus for debate; an arena in which we can construct symbolic reassurances of one kind or another for ourselves; or perhaps a battleground on which to enact struggles for power and influence. It can also easily be co-opted by governmental policy-makers, since the government is a major source of research funding as well as of honours and public recognition. I do not mean by the these comments to suggest that I and my colleagues are in any way more corrupt or flawed than anyone else. I am simply noting that academics are not exempt from the general principle that what people do and say is shaped in part by their interests. (You may remember the concept of 'producer capture' to which I referred in Chapter 8, page 128.)

Nor are social work practitioners themselves exempt from this. Practising social workers, for instance, can easily be tempted to use jargon where ordinary words would really do just as well, perhaps in order to demonstrate that they are real professionals with real expertise, like doctors or lawyers, or perhaps – uncomfortable as it is to admit it – to make themselves feel powerful in relation to service users and others by 'blinding them with science'.

Negative stereotypes

    Q: What's the difference between a social worker and a Rotweiler?
    A: Rotweilers sometimes let go.

This joke, told to me some time ago by a non-social worker, seems to me to reflect a widespread view of social workers in society at large: social workers are unwelcome and hard to get rid of. Here is another gap, this time between how social workers would like to see themselves and how they are in fact seen. The expression 'do-gooder', sometimes used about social workers in the popular press, encapsulates another part of the stereotype: social workers are seen as somewhat priggish people convinced of their own goodness. Part of this stereotype is the idea that social workers insist on imposing their own 'politically correct' standards.

If you are a social worker or a social work student, you will very likely have encountered some negative reactions to your choice of profession from friends or family, or from people you meet socially. Indeed, I have met social workers who have told me that they actually avoid saying 'social work' when asked what they do for a living.

Exercise 11.2

Assuming you are a social worker or a social work student, what negative messages have you received, if any, about your choice of profession?

What assumptions or beliefs about social work seem to lie behind those negative messages?

Why do people have these assumption or beliefs?

Comments

My guess is that you will most likely have picked up at least some negative messages about social work, if not personally then via the media. 'Child-abducting hippies' was a comment recently made to a student of mine about how social workers in general are seen. Of course there are negative stereotypes of other professions – think of accountants, psychiatrists, lawyers or estate agents – but the negative stereotypes that exist in relation to social work are, I suggest, quite pronounced.

You may feel that the media – blamed for so many things – are to blame for this too, though this begs the question as to why the media would want to perpetrate negative images of what is, after all, only one of a large number of professions, unless they were picking up on existing feelings in society at large.

You may have identified the fact that social workers are often involved in making difficult real-world decisions about matters that other people do not have to think about in any depth. For example, most people would rather not have to make choices between removing a child from a family or leaving her in a situation where she may be at risk of harm. As with other groups who have to make decisions between unpalatable alternatives – such as politicians or health service managers – the public can deal with its uncomfortable feelings about the decisions being made by blaming the decision-makers. Society, you might say, washes its hands of the hard choices between personal liberty and protection of the vulnerable, by dumping this on social workers and then blaming them when things do not work out. After all, though social workers may be characterised as interfering busy-bodies, they are also blamed often enough for failing to interfere in situations where someone subsequently gets hurt.

You might also argue that the public at large often blame social workers for problems created by the public's own unwillingness to pay more taxes. Social workers – like many other public servants – are often set up to fail by expectations that greatly exceed the resources available to meet them.

More generally social work is perhaps identified with a number of topics which most people would rather not think about, such as mental illness, disability and child abuse, so that public unease about social work is partly to do with public unease about these subjects.

Or you may have identified the reputation of social workers for using 'politically correct' language, or a certain stereotype that exists of social workers as being somewhat over-earnest, pious or self-righteous.

Many of the negative stereotypes of social work are of course unfair and in my discussion of the above exercise I have indicated some of the reasons why. But I suggest that we should not dismiss them out of hand, but actually consider them. For I suspect that many social workers would themselves to some degree share some of the public concern that social work intrudes excessively into people's privacy and imposes its own standards – some would say 'politically correct' others, as I will shortly discuss, might say 'middle class' – on vulnerable sections of society that do not necessarily share them:

> The judges of normality are present everywhere. We are in the society of the teacher-judge, the doctor-judge, the educator-judge, the 'social worker'-judge; it is on them that the universal reign of the normative is based. (Foucault, 1979: 304)

Under the cover of kindness

The ultimate gap between theory and practice would be if social work served a purpose that was *opposite* to its stated intentions and opposite to the purpose that its practitioners themselves believed themselves to be serving. *Under the Cover of Kindness* is the title of a provocative book by Leslie Margolin (1997) which questions whether social work really helps its service users at all. Since Margolin is himself a former social worker, the book is somewhat in the tradition of Thomas Szasz's (1998) or Jeffrey Masson's (1992) attacks on psychiatry, psychoanalysis and psychotherapy. Margolin proposes that social work's apparent concern for its service users, and indeed its very belief in its own benevolence, is in fact a kind of smokescreen. This 'cover of kindness' allows social work to engage in its real business: a form of surveillance of and control over elements of society who deviate from the norms that those who are powerful in society wish to impose.

Margolin refers to the concept of 'doublethink' introduced by George Orwell in *1984*, to describe the way in which social workers can hold these contradictory ideas in their minds at the same time. I mentioned earlier the deceptive way in which the phrase 'working in partnership' is sometimes used. More generally, I think of the way in which (as discussed in the last chapter) social work's coercive powers tend to be minimised in social work discourse, while elevated talk about empowerment and emancipatory values tends to be extremely prominent. For me this does give a certain uncomfortable ring of truth to the suggestion that 'kindness' is a kind of cover.

In a way, Margolin's argument is simply a scholarly restatement of the widespread public stereotype I mentioned earlier of social workers as 'interfering busy-bodies' and 'do-gooders' and it relates to the widespread unease (at least in British society) about the growth of the 'nanny state'. Social work's apparent benevolence has, Margolin's book argues, simply permitted the surveillance and control exercised by the state to be extended into 'the heretofore closed space of the home' and the 'justification of this intervention as charitable and disinterested help' (1997: 8). Whatever changes have occurred over the years in the way that social work defines itself and sees itself, this book argues that its essential nature has remained unchanged since the beginnings of professional social work in the 19th century. Even the radical, emancipatory strand in social work, which supposedly addresses issues of unequal power and structural injustice are, on Margolin's view, really simply a new kind of smokescreen. He cites, for example, the following extract from a book by Jan Fook (1986) on feminist practice as an example of a way in which social work pretends to place itself on the level of service users while in reality concealing the essential power differences that are inherent in the social worker–client relationship:

> The physical setting of the interview should be that which makes the least possible status distinction between client and worker, and encourages maximum sharing and co-operation ... [For instance] interviews conducted while both doing the supermarket shopping ..., giving the other a lift somewhere, or over lunch in the park, could provide the setting to help equalize roles, and may break down the mystique of the 'professional interview'. (Fook, 1986: 56, cited in Margolin, 1997: 169)

I have to agree that for social workers in many contexts to work in this way would indeed give a deceptive and confusing message about the nature of the relationship between social worker and client. But Margolin's book argues that the *whole enterprise* of social work is deceptive in exactly this kind of way. Whatever the language used, however it is dressed up, it all boils down to:

> People from one social class going into the homes of people belonging to another; they write biographies of these people, they judge what is normal or abnormal: they call it 'doing good'. (Margolin, 1997: 9)

Crucial to Margolin's argument, and perhaps most disturbing to us as social workers, is his contention that social workers themselves have to *believe* they are doing good for all of this to work. If this is true we cannot dismiss Margolin's argument simply by protesting our sincere good intentions, for at the core of his argument is that we do indeed genuinely believe we have good intentions and that we must do so to carry out our real function.

But what is the *purpose* of all this surveillance and control that Margolin talks about? His answer, in the tradition of Foucault, is that 'social work stabilises middle-class power by creating an observable, discussable, write-about-able poor' (Margolin, 1997: 5). This may seem at first sight rather far-fetched, as does his focus on the 'poor', as if they were the only recipients of social work services, and his rather old-fashioned assumption that social workers necessarily come from a different social class from their clients. (This may have been true in the 19th century, but it is not unusual now for social workers to be, or have been, themselves recipients of social work services.)

But it really *is* true that much of what social work is given to do – the tasks set for it by government and society – is dictated by considerations other than the best interests of service users. If you consider the way that policy is developed in relation to any of the client groups that social workers typically work with, you will find that many other agendas are also being served. In the mental health field, for instance, policy-making is influenced by the need for politicians to be seen to be addressing public perceptions that mentally ill people are dangerous and violent (even though this is in the vast majority of cases simply not true). In the children and families field, much policy is shaped by emotive responses to specific child abuse tragedies, and may result in social workers being asked to do things which are really more to do with agencies' needs to avoid blame and politicians' needs to be seen to be doing something in response to public outcry, as they are to do with the actual best interests of children.

Perhaps if we adapt Margolin's negative account of the real purpose of social work and make it something more like the following, it will seem rather more convincing:

The real purpose of social work: a negative view

Contrary to what its practitioners may like to believe, social work's primary purpose is not to serve the interests of its clients but to make the comfortable majority of people in society feel that the distressing social problems of various minorities are being managed, contained and kept away from their sight in a way that absolves them of responsibility.

Exercise 11.3

Can you think of ways in which social work might serve the interests of people other than its service users and do so in ways that actually are harmful to service users?

Comments

If you have not had much experience of social work in practice, you might find this exercise hard, but I am sorry to say that, on the basis of my own experience, I do not find it hard to think of ways in which this might happen:

- *An old person is moved from his home in response to pressure from neighbours who have lobbied the local member of parliament. He does not want to move, but neighbours find him difficult and challenging and the social work agency finds it easier to go along with this than to resist.*
- *A family are required to comply with a child protection plan which involves having to accept visits twice a day from various professionals. The plan is not clearly thought out and is actually of no use to the family: if anything it increases the parents' feeling of inadequacy and powerlessness and makes their parenting worse rather than better. But the agencies insist on the plan in the wake of critical newspaper reports about the child protection services. Each agency is anxious to be able to prove that 'everything possible is being done' even though individual practitioners may privately doubt that this is the way forward. (In a more oblique sense, the sometimes quite vicious attacks on social workers in the media that often follow child abuse tragedies in the UK suggest to me that one of the functions that social workers perform for society is providing someone to blame.)*

Finding a balance

Margolin's book begins by describing a case in America where a mother, Joy Brown, had her name placed for 10 years on a state-run child abuse register, and was thereby prevented from working in the childcare field, simply because she was momentarily distracted and her normally well-cared-for-five-year-old got onto the street, placing himself at risk from traffic. If the story is accurate, this seems officious, excessive and unnecessary behaviour on the part of the authorities. And, sadly, I can vouch for the fact that the child protection system in the UK can also sometimes be officious and even punitive in *just* this kind of way (although the instance he cites does seem quite an extreme example and I am fairly confident that no-one would be placed on a UK register for a single instance of this kind).

But Margolin undermines his own argument when he goes on to say that Joy Brown's name was placed on the register alongside those who 'torture, molest and kill children' (Margolin, 1997: 1). For this begs the question: what does he think should be done about children who *are* tortured, molested or at risk of being killed? Assuming that he agrees that there should be official intervention in at least some circumstances, who should carry it out? For after all, if this is not done by a social worker, it would still have to be done by someone doing a job that most people would identify as social work. And once we accept that social work intervention (or whatever else it might be called) is, in such extreme circumstances, justified, the question then arises as to whether it might not sometimes be better – and, indeed, less oppressive and less likely to result in the destruction of families – if social workers were to try and anticipate these kinds of problem and intervene at an earlier stage to prevent them. The more one pursues this line of argument – the more one extends it to the many other areas in which social workers operate apart from that of child protection – the more one realises that the purist position adopted by Margolin in this book simply does not work in the real world.

In a sense, this extremely negative view of social work is just as naïve and one sided as an entirely positive view which simply assumed that social work is necessarily helpful and benign simply because that is, so to speak, what it says in the job description. A more balanced position, I would suggest, is to recognise that, while social work *can* be a positive force, it also has a dark side, a side that is reflected in the negative stereotypes and jokes I mentioned earlier. In order to provide a useful service to its service users, social work needs to recognise and struggle against this dark side, rather than denying its existence or hiding it with sweeteners. In the same way, without dismissing out of hand the objectives that are set for social work, and which social workers set for themselves, it is important to recognise that there may be hidden agendas and vested interests behind them, and that fantasy – in the form of sweeteners, wishlists and decoupled thinking – may be present as well as reality in writing and talk about social work, social work theory and public policy.

Chapter summary

- **Theory and practice:** There is often a gap between social work as presented 'on paper' and social work as it is actually experienced by those doing it and/or by those receiving a social work service. I suggested that there were several ways in which the rhetoric of social work might be disconnected from the reality, and suggested the terms 'sweetening', 'decoupling' and 'wishlisting' for some of these.

(Continued)

(Continued)

- **Policy, fantasy and 'symbolic reassurance':** Public policy which social workers are required to implement is not the product of a purely rational appraisal of the facts, but of a political process in which elements of fantasy and purely symbolic gestures play a major role.
- **Other agendas:** Social work academics and social workers themselves also have their own agendas, which may also result in gaps opening up between the way social work is described and the way it actually is.
- **Negative stereotypes:** A number of negative stereotypes exist of social work. Social workers are sometimes viewed as being interfering, hard to get rid of and concerned with the imposition 'politically correct' or middle-class values.
- **Under the cover of kindness:** The most negative possible view of social work is that its proclaimed benevolence and its commitment to the socially excluded and vulnerable is a front for its real function which is one of social control.
- **Finding a balance:** The most negative viewpoint is an over-simplification, just as is a purely positive one. The need to acknowledge both positive and negative aspects.

12 | The limits of theory

- Science or art?
  - Knowledge
  - Skills
  - Values
- Reflective practice
- Looking beyond the frame
- Feedback and supervision
- Facing our shadow

This book has been based on the proposition that social workers ought to have a properly thought-out basis for what they are doing, and that they ought to be able to state what it is. My suggested definition of theory, given in Chapter 3, was '*a set of ideas or principles used to guide practice, which are sufficiently coherent that they could if necessary be made explicit in a form which was open to challenge*'.

If 'theory' can be defined in this broad sense, then social work practice should all be grounded in theory. But in most cases the theories we use are what I have called 'informal' ones and may seem so obvious and uncontroversial as not to really merit the word 'theory' at all. They are just 'common sense', as we might say. Of course there are a number of problems with 'common sense', one of them being that so-called common sense tends to incorporate the prejudices and assumptions of a particular time (at one time it was 'common sense' that women shouldn't vote in elections, for example). Another problem with 'common sense' is that it is not a reliable guide in situations where we have little personal experience. For instance, we would not be very happy to travel by air with a pilot who was completely untrained and had never flown before but assured us that flying was just common sense.

But it is also the case that there are limitations to the usefulness of 'theory'. We might not be happy to get onto a plane with a pilot who had no knowledge of flying but we would also not be very happy to get onto a plane to discover that the pilot had indeed read numerous books about flying planes, attended numerous courses, and passed many written and oral exams with the highest possible marks, *but had no previous experience of sitting at the controls of a real aeroplane*. Expertise involves practical experience as well as theory, skill as well as knowledge. It is seldom, if ever, a matter of simply knowing a theory and applying it.

The relationship between theory and practice is in fact a two-way one. Formal theory can and should inform practice, but it is in the process of testing, modifying and comparing different theories (formal and informal) in practice that social work expertise develops. A social worker who assumed that she could rely entirely on her own 'common sense' would be very limited in scope and would, in some situations, be positively dangerous. But so would a social worker who learnt and then uncritically applied one particular theoretical approach, without reflecting on whether it was always applicable, or whether it had drawbacks, or whether another approach might yield more helpful outcomes in a given situation. When people often comment sceptically that something or other is 'all very well in theory' what they are really acknowledging is that reality is never identical to the ideas and models that we use to make sense of it. Maps are often necessary to help us to find our way around but a map should never be confused with the landscape itself. The real landscape is, as I observed in the previous chapter, always more complex than any map. And maps, too, are often inaccurate, or out of date, or include material which is contentious, like frontiers or rights of way which are in dispute.

Science or art?

Social work is not, and never will be, a purely 'technical' activity. By this I mean that there will never be a body of social work theory which will tell us, simply and unambiguously, what to do in a given situation. There are several reasons for this, which can be divided up under the headings of 'knowledge', 'skills' and 'values', which I previously used in Chapter 2.

Knowledge

Social work is not an 'exact science'. In fact even the hard sciences are much less exact than we sometimes imagine. The following quote comes from a book on a branch of mathematics called Chaos Theory:

> At the moment scientists cannot even use the fundamental laws of physics to predict when the drips will fall from a leaking tap, or what the weather will be like in two weeks time. In fact it is difficult to predict very far ahead the motion of any object that feels the effect of more than two forces, let alone complicated systems involving interactions between many objects.
>
> Recently researchers in many disciplines have begun to realise that there seems to be inbuilt limits to predicting the future at all levels of complexity. (Hall, 1991: 8)

Science, for all its sophistication and power, cannot predict complex real-world phenomena like the weather with any degree of accuracy because there are simply too many 'variables'.

And if this is so in science, then it is even more so in human situations where there are so many countless variables that to try to understand what is going on, or guess what will be the outcome of various types of intervention, makes weather prediction look like child's play.

Indeed, every human situation that we encounter is unique. Donald Schön (1991: 117) quotes the psychiatrist Erik Erikson's (1958: 76) observation that every patient is 'a "series of one" who must be understood in terms of the unique experiences of his life'. The uniqueness of every situation means that we can never simply apply a rule derived from research because research is necessarily based on other situations which were never quite the same as the unique situation with which we are now faced. No theoretical model is precisely applicable in any real-life situation and even, if you choose to operate within the confines of a single theoretical model you will still be left having to make all kinds of judgements as to how to apply it in a particular case. This is true not only of social work but of life generally. Schön's (1991) book *The Reflective Practitioner*, which looks at the way that professionals really go about solving problems in practice, is not primarily about social work – in fact the main professions discussed are engineering, architecture, management, psychotherapy and town planning – but I would guess that many students of social work would identify with the following comment on the problem of applying theory to practice in a specifically social work context:

> the multiplicity of conflicting views poses a predicament for the practitioner who must choose among multiple approaches to practice or devise his own way of combining them. (Schön, 1991: 17)

What Schön helps to clarify is that, not only in social work, but in many other fields it simply is not possible to apply a rigid set of rules to problem-solving because '... the scope of technical expertise is limited by situations of uncertainty, instability, uniqueness, and conflict' (Schön, 1991: 345). Social workers are constantly faced with situations in which it is impossible to be sure how to interpret what is happening or to know for certain what the best course of action is. This does not mean that social workers are stupid, or that social work is a pointless activity – though social workers do sometimes have to deal with media accusations that one or both of these is true. On the contrary, Schön makes the point that *most* of the things that we would regard as really important in life fall into the area where it is simply not possible to know for certain what to do:

> In the varied topography of professional practice, there is a high, hard ground where practitioners can make effective use of research-based theory and technique, and there is a swampy lowland where situations are confusing 'messes' incapable of technical solution. The difficulty is that the problems of the high ground, however great their technical interest, are often relatively unimportant to clients or to the larger society, while in the swamp are the problems of greatest human concern. (Schön, 1991: 42)

Being 'in the swamp' can feel uncomfortable. We may feel that we *should* possess exact, unambiguous, unassailable knowledge and that 'uncertainty is a threat; its admission is a sign of weakness' (Schön, 1991: 69). In the UK context this fear may be understandably aggravated by the way in which social workers are so publicly pilloried when they make judgements which turn out with hindsight to have led to bad outcomes. This fear can lead to professionals persuading themselves that their level of expertise is rather higher than it really is. This is harmful on two counts. First, it can rebound on the person who makes such claims when it turns out that unrealistic expectations have been raised. Second, it is harmful to others whose own expertise is thereby diminished, particularly (in a social work context) the service user. To overrule or silence or undermine a service user's viewpoint by claiming to an expertise which you don't in fact possess is a kind of oppression. Indeed, Wilding (1982) identified 'excessive claims to expertise' as one of the characteristic ways in which professionals abuse power.

Exercise 12.1

(1) Can you think of examples, either from your own experience, or from the news, where professionals have made excessive claims to expertise, with negative consequences?
(2) Can you think of ways in which social workers might make excessive claims of expertise, with resulting harmful consequences?

Comments

First, I suspect many readers of this book will have had some personal experience of professionals making exaggerated claims to expertise in various small ways, since it is quite common. It is easy for us as professionals to fall into the habit of pretending to know more than we really do, particularly when we feel that our expertise or usefulness or status is under threat.

A recent British example of professional claims to expertise having very severe consequences is the case of Sir Roy Meadows, the eminent paediatrician, whose 'expert' evidence in the case of the solicitor Sally Clarke led to her being convicted of murder of her own babies and sent to prison. In her successful appeal it was recognised that his evidence, which effectively ruled out the possibility that they had died of natural causes, had been misleading and his claims to certainty excessive.

A famous historical example is Sigmund Freud's abandonment of his so-called Seduction Theory, that neuroses in adult life were the result of childhood sexual abuse. Unable to believe that all the stories of abuse told to him by female patients were true, he came to the conclusion that they were fantasies and built a very elaborate theory to explain this which became part of orthodox psychoanalytic thinking. Freud's refusal to believe what his patients were telling him is the basis of Jeffrey Masson's attack on the entire body of Freudian theory (Masson, 1984). Even the much more sympathetic view of Charles Rycroft (1995: 165) is that 'until Masson, most analysts underestimated [the frequency of child sexual abuse] and were predisposed to assume that patients' accounts of having been sexually abused were Phantasies'. There could hardly be a clearer example of the potential oppressiveness of excessive claims to expertise than that of psychoanalysts using 'theory' to discount their patients' disclosures of abuse.

Second, there are situations in which a social worker's opinion may have far-reaching consequences. This is perhaps particularly true in the area of child care social work where a child's entire life may be altered by decisions made by social work agencies. In a court case or in a meeting where a long-term plan for a child is being decided, a social worker who claimed to possess certain knowledge, or claimed to have the backing of research might well alter the final decision. So it is important that social workers clearly differentiate between fact, opinion and mere guesswork. These decisions always do have to be made on imperfect information – it is almost never possible to be 100 per cent certain – but we should be honest about this.

Skills

I have already discussed the fact that each situation encountered by a social worker is unique. You will encounter cases with many similarities to one another, but you will never encounter *exactly* the same combination of circumstances more than once. I noted that this sets limits to the extent that we can simply apply rules or procedures derived from research, or from past experience, to new situations.

But it is also the case that every *social worker* is unique. As we deal with new situations we each bring our own unique combination of personality characteristics and skills. This means that what works well for one social worker will not necessarily work for another, *even if they were faced with precisely the same circumstances.* This again limits the extent to which rigid rules can be developed as to how to operate. Insofar as we each have to find our own way of practising, social work is as much 'art' as 'science.'

Values

Another very important reason why social work can never be a purely 'technical' activity is that almost all of the important decisions that are made by social workers have a 'values' component as well as a 'knowledge' component. Earlier in this book, in Exercise 2.2 (page 20), I looked at the case of an elderly person, Alice Young, whose neighbours felt she was not safe in her own home. In this case any decision as to what to do about the situation certainly contained a 'knowledge' component, which would include, for instance, an assessment of the degree of risk to Alice in her own home and an assessment of her level of mental functioning, but it would also have to include a 'values' component. However detailed our knowledge, a judgement would have to be made on what constituted an *acceptable* level of risk and on the extent to which Alice was *entitled* to make her own decisions about risk.

Reflective practice

To sum up the discussion so far, social work is not a purely technical activity. It is not an activity which can be, or could be, carried out simply by following rules derived from theory, for the following reasons:

- Social work involves dealing with inherently uncertain situations.
- Each situation is unique.
- Each social worker brings different things to each situation.
- Each situation requires that value questions – not merely knowledge questions – are addressed.

This is not to say that social workers should feel free to ignore formal theory or the findings of research in their practice – far from it – but my point is that we cannot expect to take a blue-print from research or from theory and apply it in a mechanistic fashion. We also cannot expect to be 'experts' in the human and social sphere in the sense that, say, a washing machine repairman, is an expert on the workings of washing machines. A social worker who does claim to have that kind of precise technical knowledge (other than in certain 'technical' areas, such as knowledge of the benefits system) will be guilty of making excessive claims to expertise. The expertise of a good social worker, like that of many other professionals, does not reside simply in factual knowledge but also (and often mainly) in an ability to practice in a reflective way. Central to this is a willingness to recognise the limits of what you know, to live with uncertainty and to be open to new possibilities. Being prepared and able to 'reflect' may be one of the most useful things that we can bring to many situations, although it is, by its nature, not an easy skill to describe:

> Developing a capacity for critical reflection is much more than simply learning procedures or achieving particular 'competencies'. Part of the process of becoming a reflective practitioner is the adoption of a critical and informed stance towards practice. This can only come about through doing the practice, reflecting on it through dialogue and questioning, and changing the practice in the light of reflection. (Banks, 2001: 162)

Sarah Banks could have added that the process of developing a capacity for critical reflection, by its nature, cannot really be acquired by reading a book. Like riding a bicycle or learning to swim, it is something that can, in the end, only be learned 'on the job'. But, unlike riding a bicycle, it is a self-conscious process, requiring the social worker to engage in a kind of dialogue. Some of the elements of that process I would summarise as follows:

- Actively testing theoretical ideas and research findings against your own experience as a practitioner.
- Being clear about the theories behind your actions, so that you can test their usefulness by considering subsequent events.
- Checking out and challenging the assumptions on which you base your work (your 'frames' – see below).
- Noticing and challenging the assumptions ('frames') within which your agency tends to operate.
- Seeking feedback from others, including service users and colleagues. This is often best seen as a two-way process. For instance, one of the really valuable roles that a social work student on placement can perform for the host agency is asking questions.

↗ 'Technical areas' within social work

As I have said that social work is not simply a technical activity, I should add the caveat that there are *elements* of knowledge that social workers may apply which could indeed be described as technical. These are areas where precise knowledge is possible and where a social worker's possession of precise knowledge may well be extremely useful to service users. For example:

- Understanding of the benefits system.
- Understanding of housing law/immigration law/childcare law and so on.
- Understanding of agency and multi-agency processes, such as the adoption approval process or the local multi-agency child protection system.
- Knowledge of research on the outcomes of specific types of intervention.

Looking beyond the frame

Schön (1991) suggests that how we understand a situation, and how we respond to it, largely depends on the 'frame' in which we choose to see it. It is quite easy to forget that we are seeing things through one particular 'frame' and to come to think of our particular way of seeing as being the *only* way. One of the aims of reflective practice is to become aware of our own frames and therefore also aware of the possibility of alternatives. When a person becomes aware of the frames he is using, he is able to notice 'the values and norms to which he has given priority, and those he has given less importance, or left out of account altogether.' (Schön, 1991: 310). The opposite of a reflective practitioner is one who does things in a certain way 'because that's how we always do it'. A reflective practitioner is open to the possibility that there may be completely different ways of looking at things which could turn out to be more useful than the ones he is now using.

Here is an example. When the community care reforms of the 1990s came in, social workers were encouraged to stop thinking in terms of slotting service users into existing services (as in 'Mr Jones is a day centre case') and instead think of their service users' *actual individual needs* (as in 'Mr Jones and his wife need a break from one another, and Mr Jones could do with some company in a context where he can be physically cared for'). The theory was that, rather than simply applying for a day centre place for Mr Jones, the social worker would then seek funding for an individual package of care tailored to meet Mr Jones' particular individual needs. In practice things have not always worked out like that (not least, as I discussed in the previous chapter, because of a less well-publicised aspect of the community care reforms: an urgent requirement to rein in expenditure and ration resources) but you can see that the original idea was to encourage social workers to move outside a particular narrow frame and look at things in another way. Exercise 12.2 provides another illustration.

Exercise 12.2

Jane is a social worker in an English child protection team. Asked to define her job she says: 'Basically my job is to identify situations where a child is at risk of mistreatment, and then to take steps either to remove that risk, or – failing that – to remove the child from the risky situation.'

Can you see any ways in which this definition of her role might be restricting? And can you think of other frames which Jane might apply to her work?

Comments

In one sense, Jane's definition of her job is accurate. Under the Children Act, 1989 child protection social workers are required to step in where children are at risk of significant harm and try to prevent that harm, with the physical removal of children available as a last resort.

(Continued)

(Continued)

But the precise way in which Jane conceptualises (or 'frames') her task, is rather static (as opposed to dynamic). By this I mean that she seems to assume that the risk is a 'given' – something fixed that is just 'out there' – and that her only options are to physically remove the source of the risk, or physically remove the child. Perhaps this particular frame will make Jane rather prone to 'solutions' that involve the physical removal of children into care, or the physical removal from families of adults alleged to be abusive?

The fact is that much of what we identify as child maltreatment is about unhappy family relationships (for instance, relationships in which a child has become the brunt of anger, or disappointment, or has become a scapegoat for other difficulties in a family). And many carers who we identify as abusive are also very important to the children they are mistreating. It is not always – or even often – a good solution to break up a family.

If Jane reframed her job and described it as follows, perhaps she would be less inclined to think in terms of physical removal of family members (whether victim or alleged abuser) and more in terms of helping a family as a whole change the way it operated:

My job is to identify situations where patterns of family relationships are resulting in children being treated in ways that are harmful to them – and helping the family relate to one another in different ways which will be less harmful.

This in itself is only another way of framing the task and you will doubtless be able to think of objections to this one also. My point is that it is a different frame and will tend to result in a different approach to the job.

↗ 'Frames' and therapeutic work

I am asking you here to look at the frames within which we operate as social workers, and I am suggesting that it is important to try to:

(1) recognise our own frames and their limitations, and
(2) remain open to the possibility that other frames exist that might be more useful.

It occurs to me that one of the main aims of most kinds of therapeutic work is to help clients to do something similar. Psychodynamic therapists seek to help their clients understand problems in terms of the past, thus reframing them. Solution-focussed therapists seek to help clients to see themselves as separate from their 'problem' rather than necessarily inside it and to reframe the therapeutic process itself from being an exploration of problems to an exploration of problem-solving. Family therapists and marital counsellors typically try to get families to 'reframe' their difficulties in ways that will help them to move on.

(Continued)

(Continued)

Another kind of 'reframing' was contained in the 'narrative' approach of Michael White (White and Epston, 1990) which I briefly mentioned in Chapter 5. He argues that people have 'dominant stories' to describe their own lives, but that, there are always aspects of their experience – 'unique outcomes' – which contradict these dominant stories. The therapist tries to encourage the client to build these unique outcomes into new dominant stories.

The frames within which social workers can become confined may be of several overlapping forms which we could sum up as:

- *Personal.* We each have our own individual way of seeing and understanding the world. Everyone has his or her own assumptions and characteristic habits of thought. What is perhaps harder to acknowledge is that, for each one of us, our preferred ways of working are influenced by our own needs and wants and fears.
- *Organisational.* Agencies may impose procedures that will tend to make us view the world of service users in a particular way. For instance, statutory social work agencies commonly have a rather complex and formal assessment procedure, which is supposed to be carried out before an intervention is decided upon. Arguably, this results in a rather static and external way of understanding the lives of service users, since it assumes that we can collect together a picture of their 'needs' and that this is a separate process from trying to meet those needs.
- *Cultural.* As well as formal procedures, an informal culture exists within any agency that contains certain assumptions about (for instance) the nature of the working relationship between the agency's social workers and service users. In the context of a busy agency with a demanding workload and many organisational pressures and demands to meet, it is very easy to fall into a particular way of working – 'It's just how we've always done things' – which ceases to be questioned or examined. As a student on placement in an agency, or as a new member of staff, you may well observe social workers going about things in ways which seem odd, or unhelpful, or even discriminatory or oppressive. It is easy to assume that, as a relatively inexperienced student, you must simply be missing something. But in fact it may well be that the *agency* is missing something. The agency's staff may no longer see what they are doing because they have grown accustomed to it.
- *Theoretical.* One of the reasons that it is important to be familiar with a range of different theoretical perspectives is that they challenge our own frames and offer alternatives. Indeed each theoretical perspective *is* a frame – the various frames on offer challenge one another.

To take up the last point, you might notice for instance, how the 'future-orientated' or 'solution-focussed' approaches discussed in Chapter 5 challenge the assumption that to solve a problem we necessarily have to understand its causes, the latter assumption being characteristic of psychodynamic models, including the model offered by attachment theory. By contrast, attachment theory (and other psychodynamic approaches) challenge the commonplace notion that people can do and be whatever they want 'if only they make their mind up to it'. Attachment theory suggests that we all carry baggage from the past which we cannot simply discard at will *because it is in itself a frame through which we see and understand the world.*

To give another example of how one 'frame' may challenge others: family systems approaches challenge the notion that we can understand an individual's behaviour purely in terms of the psychology of that individual, suggesting that we can only make sense of individual functioning in the context of the groups of which they are part. Likewise group work theory challenges the assumption that individual or family casework is necessarily the best way to approach problems and the radical political perspective that lies behind the idea of empowerment suggests that what may *appear* to be individual problems are in fact simply symptoms of structural injustices and that, by casting them as individual problems we may be colluding with those injustices. In the previous chapter I offered a frame which challenges the value of social work itself.

Feedback and supervision

One way of reflecting on practice is to get someone else to give you feedback. Feedback from anyone who has been in a position to observe your work is potentially useful, the most obvious source being of course service users, since they are the people for whose benefit you are supposed to be working. Service users themselves only offer a partial view and we should be wary of the assumption that being liked is necessary the same thing as being effective. (I am not sure whether I am necessarily able to accurately judge every aspect of the work of my dentist – for all I know he drills my teeth completely unnecessarily – but I can certainly vouch for the fact that he has a reassuring manner and is good at explaining things.) We should also be aware that the differences in power between social workers and service users may mean that feedback is not always completely accurate. Your clients may feel the need to placate you and to keep in your good books, or they may give excessively negative feedback to punish you. But feedback from any source has to be handled with caution.

One of the main sources of feedback in social work comes from supervision. Professional supervision is something that many professions could benefit from, but which happens to be more highly developed in social work than in most other professions. Put at its simplest, social work supervision consists of a period of time in which a social worker, or sometimes a group of social workers, discuss their work with someone else. Typically in social work this is with the social worker's immediate line manager. This differs from the professional supervision, which, for instance, a private therapist might buy in from another therapist, and it has some advantages but also a number of disadvantages, in that the line manager has two distinct roles in a supervision session, and these roles can clash, just as a social worker's different roles in work with service users can clash.

Your line manager, in her capacity as manager, is accountable for your work and must therefore check that you have done the work in the way that she wants, and that your performance is (in her view) adequate. She must also assess your workload vis-a-vis other team members and (at times) give you specific instructions as to what to do. Your line manager may also be the first person you need to talk to if you feel that there is a need for additional resources to be provided by your agency in the form of money and services.

In her capacity as your professional supervisor, on the other hand, your line manager should be providing you with a space to reflect on your work, clarify your own thinking, develop plans for the future and consider any obstacles (including your personal feelings) which are getting in the way for you. She should also be considering your own needs, insofar as they effect the job you do, and be trying to address those needs. This is a complex role, which can include an *educational* element (particularly, if the supervisee is much less experienced than the supervisor) but also a *supportive* element that at times borders on a form of counselling. The latter would apply, for example, in situations where a case is arousing very strong feelings for you which you need to unravel into order to clarify what you are doing. In some of the more emotive areas in which social work operates, this may be a significant part of supervision.

It is particularly this last element that at times sits uncomfortably with a line manager relationship. On the whole we want our *line manager* to form a good impression of our work and our capabilities – indeed, things like career progression, salary scales and so on may depend on it – and yet to get the most out of *professional supervision*, we may at times need to share our self-doubts, our fears and our awareness of areas of practice which we are not so good at. In my experience, provided that a reasonable relationship of trust has been established between supervisor and supervisee, this tension between roles need not present insurmountable problems. We all are vulnerable and the kinds of situations that social workers deal with arouse strong feelings in all of us. So a good supervisor should be able to view a social worker's willingness to be honest about her own uncertainties in a positive light rather than as a sign of weakness (though we have to recognise as well that sometimes we really may not *be* up to the job.)

However, although there are elements of a counselling role in good professional supervision, a supervisor/line manager is not there as a counsellor or therapist for social work staff, and there is a point beyond which the supervision session ceases to be an appropriate forum for a social worker to discuss her own feelings and issues. Most social work agencies will have separate counselling services for the use of staff when such a point has been reached.

A supervisor also cannot ever be the font of all wisdom:

> In all the helping professions there are many who are waiting for the perfect supervisor. The person who will make the confusion clear, the complex understandable, absolve the guilt, rebuild our self-worth and magically remove the pain and distress. Inevitably there is much disappointment, for such supervisors do not exist. (Hawkins and Shohet, 1996: viii)

Nor, of course, do perfect social workers exist. Our service users have to make do with what we are able to offer within our own limitations. But just as service users are entitled to expect certain minimum standards from social workers, and should be entitled to seek redress if those minimum standards aren't met, so a social worker is entitled to expect certain minimum standards from her supervisor. It is worth thinking about what you would want those standards to be and what standards you think a supervisor should be able to expect in return.

Facing our shadow

In the previous chapter, I discussed the 'dark side' of social work. I pointed out that social work is not just about being kind and helpful and empowering and good. There is some truth in the popular stereotype of social workers as 'interfering busy-bodies'. Social work can indeed also be about interfering in people's lives, oppressing those who are already down, taking away people's confidence in their ability to control their own lives. I argued that we should face this fact and not attempt to paper it over with mere rhetoric, for sadly oppression can quite easily be perpetrated in the name of 'anti-oppressive practice' and power can quite easily be abused in the name of 'empowerment'.

I want to bring this book to a close by pointing out that we should not deceive ourselves into thinking that this 'dark side' is necessarily located 'out there' – in the bureaucracy; in the system – and that we ourselves as individuals are necessarily free of it. The dark side is, in part, inside ourselves. In a discussion on the motivation of people in the helping professions Peter Hawkins and Robin Shohet (2000) take the idea of the 'shadow' from Jungian psychology to refer to the parts of ourselves which we exclude from our social persona, and are reluctant to own or to own up to but which nevertheless exist (for a brief explanation of the concept, see Stevens [1990: 43–6]). Our motives for going into a job such as social work are complex and, whatever we might like to believe, are never simply pure and unalloyed altruism. Our less 'pure' motives may include:

- Enjoyment of power, or of the feeling of importance that comes from having authority, or from having others dependent on us.
- A need to be seen as 'good' (or 'strong', or 'tough', or 'competent', or 'heroic', or 'wonderful').
- The reassurance that comes from being with others whose problems are more severe than our own (and the sense of mastery that comes from being able to offer help).
- A desire for praise or the need to be liked.
- A need to feel indispensable.
- A need to assuage guilt.
- A need to refight old battles or to find an arena in which to explore issues which we ourselves have never resolved in our personal life.

Once we are in the job, our day-to-day actions and decisions will be influenced too by other, less than noble motives including some of those listed above but also things such as:

- Avoiding blame.
- Trying to please or impress people whose opinion we value.
- Avoiding situations that we find frightening or uncomfortable.
- Punishing people who have caused us distress.
- Getting home on time.

We may be reluctant to admit to some of these kinds of motive, even to ourselves. Who, for instance, wants to think of themselves as someone who takes pleasure in power? And yet we all do enjoy it to some extent. It is not so surprising that, in an uncertain, dangerous world, we like the feeling of having some control. The point is that it is not so much *having* these needs as the *denial* of them that is likely to be harmful to our practice. 'A willingness to examine our motives, "good" or "bad", pure or otherwise, is a prerequisite for being an effective helper' (Hawkins and Shohet, 2000: 9). It is, for one thing, essential if we are to be able to offer the quality of *genuineness* which Rogers identified as so important (see Chapter 5). But it is essential too to our decision-making, not only in a 'direct change agent' role but in all the roles that social workers play, that we have a sense of where we are coming from. For example, if a social worker is involved in a decision-making process about which service users should have access to some limited resource – let us say a place in a newly established group home – she needs to be aware of the personal feelings she may have towards those service users which might colour her judgement. A social worker who has strongly punitive feelings towards a particular client, but was unable to acknowledge them even to herself, is potentially dangerous, as is a social worker who is unable to see that she over-identifies with a particular service user.

Self-awareness lies at the core of good reflective practice, as does an ability to look at what we do 'from outside'. And, in spite of the many limitations of formal 'theory', one of its great benefits is that it helps us to do this, by providing frames to view the world through other than those we have constructed for ourselves, or have absorbed unthinkingly from the society that surrounds us.

Chapter summary

This chapter has explored the idea of 'reflective practice' and looked at ways of reflecting on practice, including the use of theoretical ideas to challenge your own thinking and to challenge other theoretical ideas, obtaining feedback from service users and carers, and the use of supervision. The following headings were covered:

- **Science or art?** Social work is not an exact science and will never be an activity that could be performed satisfactorily simply by mechanically applying rules.
- **Reflective practice:** The importance of self-awareness and an ability to think critically about our own assumptions and about the theories that we apply.
- **Looking beyond the frame:** 'Frames' as sets of assumptions, the way that we can be trapped in particular frames and the ways in which one frame can be used to challenge another.
- **Feedback and supervision:** Feedback as a form of reflection, supervision as a form of feedback and the nature of supervision in social work.
- **Facing our shadow:** Recognising our own less noble motives and making allowance for them.

References

Adams, R. (2003) *Social Work and Empowerment,* 3rd edn. Basingstoke: Palgrave.

Adkins, A., Awsumb, C., Noblitt, G. and Richards, P. (1999) *Working Together? Grounded Perspectives on Interagency Collaboration.* Cresskills, NJ: Hampton Press.

Ainsworth, M., Blehar, M., Aters, E. and Wall, S. (1978) *Patterns of Attachment: A Psychological Study of the Strange Situation.* Hillside, NJ: Laurence Erlbaum.

Bailey, R. and Brake, M. (1975) 'Social work in the welfare state' in R. Bailey and M. Brake (eds) *Radical Social Work.* London: Edward Arnold. pp. 1–12.

Bandura, A (1977) *Social Learning Theory.* Englewood Cliffs, NJ: Prentice-Hall.

Banks, S. (2001) *Ethics and Values in Social Work,* 2nd edn. Basingstoke: Palgrave.

Bateman, N, (2000) *Advocacy Skills for Health and Social Care Professionals.* London: Jessica Kingsley.

Becker, H.S. (1996) *Outsiders: Studies in the Sociology of Deviance.* New York: Free Press.

Beckett, C. (2003) 'The language of siege: military metaphors in the everyday language of social work', *British Journal of Social Work,* 33 (5): 625–39.

Beckett, C. and McKeigue, B. (2003) 'Children in limbo: cases where care proceedings have taken two years or more,' *Adoption and Fostering,* 27 (3): 31–40.

Beckett, C. and Maynard, A. (2005) *Values and Ethics in Social Work: An Introduction.* London: Sage.

Beutler, L., Machado, P. and Neufeldt, S. (1994) 'Therapist variables', in A. Bergin and S. Garfield (eds) *Handbook of Psychotherapy and Behavioural Change.* New York: John Wiley & Sons. pp. 229–69.

Bowlby, J. (1998) *Attachment, Separation and Loss,* 3 vols. London: Pimlico.

Brandon, D. (1991) *Innovation without Change? Consumer Power in Psychiatric Services.* Basingstoke: Macmillan.

Brandon, D. and Brandon, T. (2001) *Advocacy in Social Work.* Birmingham: Venture Press.

Braye. S. (2000) 'Participation and involvement in social care: an overview', in H. Kemshall and R. Littlechild (eds) *User Involvement and Participation in Social Care: Researching Informing Practice.* London: Jessica Kingsley. pp. 9–28.

Burns, P. (1994) Pro-social practices in community corrections, honours thesis, Monash University, Melbourne.

Butler-Sloss, Lord Justice E. (1987) *Report of the Inquiry into Child Abuse in Cleveland.* London: HMSO.

Caplan, G. (1961) *An Approach to Community Mental Health.* New York: Grune and Stratton.

Carr, A. (2000) *Family Therapy: Concepts, Process and Practice.* Chichester: Wiley.

Crittenden, P. (2000) 'A dynamic-maturational approach to continuity and change in patterns of attachment', in P. Crittenden and A. Clausson (eds) *The Organization of Attachment Relationships: Maturation, Culture and Context,* New York: Cambridge University Press. pp. 343–57.

De Jong, P. and Berg, I.K. (2001) 'Co-constructing cooperation with mandated clients', *Social Work,* 46 (4): 361–74.

de Shazer, S. (1985) *Keys to Solution in Brief Therapy.* New York: W.W. Norton.

de Shazer, S. (1988) *Clues: Investigating Solutions in Brief Therapy.* New York: W.W. Norton.

Delaney, R. (1998) *Fostering Changes: Treating Attachment-Disordered Children.* Oklahoma City, OK: Wood W. Barnes.

Department for Constitutional Affairs (formerly Lord Chancellor's Department) (1992–2003) *Judicial Statistics, Annual Reports.* London: Department for Constitutional Affairs (formerly Lord Chancellor's Department).

Department of Health (1995) *Child Protection: Messages from Research.* London: HMSO.

Department of Health (1996) *Community Care (Direct Payments). Act, 1996: Policy and Practice Guidance.* London: Stationery Office.

Department of Health (1999a) *Working Together to Safeguard Children.* London: Stationery Office.

Department of Health (1999b) *Effective Care Co-ordination in Mental Health Services: Modernising the Care Programme Approach.* London: Stationery Office.

Department of Health (1999c) *National Service Framework for Mental Health.* London: Stationery Office.

Department of Health (2000) *Framework for the Assessment of Children in Need and their Families.* London: Stationery Office.

Department of Health (2002) *Single Assessment Framework for Older People* (HSC 2002/001/LAC(2002)1). London: Department of Health.

Department for Education and Skills (2003) *Every Child Matters.* London: Stationery Office.

Di Clementi, C. (1991) 'Motivational Interviewing and the Stages of Change', in S. Rollnick *Motivational Interviewing.* London: Guilford Press. pp. 191–202.

Doel, M. (2000) 'Groupwork' entry, in M. Davies (ed.) *The Blackwell Encyclopaedia of Social Work.* Oxford: Blackwell. pp. 148–50.

Doel, M. and Marsh, P. (1992) *Task-Centred Social Work.* Brookfield, VT: Ashgate.

Douglas, T. (2000) *Basic Groupwork,* 2nd edn. London: Routledge.

Downrie, R.S. and Telfer, E. (1980) *Caring and Curing: a Philosophy of Medicine and Social Work.* London: Methuen.

Edelman, M. (1985) *The Symbolic Uses of Politics.* Chicago, IL: University of Illinois Press.

Erikson, E. (1958) 'The nature of clinical evidence', in D. Lerner (ed.) *Evidence and Inference.* Glencoe, IL: The Free Press of Glencoe. pp. 66–94.

Fahlberg, V. (1981) *Helping Children When They Must Move.* London: BAAF.

Fahlberg, V. (1994) *A Child's Journey through Placement.* London: BAAF.

Fook, J. (1986) 'Feminist contributions to casework practice', in H. Marchant and B. Wearing (eds) *Gender Reclaimed: Women in Social Work.* Sydney: Hale and Iremonger. pp. 54–63.

Fook, J. (2002) *Social Work: Critical Theory and Practice.* London: Sage.

Foucault, M. (1972) *The Archaeology of Knowledge.* London: Tavistock.

Foucault, M. (1979) *Discipline and Punish.* Harmondsworth: Penguin.

Foucault, M. (1980) 'Truth and power', in M. Foucault *Power/Knowledge.* Hemel Hempstead: Harvester Wheatsheaf. pp. 109–33.

Freddolino, P., Moxley, D. and Hyduk, C. (2004) 'A differential model of advocacy in social work practice', *Families in Society,* 85 (1): 119–28.

French, J. and Raven, B. (1959) 'The bases of social power', in D. Cartwright (ed.) *Studies in Social Power.* Ann Arbor, MI: Institute of Social Research.

Friere, P. (1986) *Pedagogy of the Oppressed.* Harmondsworth: Penguin.

Gardner, F. (2001) *Self-harm: A Psychotherapeutic Perspective.* Hove: Brunner Routledge.

Gibbons, J., Gallagher, B., Bell, C. and Gordon, D. (1995) *Development after Physical Abuse in Early Childhood.* London: HMSO.

Hall, N. (1991) *The New Scientist Guide to Chaos.* Harmondsworth: Penguin.

Harlow, H. (1963) 'The maternal affectional system', in B.M. Foss (ed.) *Determinants of Human Behaviour.* London: Methuen. pp. 3–29.

Hawkins, L., Fook, J. and Ryan, M. (2001) 'Social workers' use of the language of social justice', *British Journal of Social Work,* 31 (1): 1–13.

Hawkins, P. and Shohet, R. (1996) 'Series editors' preface', in A. Brown and I. Bourne (eds) *The Social Work Supervisor.* Buckingham: Open University Press. pp. viii–xii.

Hawkins, P. and Shohet, R. (2000) *Supervision in the Helping Professions.* Buckingham: Open University Press.

Healy, K. (2005) *Social Work Theories in Context.* Basingstoke: Palgrave.

Henderson, P. (2000) 'Community work', in M. Davies (ed.) *Blackwell Encyclopaedia of Social Work.* Oxford: Blackwell. pp. 72–4.

Howarth, J. and Morrison, T. (2000) 'Assessment of parental motivation to change', in J. Howarth (ed.) *The Child's World: Assessing Children in Need.* London: Department of Health. pp. 77–90.

Howe, D. (1989) *The Consumer's View of Family Therapy*. London: Gower.

Howe, D., Brandon, M., Hinings, D. and Schofield, G. (1999) *Attachment Theory, Child Maltreatment and Family Support*. London: Macmilan.

James, R. and Gilliland, B. (2005) *Crisis Intervention Strategies*, 5th edn. Belmont, CA: Brooks/Cole.

Jones, C. (1996) 'Anti-intellectualism and the peculiarities of British social work', in B. Parton (ed.) *Social Theory, Social Change and Social Work*. London: Routledge. pp. 190–210.

Kanel, K. (2003) *A Guide to Crisis Intervention*. Pacific Grove, CA: Brooks/Cole.

La Fontaine, J. (1998) *Speak of the Devil: Tales of Satanic Abuse in Contemporary England*. Cambridge: Cambridge University Press.

Laming, Lord H. (2003) *The Victoria Climbié Inquiry*. London: Stationery Office.

Lewis, J. and Glennerster, H. (1996) *Implementing the New Community Care*. Buckingham: Open University Press.

McKeigue, B. and Beckett, C. (2004) 'Care proceedings under the 1989 Children Act: rhetoric and reality', *British Journal of Social Work*, 34 (6): 831–49.

Madanes, C. (1981) *Strategic Family Therapy*. San Francisco, CA: Jossey Bass.

Margolin, L. (1997) *Under the Cover of Kindness: The Invention of Social Work*. Charlottesville, VA: University of Virginia Press.

Masson, J. (1984) *The Assault on Truth*. New York: Farrar, Strauss and Giroux.

Masson, J. (1990) *Against Therapy*. London: Fontana.

Masson, J. (1992) *Against Therapy*. London: Fontana.

Minuchin, S., Lee, Y. and Simon, G. (1996) *Mastering Family Therapy: Journeys of Growth and Transformation*. Chichester: John Wiley.

Myers, J. (ed.) (1994) *The Backlash: Child Protection under Fire*. Thousand Oaks, CA: Sage.

Office for National Statistics (ONS) (1996) *Young Carers and their Families*. London: Stationery Office.

Orwell, G. (1993) *Nineteen Eighty-Four*. London: Methuen.

Parton, N. (1991) *Governing the Family; Childcare, Child Protection and the State*. Basingstoke: Macmillan.

Parton, N. and O'Byrne, P. (2000) *Constructive Social Work: Towards a New Practice*. Basingstoke: Macmillan.

Payne, M. (1997) 'Task-centred practice within the politics of social work theory', *Issues in Social Work Education*, 17 (2): 48–65.

Phillips, J. (2001) *Groupwork in Social Care: Planning and Setting Up Groups*. London: Jessica Kingsley.

Pithouse, A. (1998) *Social Work: The Social Organisation of an Invisible Trade*. Aldershot: Ashgate.

PIU (Performance and Innovation Unit) (2000) *Prime Minister's Review on Adoption*. London: Cabinet Office.

Popple, K. (1994) 'Towards a progressive community work praxis', in S. Jacobs and K. Popple (eds) *Community Work in the 1990s*. Nottingham: Spokesman. pp. 24–36.

Preston-Shoot, M. (1987) *Effective Groupwork*. Basingstoke: Macmillan.

Raven, B. (1993) 'The bases of power: origins and recent developments', *Journal of Social Issues*, 49 (4): 227–51.

Regan, S. (2001) 'When forms fail the reality test,' *Community Care*, 25–31 October: 36–7.

Reid, W. (1997) 'Research on task-centered practice', *Social Work Research*, 21 (3): 132–7.

Reid, W. and Epstein, L. (1972) *Task-Centred Casework*. New York: Columbia University Press.

Reimers, S. and Treacher, A. (1995) *Introducing User-friendly Family Therapy*. London: Routledge.

Rogers, C. (1946) 'Significant aspects of client-centred therapy', *American Psychologist*, 1: 415–22.

Rogers, C. (1951) *Client-centred Therapy*. London: Constable.

Rogers, C. (1967) *On Becoming a Person: A Therapist's View of Psychotherapy*. London: Constable.

Rooney, R. (1992) *Strategies for Work with Involuntary Clients*. New York: Columbia University Press.

Rowe, J. and Lambert, L. (1973) *Children Who Wait: a Study of Children Needing Substitute Families*. London: Association of British Adoption and Fostering Agencies.

Rycroft, C. (1995) *A Critical Dictionary of Psychoanalysis*, 2nd edn. Harmondsworth: Penguin.

Schneider, R. and Lester, L. (2001) *Social Work Advocacy: A New Framework for Action*. Stamford, CA: Brooks/Cole.

Schön, D. (1991) *The Reflective Practitioner: How Professionals Think in Action*. Aldershot: Arena.

Schore, A. (1999) *Affect Regulation and the Origin of the Self: The Neurobiology of Emotional Development*. Mahwah, NJ: Lawrence Erlbaum.

Seligman, M. (1975) *Helplessness: On Depression, Development and Death*. San Francisco, CA: Freeman.

Sheldon, B. (1995) *Cognitive-behavioural Therapy: Research, Practice and Philosophy*. London: Routledge.

Sheldrick, C. (1998) 'Child psychiatrists in court: their contribution as experts in care proceedings', *Journal of Forensic Psychiatry*, 9 (2): 249–66.

Sibeon, R. (1989) 'Comments on the structure and form of social work knowledge', *Social Work and Social Sciences Review*, 1 (1): 29–44.

Skinner, B.F. (1974) *About Behaviourism*. London: Jonathan Cape.

Smith, A. (1996) *An Inquiry into the Nature and Causes of the Wealth of Nations*. Chicago, IL: Chicago University Press.

Stevens, A. (1990) *On Jung*. Harmondsworth: Penguin.

Szasz, T. (1998) *Cruel Compassion: Psychiatric Control of Society's Unwanted*. New York: Syracuse University Press.

Thatcher, M. (1987) 'Aids, education and the year 2000!' *Women's Own*, 31 October: 8–10. Available at: www.margaretthatcher.com (accessed April 2005).

Thompson, N. (2000) *Understanding Social Work: Preparing for Practice*. Basingstoke: Macmillan.

Thompson, N. (2001) *Anti-discriminatory Practice*, 3rd edn. Basingstoke: Palgrave.

Trevithick, P. (2000) *Social Work Skills: A Practice Handbook*. Buckingham: Open University Press.

Trevithick, P. (2003) 'Effective relationship-based practice: a theoretical exploration', *Journal of Social Work Practice*, 17 (2): 163–76.

Trotter, C. (1999) *Working with Involuntary Clients*. London: Sage.

Trotter, C. (2004) *Helping Abused Children and their Families*. London: Sage.

Walker, S. and Beckett, C. (2003) *Social Work Assessment and Intervention*. Lyme Regis: Russell House.

Ward, A. (2003) 'The core framework', in A. Ward, K. Kasinski, J. Pooley and A. Worthington (eds) *Therapeutic Communities for Children and Young People*. London: Jessica Kingsley. pp. 21–42.

White, M. and Epston, D. (1990) *Narrative Means to Therapeutic Ends*. New York: Norton.

Wilding, P. (1982) *Professional Power and Social Welfare*. London: Routledge & Kegan Paul.

Young, P.V. (1935) *Interviewing in Social Work*. New York: McGraw-Hill.

Web references

International Federation of Social Workers: www.ifsw.org
Youth Justice Board: www.youth-justice-board.gov.uk
National Statistics: www.statistics.gov.uk

Index